32·00

GU00949790

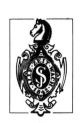

JOHN S. ROYLANCE
5 SOUTHGATE ROAD
TENTERDEN
KENT
TN30 7BS
0580 765267/762332

J. W. Paulley   H. E. Pelser

Psychological Managements for Psychosomatic Disorders

With Contributions by
R. B. Coles   K. C. Draper   U. Gieler
H. A. Ripman   R. H. Seville   U. Stangier

Foreword by J. J. Groen

Springer-Verlag Berlin Heidelberg New York
London Paris Tokyo Hong Kong

J. W. Paulley, MD, FRCP, DSc (Hon)
Formerly Consultant Physician to the Ipswich Hospitals
51, Anglesea Road, Ipswich, IPI 3PJ, UK

H. E. Pelser, MD
Formerly Senior Physician and Head Endocrinological Outpatient
Department Amsterdam University Hospital, Wilhelmina Gasthuis
Velazquezstraat 13, 1077 NG Amsterdam, The Netherlands

ISBN 3-540-19298-0 Springer-Verlag Berlin Heidelberg New York
ISBN 0-387-19298-0 Springer-Verlag New York Berlin Heidelberg

Library of Congress Cataloging-in-Publication Data. Paulley, J. W., 1918–. Psychological managements for psychosomatic disorders / J. W. Paulley, H. E. Pelser; with contributions by R. B. Coles… (et al.). p. cm. Bibliography: p. ISBN 0-387-19298-0 (U.S.) 1. Medicine, Psychosomatic. I. Pelser, H. E. (Henk E.) II. Title. RC49.P38 1989 616.08 – dc19 89-5873

© Springer-Verlag Berlin Heidelberg 1989
Printed in the United States of America

Typesetting: Elsner & Behrens GmbH, Oftersheim
2119/3140-543210 – Printed on acid-free paper

Foreword

It is a privilege to introduce this unusual book.

In a time when most docotrs practise medicine as a technical application of the natural sciences, the authors, both experienced clinicians, combine the use of modern techniques with human understanding and psychological management of their patients in the practice of internal medicine.

Many of these patients suffer from "psychosomatic disorders", i.e. diseases in which emotional stresses play a major role in the production of the symptoms and/or signs. But just because such a large proportion of all illnesses seen by physicians fall within this category (whether functional or organic), this book is not only a guide to the theory of psychosomatic medicine; it describes the way in which the authors deal with patients in their daily practice. Based on many years of clinical experience and a critical appraisal of the literature, they have developed and tested an approach to what they describe as "psychological management". This is partly based on psychological and psychiatric principles but differs from specialised "psychotherapy" and can be learned and practised by physicians in combination with their technical medical treatment. Extensive attention is paid to the stresses, ambivalences and incompatibilities which the patients encounter in their communication with the key figures in their family and at work, and to which they have unsuccesfully tried to adapt without having been able to solve the problems actively. The authors' method is a further development of the art of history taking, with more attention given to sympathetic and understanding questioning and listening and the non-verbal signs of communication than to precisely focused advice or prescription. Their knowledge, accumulated over the course of years, of the *specific* problems which seem to precede the onset of the different psychosomatic disorders is presented at length and illustrated by numerous case histories.

The style of the book is highly personal; the literature is critically confronted with the personal experience of the authors. It is therefore not a formal, scholastic text and does not present the reader with a consensus of generally accepted opinions. On the contrary, its contents are based on personal opinions derived from personal, practical experience. It stimulates, even challenges the reader to compare his or her own knowledge critically with that of the authors. It is not an elementary textbook for students but a guide for practising physicians who want to be (or become) better doctors and do not fear, but may even enjoy critical controversies.

The book covers, then, the whole field of internal medicine. It also offers valuable chapters on the general methodology of psychosomatic practice. The chapters on the psychosomatic aspects of dermatology, obstetrics and gynaecology have been written by experts in these fields. The collaboration of authors from Great Britain, The Netherlands and West Germany is a special feature.

Amsterdam, June 1989

J. J. Groen, M.D., F.R.C.P., F.R.C.Psych., F.A.C.P., F.I.C.P.M., Emeritus Professor of Medicine and Psychobiological Research, Universities of Jerusalem, Israel, and Leiden, The Netherlands.

Contents

List of Contributors

R. B. Coles, OBE, MB, FRCP
Formerly Consultant Dermatologist
Northampton General Hospital
461, Wellingborough Road, Northampton NN3 3HW, UK

K. C. Draper, MB, BChir
Medical Gynaecologist, The Institute of Psychosexual Medicine
11, Chandos Street, London W1, UK

U. Gieler, MD
Medizinisches Zentrum für Hautkrankheiten
Klinikum der Philipps-Universität
Deutschhausstrasse 9, D-3550 Marburg
Federal Republic of Germany

J. W. Paulley, MD, FRCP, DSc (Hon)
Formerly Consultant Physician to the Ipswich Hospitals
51, Anglesea Road, Ipswich IPI 3PJ, UK

H. E. Pelser, MD
Formerly Senior Physician and Head Endocrinological Outpatient
Department Amsterdam University Hospital, Wilhelmina Gasthuis
Velazquezstraat 13, 1077 N.G. Amsterdam, The Netherlands

H. A. Ripman, FRCS, FRCOG
Formerly Consultant Obstetrician and Gynaecologist
Ipswich Hospitals
51, Anglesea Road, Ipswich IPI 3PJ, UK

R. H. Seville, MD, FRCP
Formerly Consultant Dermatologist, Royal Infirmary, Lancaster
2, Hayfell Grove, Hest Bank, Lancaster LA2 6DT, UK

U. Stangier, Dipl.-Psych., Dr. rer. nat.
Medizinisches Zentrum für Hautkrankheiten
Klinikum der Philipps-Universität
Deutschhausstrasse 9, D-3550 Marburg
Federal Republic of Germany

Abbreviations

ACTH	adrenocorticotrophic hormone
AI	autoimmune
AIDS	acquired immune deficiency syndrome
ANF	anti-nuclear factor
AN	anorexia nervosa
BP	blood pressure
CAT	computerised axial tomography
CCU	coronary care unit
CLP	consultation liaison psychiatry
CNS	central nervous system
CSF	cerebrospinal fluid
CVP	central venous pressure
DU	duodenal ulcer
EB	Epstein-Barr
ECG	electrocardiogram
ECHO(virus)	enterocytopathogenic human orphan
ECT	electroconvulsive treatment
EEG	electroencephalogram
ENT	ear, nose, throat
ESR	erythrocyte sedimentation rate
FSH	follicle-stimulating hormone
GBS	Guillain-Barré syndrome
GP	general practitioner
HLA	human lymphocyte antigen
IBD	inflammatory bowel disease
IBS	irritable bowel syndrome
IC	interstitial cystitis
ICU	intensive care unit
IHD	ischaemic heart disease
IUCD	intra-uterine contraceptive device

MCT	mixed connective tissue (disease)
MI	myocardial infarction
MS	multiple sclerosis
NCO	non-commissioned officer
OED	Oxford English dictionary
PAN	polyarteritis nodosa
PID	prolapsed intervertebral disc
PM	psychosomatic medicine
PMT	premenstrual tension
RA	rheumatoid arthritis
RAF	Royal Air Force
RNP	ribonucleoprotein
SAH	subarachnoid haemorrhage
SLE	systemic lupus erythematosus
TAT	Thematic Aperception Test
TIA	transient ischaemic attack
TRH	thyroid releasing hormone
TSH	thyrotrophin stimulating hormone
UC	ulcerative colitis
UCH	University College Hospital
WBC	white blood count (cell)

1 Introduction

This book concerns the psychological management of psychosomatic disorders, by which we mean physical disorders in whose pathogenesis emotional stress has had a *major* role. In one hour we had no difficulty in listing 130 of them. About 80 of these have been included, especially the more common ones, or those in which definitive forms of psychological management can bring remission or worthwhile amelioration.

The book is *not* about somatopsychic disorders (a term applied to mental illness or psychiatric states induced by physical causes such as injuries, amputations, drugs, abnormalities in biochemistry or endocrine function), which are properly the business of every clinician or psychiatrist. For a comprehensive review of these readers are referred to a recent book [1]. The topic is also discussed in Chap. 2.

We have had to restrict references to past research and theory in order to find space for more detailed descriptions of psychological management than those attempted since Dunbar [2] and Weiss and English [3] some 40 years ago. Readers who wish to fill this gap are advised to consult the extensive reviews by Weiner [4], von Uexkull [5] and Taylor [6]. In view of this vast store of work and knowledge, it is perhaps surprising that so few practical applications for the benefit of patients with psychosomatic disorders have emerged. Even the most recent of these excellent books [6] is disappointing in this respect.

Young doctors and students are often aware that emotional factors appear to have played a part in the onset or relapse of a patient's illness, but when they seek guidance about psychological management, they are unable to find any. This may be because books which claim to deal with "the psychosomatic approach" and "whole person medicine" [7–9] either have confused the reader with much that is not psychosomatic at all or are profuse with generalisations, while lacking the details of management without which a doctor responsible for a patient with a psychosomatic disorder is likely to fail or suffer needless frustration.

It may be queried whether such management techniques can be transmitted through the written or spoken word or whether they must be experienced. One example should suffice in reply. In 1952 during a brief visit to Amsterdam, members of Professor Groen's unit were able to pass on to one of us (J.W.P.) the essentials of psychological management of asthma. Previously, J.W.P.'s asthmatic patients responded poorly to treatment and needed repeated re-admission; their passive-aggressive behaviour irritated him and the staff. Subsequently, management of asthma became a gratifying experience and a challenge to be overcome rather than a recurrent cause of frustration and anxiety.

The interested reader should not be put off if some of the finer aspects of verbal and non-verbal communication and management are not immediately obvious. Few students are able to distinguish difficult heart sounds until they have heard them several times and their ears have become attuned; similarly, considerable experience of palpation is necessary before one is able to feel a soft spleen.

Although this book has not been written for liaison psychiatrists, whose work involves them with many disorders other than psychosomatic ones, some may find parts of it useful. It is unfortunate that they will always be unable to see more than a fraction of the people with psychosomatic disorders needing help, because there are so many.

The book will also discuss why an unnecessary degree of therapeutic nihilism has developed over the past 25 years after much early promise, and will attempt to correct it. Part of the reason is that interpretative psychotherapy or management has for years been dismissed as too time consuming, too costly or unproven; this ignores the effectiveness of brief psychotherapy for psychosomatic disorders which at first surprised Dunbar [2] and has been confirmed by many authorities. The books by Dunbar [2] and Weiss and English [3] are still more relevant to the relief of patients than many written since. They are especially good on psychosomatic history taking, and it is sad that they are now not widely read. This may be because they were too long, or because they were written from a psychoanalytic viewpoint, thereby deterring those untutored in psychoanalytic concepts and language. Thus what were essentially fairly simple things about feelings and emotions were made to appear complex.

It is our view and that of others [10] including Dunbar that some psychosomatic disorders are linked by a similar and overlapping psychopathogenesis, and that each group requires its own distinctive interviewing technique and subsequent psychological management. For example management for the AI diseases differs greatly from that for disorders associated with "uptight" (tense) personalities such as migraine, aphthous ulcers, IBS backache and intervertebral disc problems. Quite different again is the management appropriate for asthma and vasomotor rhinitis, disorders sharing overlapping pathogenesis. This may appear unorthodox, but this book will attempt to explain the reasons for the value of a well honed and precisely directed approach both in diagnosis and in subsequent treatment. For example, the approach needed to promote remission in a patient with ulcerative colitis would be useless for an asthmatic and might even bring on status. Nor would it confer any benefit to a migraine or RA sufferer. The reasons for this are still not understood, even by many liaison psychiatrists. Equally, standard psychotherapy effective for some psychoneuroses has been found to be of limited value in the relief of psychosomatic disorders [11–13]. Both of the above factors contributed to the pessimism about the value of psychotherapy or psychological management using basic psychodynamic concepts which set in about 1960 and which still continues today. The wide range of cases we shall describe will show that this pessimism was premature and unwarranted.

Therefore, this book in many ways may be compared to a manual of operative surgery with differing approaches and managements instead of operations. Both require sufficiently detailed guidance of what to do for a reader to be able to test the recommendations for himself. Then, just like the surgeon who seeks to improve on the operative technique he has learned, the clinician undertaking the psychological management of psychosomatic disorders will develop approaches of his or her own.

The guidance the book offers will be supported by earlier reports where available, and illustrated by case histories and transcripts. It is hoped in this way to give the interested clinician or practitioner a bench mark to aim at, which to date has been lacking.

Most doctors think all psychological work involves the expenditure of additional time. This is a misconception. The psychological managements recommended for most disorders described in the book may be carried out simultaneously with standard medical managements, and many such are notorious for the amount of general practitioner and hospital time and costly investigations they take up. Effective psychological management reduces both in the long run. Even in the minority of disorders which call for work at greater depth, e.g. MS (Chap. 9), Crohn's disease (Chap 6), RA and AI diseases (Chap 10), which are disabling and refractory, and make heavy demands on the time and skills of all care givers in any case. Any additional time initially spent on this restricted group is soon repaid in lessened morbidity or remission.

The research and teachings of the Balints and others [14, 15] on brief psychotherapeutic intervention in general practice have undoubtedly benefited many patients by enhancing their doctor's sensitivity to interactions in the "here and now". The techniques of "tuning-in", "flash" or focal therapy are clearly relevant to all disorders, psychosomatic or otherwise, but fall short, just as psychoanalysis does, of providing the rather precise tools a doctor needs to treat psychosomatic disorders effectively in the time normally available. It would be dangerous to deprive previously diagnosed patients presenting with new symptoms of a standard if streamlined medical history and examination. How this may be achieved in a busy outpatient clinic or GP's surgery will be discussed in Chap 5.

Throughout this book we shall stress the importance of matching competent orthodox medical management with competent psychological management. Without the former, a doctor's efforts will be frustrated by the patient's unconscious resistance. Obvious examples are patients exhibiting so-called non-compliance – an insensitive term – in taking drugs, or those who for no apparent reason do not get better or frequently relapse.

Chapter 2 will explain what is a psychosomatic disorder and what is not, because there is still much confusion about the definition. It will translate some of the jargon used in the psychosomatic field such as "typicality", "specificity" and "syndrome shift". The implications of multicausality will be discussed, and the tendency of psychosomatic patients to "scatter" or "split" their various therapists to their own detriment [16]. The traps which this sets for GPs, hospital doctors, nurses, dietitians, physiotherapists, social workers, etc. are many, and unless understood better than they are today, patients with psychosomatic disorders will continue to suffer as a result. From this it follows that the *therapeutic team,* both inside and outside hospital, is of paramount importance. Attention will also be given to the "placebo effect". Chapter 3 discusses who is best suited to treat a particular patient.

Chapter 4 will deal with the few essential psychodynamic concepts and mechanisms which doctors or therapists hoping to treat psychosomatic patients effectively, need to know.

Chapter 5 will cover history taking, spacing of interviews and termination. The importance of the first appointment and how it is made will be emphasised, as well as the ways in which the psychosomatic interview differs from the standard medical or psychiatric one. Attention will be drawn to forms of non-verbal communication, which are all important with psychosomatic patients who share a common difficulty in expressing their emotions.

Suggestions will be offered about "facilitations" which can be used to help these patients express their feelings, sometimes for the first time in their lives. The question of touching the patient will be considered and the problem that it poses for young doctors, and mention will be made of those disorders in which "touching" should be avoided. Why joint interviews with spouses or partners can be valuable in some psychosomatic disorders and not others will be discussed.

The clinical chapters follow system by system. Only those psychosomatic disorders have been included which in our or other people's experience have been found to remit or improve with psychological management. Many other disorders are predominantly psychosomatic in pathogenesis, but psychological management is not appropriate for them because the somatic result is irreversible, for example acute appendicitis, pernicious anaemia, alopecia totalis, or is of such small benefit that it is not worthwhile for the patient or doctor. Two chapters have been written by invited specialists. A chapter on anorexia (bulimia) nervosa has also been included, although by Halliday's and our definition it is not a true psychosomatic disorder because the link between psyche and soma is fully within the patient's consciousness. However, we felt we should include it because it is such a problem for general practitioners and physicians, and it is generally thought of as "psychosomatic". Chapter 18 is addressed mainly to those who have the responsibility of teaching psychosomatic medicine rather than young doctors and students themselves. It looks critically at some philosophical blind alleys which have failed to benefit patients in the last 25 years. Suggestions for the future include possible ways of transmitting to young doctors some of the hard-won clinical experience of the pioneers in the psychological management of true psychosomatic disorders. It urges more work with patients, less armchair philosophy and the abandonment of imprecise labels such as "illness behaviour".

References

1. Lader MH (1983) Mental disorders and somatic illness. Cambridge University Press, Cambridge (Handbook of psychiatry 2)
2. Dunbar F (1943) Psychosomatic diagnosis. Hoeber, New York
3. Weiss E, English OS (1949) Psychosomatic medicine. Saunders, Philadelphia
4. Weiner H (1977) Psychobiology and human disease. Elsevier, New York
5. Uexkull T von (1981) Lehrbuch der psychosomatischen Medizin. Urban and Schwarzenberg, München
6. Taylor CJ (1987) Psychosomatic medicine and contemporary psychoanalysis. International University Press, Madison
7. Haynes SN, Gannon L (1981) Psychosomatic disorders: a psychophysiological approach to etiology and treatment. Praegar, New York
8. Christie M, Mellett P (1986) The psychosomatic approach. Contemporary practice of whole-person care. Wiley, Chichester
9. Creed F, Pfeffer JM (1985) Medicine and psychiatry: a practical approach. Pitman, London
10. Groen J (1950) Emotional factors in the etiology of internal diseases. J M Sinai Hosp NY 17:71–89

11. Ruesch J (1948) The infantile personality: the core problem of psychosomatic medicine. Psychosom Med 10:134–144
12. Sifneos PE (1973) The prevalence of "alexithymic" characteristics in psychosomatic patients. Psychother Psychosom 22:255–262
13. Nemiah JC (1973) Psychology and psychosomatic illness: reflections on theory and research methodology. Psychother Psychosom 22:106–111
14. Balint M (1964) The doctor, his patient and the illness, 2nd edn. Pitman, London
15. Balint E, Norell JS (1973) Six minutes for the patient. Tavistock, London
16. Winnicott DW (1966) Psychosomatic illness in its positive and negative aspects. Int J Psychoanal 47:510–516

2 Definitions and Terms

Some authors have recently used the term *psychosomatic* to cover topics ranging from the *normal* stresses of *normal* events such as birth and dying to the newer one of genetic counselling [1]. Even benzodiazepines for anxiety and insomnia have been included and other psychological problems such as those arising from renal dialysis [2]. While these are the legitimate business of all doctors, they are not psychosomatic. The umbrella term *psychosomatic* has also been used recently to include behavioural disorders such as alcoholism and other addictions and much else that is properly in the province of social medicine and psychiatry [3, 4]. The adverse affects of such confusion will be discussed in later chapters. Instead we prefer Halliday's 1937 [5] definition and our own modification. Halliday said,

> Psychosomatic illness ... connotes both an aetiology and a mechanism ... the agents which provoked the reaction of illness were of a special kind being neither phsysical nor chemical, nor microorganic but psychological – as for example, the loss of a beloved object ... As regards the mechanism ... the external agent is encountered by the individual not directly by the outer or inner surfaces of the body, such as skin or mucous membranes, but *indirectly* [our italics] via the special senses and integrating mechanisms of the diencephalon, autonomic nervous system, and endocrine glands. This triad is sometimes called the psycho-neuro-endocrine system or the "bodily mechanisms of emotion".

To us a psychosomatic disorder is one in which emotional factors are a major aetiological determinant, of which the patient is unconscious or only partly conscious; the pathway through which Mind (psyche) affects the Body (soma) causing dysfunction or structural damage is wholly unconscious. The link is always internal, psycho-neuro-endocrinological, psycho-neuro-immunological, via the autonomic nervous system or via striated muscle innervated by the voluntary nervous system, as for example disorders of motor co-ordination (breathing and swallowing) and of muscular tone and posture.

Behavioural disorders such as addictions, alcoholism, smoking, drugs, etc. are not psychosomatic because the individual is wholly aware of his actions, and that they are the cause of the somatic symptoms, i.e. the link between psyche and soma is conscious and external. Similarly, hair balls (bezoars) are not psychosomatic nor is dermatitis artefacta. The chewing of hair or excoriation is also external and conscious. However, there are other physical abnormalities arising from things that patients do consciously in which habit, cultural pressures and fashion arc more important than any underlying psychological disturbances or neurosis, e.g. "joggers' nipple", "disco deafness", "pop acne" (when long hair of the 1960s hid the face). What is, or what is not, a truly psychosomatic disorder is of some importance when it comes to prognosis. Why this is so is explained at the end of Chap. 3.

2.1 Somatopsychic Presentations

As stated in Chap. 1, psychiatric states secondary to chemical and hormonal changes and to toxins, drugs, infections and brain damage from tumours and encephalopathies are very common. They pose the hazard of treating the psychiatric presentation with psychotropic drugs or ECT instead of the underlying cause, which may then be masked and remain undiagnosed even until autopsy.

A question then often asked is whether these psychiatric or mood states, induced somato-psychically for one of the above reasons, can in turn promote a psychosomatic disorder? In practice this occurs very rarely, but it can do so occasionally, for example, hyperventilation and vasomotor changes resulting from fear and anxiety, or MI and heart failure seen in mania or hypomania as a result of the intense hyperactivity.

On the other side of the coin, the somatic components of many psychosomatic disorders, particularly those causing fatigue from pain, weakness or sleeplessness, may themselves provoke anxiety or depression, and thereby tend to compound the underlying emotional state which provoked the psychosomatic disorder in the first place, e.g. AI disorders (Chap. 10).

However, we feel that too much has been made of such niceties by some defenders of "holistic purity" against what they see as the heresy of Cartesian dualism. Bernard Engel [6] recently made the point that the two concepts are not mutually exclusive, and one may be valid without affecting the other. Nevertheless, the debate continues to fog essential issues and is one reason for the delayed provision of the modest but often effective psychological help awaited by millions of sufferers from psychosomatic diseases all over the world. For further comment see Chap. 18.

2.2 Profiles and Associated Hypotheses

After 12 years of research Dunbar, in co-operation with the Departments of Medicine, Surgery and Psychiatry of the Presbyterian Medical Center, Columbia University, New York, published her findings [7]. Her studies centred on patients categorised into four groups by disorder: (a) those with fractures (accident prone), (b) cardiovascular, (c) rheumatic and (d) diabetic. On p.142 she stated:

> It is probably useful to note only that ... the personality picture we associate with each syndrome ... was more specific than any of us anticipated at the outset ... the different groups showed marked differences in family and environmental history, especially sphere of conflict, taken in ways of dealing with difficulties (including action, speech, and fantasy).

She adopted the term *profile* for each group.

Alexander [8] and his colleagues at the Institute of Psychoanalysis in Chicago working at the same time as Dunbar came to a similar conclusion regarding seven disorders found to have a substantial emotional determinant in their causation: neurodermatitis, hypertension, RA, peptic ulcer, UC, asthma and thyrotoxicosis. Alexander reported distinctly differing unconscious constellations of conflict in each disorder. His formulations were subsequently validated [9] in prospective blind trials by himself and his colleagues at a level of probability better than chance and also better than by physicians untrained in psychodynamic concepts and not cognisant with Alexander's formulations. Comparable research by Ring [10] also supported the validity of *specificity,* the term given to this degree of congruity. However, as one dictionary meaning of the word is "pertaining to and no other", we and others prefer the term *typicality,* which is semantically less absolute.

Alexander did not claim, as some critics have alleged, that the personality profiles described were unique to the disease in question, nor was he unaware that the pathogenesis involved is a non-linear chain of responses and interaction. Indeed, he has been credited [11, 12] with having made comprehensive statements about multiple factors having a role in pathogenesis. Dunbar was also clear about this. Thus these criticisms made by their opponents are not valid, yet it is these criticisms which have come to be believed. This situation arose as a result of parrot-like recitation by those remote from day-to-day care of patients and antipathetic to psychodynamic mechanisms and interpretative psychotherapy. As a result advances in the clinical application of psychosomatic medicine have been retarded.

At the 1st European Conference on Psychosomatic Research (London 1955), one of us (J.W.P.) while touching on *superstability* suggested that the methods a person uses, or perhaps more importantly *fails* to use, to communicate his inner feelings to the world may confer *specificity* much as some families of bacteria share the same group antigen ("O") but have differing surface "H" antigens which confer specificity, and added that investigators with an orthodox psychological training tend to dig deeply, "brushing aside superficial layers of soil". Thereby, inventories and psychological tests for obsessionality, aggressivity, etc., and other deeper aspects of personality have failed to show significant differences between psychosomatoses or psychoneuroses, a finding often misused by critics of specificity. However, the concept is again much alive [13, 14], e.g. "There *is* specificity, what is at issue is its nature" [14], and Bastiaans [13] on the implications of the concept in treatment: "these important findings have not irradiated sufficiently in teaching and international literature." In clarifying our 1955 hypothesis, it is thought that coping mechanisms confer the typicality/specificity.

Coping mechanisms are ways by which individuals seek to evade or ameliorate tension arising from emotional conflicts, personal or situational. These mechanisms may be partly inherited but as the later clinical chapters will illustrate are mostly acquired in infancy and childhood as a result of emotional interaction with key figures. Examples include striving to relieve the insecurity of disapproval, the asthmatic's passive-aggressive response to domination or rejection, activity to fend off guilt over loss, and the giving-up response as the only way by which a particular child can avoid the terrifying fear of separation from a dominating parent habitually threatening withdrawal of love at any gesture of independence. However, coping mechanisms such as these inevitably become less and less effective in adolescence, or later, when the psychosomatic patient, lacking the ability of emotional expression of the psychoneurotic, gets "stuck" with the tension, and somatic dysfunction or structural damage results. A healthy person may be likened to someone in a room with many doors by which he or she may escape when feeling emotionally threatened. By contrast, the psychosomatic patient's room has few doors and when one or more of these, such as acting out, are closed for some reason – the psychoneurosis being no longer acceptable socially or economically – or blocked by psychotropic drugs, then the door of psychosomatic emotional release is often the only way open to him or her.

Taylor [12] in a useful recent book has proposed that diseases may be viewed as disorders of psychological regulation. Although the concept is based on the Object Relation Theory previously advanced by psychoanalysts [15–17], it was the work of Mirsky on DU [18] (Chap. 6) and that of Bowlby [19], Hofer [20] and others working with animals that has provided the psychobiological basis for it.

Taylor's *internal* (self) *regulators* seem indistinguishable from what we have called coping mechanisms, both being acquired, learned or programmed in infancy and childhood in the interactions between child and mother, and then early surrogates such as father, grandparents, siblings and later other key figures, uncles, aunts, teachers, etc. Both mechanisms are directed at restoration of homeostatic equilibrium when it has been disturbed by internal and/or external emotional stress.

However, no individual's internal regulators or coping mechanisms, however efficient, are enough on their own without some support from external regulators. People whose self regulators lack flexibility or are defective in other ways are proportionately more dependent on external regulators for emotional equilibrium, but because of that dependence are vulnerable, as illustrated by many patients' case histories in this book. For example, it is common for people who have suffered severe emotional deprivation in childhood to find their first happiness with marriage in the love of a spouse, and later of their children. One way of pointing this out to them is to suggest that their spouses and children "count double" compared with an average person, and for them even minor illnesses in the family, feelings of alienation or seeing the children growing up and leaving home can be especially threatening and frequently provoke psychosomatic disorders if they are also *superstable* subjects. The most important external regulators are the family, followed by friends, neighbours, work and club mates and if they take ill, a physician or nurse. Therefore doctors who suddenly tell these dependent patients that they need no more treatment, or go on holiday without warning them, or pass them on to someone else without working through termination (Chap. 5) often provoke relapses, e.g. UC, asthma, MS, RA and AI disease. Taylor also makes the perceptive suggestion that the placebo is regarded as a transitional object representing whichever significant person the doctor prescribing it stands for in the transference. However, in the long term placebos like "alternative" medical remedies to which psychosomatic patients become much attached only serve to compound their damaging coping mechanisms (deficient internal regulators). Doctors treating them should be trying to help them change these rather than reinforcing them by unwise prescribing, e.g. of tranquillizers.

However, as we have pointed out elsewhere, any effective psychological management depends on a doctor being able to "hold" his patient long enough in the therapeutic situation. This applies especially to these superstable psychosomatic subjects. In the short term it is necessary for doctors to be tolerant of their patients' foibles, challenges and "bolts for freedom" while at the same time tactfully pointing out what they are doing. It is also important to recognise that most patients are unable to modify their internal regulators (coping mechanisms) without a sufficient passage of time (measured in months and often years). In our experience of psychosomatic patients this seems to be more important than the fequency or even the length of therapeutic interviews.

Attitudes and conscious emotions specific to certain bodily diseases were described by Grace and Graham in 1952 [21]. Later Graham and his co-workers [22] described 18 diseases in which predictive studies supported the specificity of the attitude-response hypothesis. An attitude is what patients felt was happening to them and what they wanted to do about that particular situation at the time the symptoms occurred. For example, vasomotor rhinitis occurred in 12 patients when faced with a situation which they wished would go away, or which they did not want to do anything about. This is not unlike the provocative feeling of *frustration* which so commonly precedes sneezing attacks and nasal congestion, or *rejection* before asthma, while their description of attitudes before migraine, e.g. "I had to get it done – I had to meet a deadline", could have come from our own section on the subject.

What people feel consciously about situations is certainly relevant to the advent of many disorders mentioned by Graham and also described in this book. However, patients are often *wholly unaware* of the relationship between what they feel emotionally and their particular somatic presentation. Helping them become aware is often their first step to recovery (see in cases of UC and IBS in Chap. 6 and hyperventilation in Chap. 7). However, in many disorders modification of inflexible attitudes cannot be achieved without at the same time bringing into consciousness the unconscious coping mechanisms from which they arise.

2.3 Typicality of Life Events and Situations

In practice it is found that the same, or similar, events or situations are recurrently provocative of a particular psychosomatic illness, whereas others are not. Thus, it is the *coping mechanism* which selects the provocative event or situation. An understanding of this other aspect of *typicality* is invaluable in management as outlined in the clinical chapters. It also explains why some people suffer syndrome shifts in response to differing life events, situations or stresses, e.g. migraine → IBS dropped shoulder syndrome → PID, or DU → IHD, or UC → MS.

2.4 Multicausality

As already pointed out proponents of specificity have never claimed that disease is not multicausal. Diathesis is the old term for what is now a growing understanding of inherited disposition through measureable markers such as HLA tissue antigens and serology in AI diseases. However, because few hereditary diseases present at the moment of conception, other factors such as age, temperature, infection or indeed emotional stress may be involved before a disease becomes clinically manifest; sometimes it is only one of identical twins who develops a disease such as RA or MS.

French and Alexander [9] and others quoted, including ourselves, have offered evidence that the "psychological factor" is often the major determinant in many disorders; in others such as tuberculosis in which it is also influential [23, 24] the main determinant must be the tubercle bacillus itself. Similarly, other opportunist infections do not occur or are suppressed when an individual is immunologically competent. Accumulating evidence that immunological competence may either be depressed or so distorted as to attack "self" following the stress of loss and mourning will be presented in Chap. 10.

A major extension to our understanding of multicausality was Mirsky's study [18] on the aetiology of DU. He showed one factor to be genetically determined: the secretion level of pepsinogen-1, which was set from birth. (The quality of protective mucus has recently been thought to be another factor.) Mirsky's second factor was multiple within itself, being dependent on the interaction between infants with strong oral cravings and the mother, e.g. their influence on her, and her influences on them via her response. The outcome of that interaction was reflected physiologically in levels of gastric secretion and later psychologically in patterns of behaviour. Thirdly, he drew attention to a social parameter. In other words, if such a predisposed individual's environment was sufficiently supportive he or she could be expected to avoid both maximal gastric secretion and an ulcer, but when high demands from either the domestic or work environment, or both, were not met, he or she would be at risk of developing a DU . (See Chap. 6 for reasons why only selected cases of DU are likely to respond to psychological management.) Most other psychosomatic disorders which are included in this book are less complex and more amenable to psychological management. That is because the somatic aspect is readily reversible, and the psyche is the major determinant. Multicausality, however, will be present to a greater or lesser degree in all of them.

2.5 Syndrome Shift

Clinicians working in the psychosomatic field have noted that patients may switch from one psychosomatic presentation to another, or from a psychosomatic disorder to a psychoneurosis or psychosis, and vice versa [25–27] (see examples of UC, asthma and MS in later chapters). Such changes of direction may then occur in response to a different life situation, or when psychotherapy is pressed too fast, at too great a depth or with premature interpretation, before a patient has had sufficient time to move his emotional stance and accept that the way he has coped with certain stressful emotions hitherto had been inadequate, somatically damaging and contributory to his illness.

Twenty years ago some doctors and therapists expressed worries about promoting syndrome shift from a psychosomatic disorder, such as asthma, to a psychosis or anxiety state. At that time Thomas Main expressed the view that the latter condition was easier to treat than the original psychosomatic disorder. We concur with this, and in any case experience has shown that shifts to psychosis are very rare (e.g. one out of approximately 2000 patients with UC seen by one of us, J.W.P., over 40 years).

When patients receiving psychological management/psychotherapy for such disorders as MS, AI diseases and UC begin to complain of feelings of depression and anxiety, it is a sign of progress, even if they at first say they would prefer their psychosomatic disorder to these uncomfortable feelings. The doctor must empathise with their distress and at the same time explain that both depression and anxiety are forms of emotional expression which they had previously been unable to use. He makes use of this chink in their armour, first by facilitating their expressions of anger, guilt, self-pity, fears of retribution, panic at separation, etc. and then by accepting them on behalf of whichever or their significant figures he stands for in the transference enables change to occur in coping patterns previously somatically damaging.

2.6 Superstability

We are grateful to Bastiaans of Amsterdam for first introducing us to the term *superstable*. This describes so clearly the characteristic shared by all patients with psychosomatic disorders, some more than others, of concealing or denying sensitive feelings and preserving as far as possible an external facade of excessive stability in circumstances of emotional stress which in most other people would evoke an appropriate expression of affect. However, Wretmark [28] cites Sjöbring as an earlier user of the term [29].

Ruesch [30] in 1948 made the same observation and later said that poverty of emotional expression was the common denominator of all psychosomatic disorders and remarked on these patients' difficulty or inability to fantasise, free associate and present dreams.

Essentially, the same point was made in 1963 by Marty and de M'Uzan [31]. *Pensée opératoire* and *basic representative inhibition* were their description of this form of mental functioning, which distinguishes the psychosomatic from the psychoneurotic patient.

> The psychosomatic symptom ... in the consequence of an incapacity, more or less marked, to elaborate conflicts on a mental level ... The appearances of considerable fantasy activity is in a psychosomatic patient the sign of a process of recovery ... The patient with pensée opératoire *appears to be the witness rather* than the actor of his or her own existence.

For example, a patient would say: "People think my sister is unkind to me" rather than: "I think my sister is unkind to me," and make frequent use of clichés: "My mother always says ..."

2.7 Alexithymia

In 1972 *alexithymia* was the term proposed by Sifneos [32] and then adopted by Nemiah [33] for the same shared characteristic of all patients with psychosomatic disorders. Nemiah wrote: "They [patients] came out of [psycho]therapy as incapable of experiencing and describing affect and fantasy as when they entered it."

Sifneos and Nemiah initially suggested that this characteristic might be partly due to a physical or biochemical defect. We and others disagreed on the grounds that this did not accord with the ability of such patients to overcome the alleged "defect" when helped to do so by the facilitating techniques and management described later. Sifneos now seems to accept that the defect is not physically based, but thinks as we do that it is due to a failure to *learn* to express emotions in childhood from equally undemonstrative parents, or because the child is discouraged from showing emotion, or feels it is too dangerous to do so. (See case histories in chapters on UC, Crohn's disease, hypertension, and MS.)

2.8 Hypochondriasis

The term *hypochondriasis,* first used by Galen about 350 B.C., has recently been described by Lipsitt [34] as "a diagnosis in search of a disease". He added: "Our persistence in trying to retain such terms may lead not only to further inappropriate application ... but worse to a stifling of investigations into complex conditions." *Functional illness* replaced hypochondriasis as the favoured name for a group of diseases which doctors found difficult to explain or treat.

In 1951 *the sick role* was put forward by Parsons [35] to explain the sociological implications of this problem. *Illness behaviour* was subsequently coined by Mechanic [36] and later endorsed by Pilowski [37, 38] to replace *hypochondriasis,* which was rejected "as a very imprecise term". However, none of these new labels was any more precise than the old ones, and nor was the term *abnormal illness behaviour,* added by Pilowsky in 1969 [38].

Clearly, the introduction of such labels does not help a single patient to get better, and Mayou [39] acknowledged that "it is essential to realise that illness behaviour does not refer to a theory but is a portmanteau term". However, despite the widespread recognition that pseudodiagnostic pigeonholes have bedevilled constructive thought in medicine for far too long, another has recently appeared.

This latest addition is *somatization* [40, 43]. Those who suffer from it are deemed by psychiatrists and behavioural scientists who use the term, to have a "somatoform" or "somatization" disorder [41, 42, 44]. Advocates of the concept seem as unconcerned about precision in clinical diagnosis, or the need for knowledge of the psychosomatic medical literature and seminal studies on definitive pathology and psychopathology of the psychosomatic disorders which they lump together, as were earlier supporters of the *sick role* or *illness behaviour.* They seem blind to the full range of manifestations of the hyperventilation syndrome, and their failure to quote White and Hahn [45], Weiss and English [46] or Lum [47] "on the tip of the iceberg", suggests that they have not read them. Articles on somatization do not mention the phenomenon of syndrome shift, which is so relevant to an understanding of the various somatic pathologies as well as the psychopathologies of the common afflictions which feature prominently in articles on the so-called somatization disorder. (Syndrome shift is described in this chapter and examples of cases may be found in chapters on the alimentary tract, respiratory tract, the central nervous system, the musculoskeletal system, and urological disorders.)

It is clear however, that much responsibility for the growth of these portmanteau labels lies with clinicians who refer patients to psychiatrists prematurely. Their failure to distinguish the underlying somatic basis of many of these patients' symptoms may be related to a decline in the importance attached to history taking and doing a complete physical examination as ultraspecialties and sophisticated investigations have multiplied. As many as 40 years ago chest physicians could be heard to refer to their stethoscopes as "guessing tubes", yet these may still provide a clinician with an attuned ear with the first pointer to previously unsuspected hyperventilation.

The result is that clinicians are only too willing to pass on patients who make up a large subsection of the population, the 10%–20% with afflictions such as musculoskeletal pain, migrainous headaches, IBS and pseudo-cystitis, in whom they have been unable to find "a physiologic explanation of their symptoms", especially if at the same time they rid themselves of patients who not only baffle them, but also irritate them by their tense, "uptight", rather obsessional attitudes and ill-concealed dissatisfaction. The fault of the psychiatrists, on the other hand, is their trusting acceptance of clinicians' assurances that there is no pathophysiological explanation. Examples of disorders in which flawed diagnoses (e.g. "Headache, CAT scan negative") and inept management are very common can be found in the sections on IBS (Chap. 6), hyperventilation (Chap. 7), chest pain and palpitations (Chap. 8), head and face pain (Chap. 9), arm and back pain (Chap. 12) and bladder symptoms (Chap. 13).

The label *illness behaviour* has been applied to delayed recovery from life-threatening experiences such as MI or bypass surgery, yet doctors have long been aware of the reasons for this, which have to be identified before management can be effective. These include cultural and parental views on illness and attitudes of spouses, workmates and union secretaries as well as of the caregivers. What is less understood is the typical psychopathology of MI, containing within it the implicit fears of inability to work and what is felt to be a loss of social recognition. This is far more relevant than labels like *abnormal illness behaviour* or *somatization,* yet continues to be neglected.

Abnormal illness behaviour has also been applied to those patients found to have "lily white" appendices at appendectomy and who remain symptomatic for months afterwards [49, 50]. In practice nearly all of these are misdiagnosed cases of IBS and require quite specific forms of psychological management. The recommendation to look into these patients' social relationship and adjustment is much too vague for any doctor to be able to treat them effectively in the time normally available.

In the last chapter of this book we shall draw attention to other blind alleys into which psychosomatic medicine has blundered and which continue to block progress. We suggest that there may be some residual value in retaining the term *hypochondriac* to describe a small but recognisable group of chronic complainers who seem to "enjoy" their maladies and associated trappings, tests, drugs, exotic treatments and being the centre of scientific attention. In contrast patients with disease phobias live in perpetual terror that they are going to die, whereas the group we have mentioned love to indulge their foibles for diets, keeping out of draughts, etc. Mr. Woodhouse in Jane Austen's *Emma* [51] is an excellent example.

An egg boiled soft is not unwholesome ... Opening the windows! but surely, Mr. Churchill, nobody would think of opening windows at Randalls. Nobody would be so imprudent ... The dews of a summer evening are what I would not expose any lady to [– or himself!]

2.9 Placebo Effect

Most doctors and students are well aware to the placebo phenomenon in relation to prescribed pills or medicine. Kurland [52] said, "The placebo reaction is generally accepted to be a manifestation of suggestion." Thomas Jefferson [53] wrote to Dr. Casper Wistar in 1807, "One of the most successful physicians I have ever known has assured me that he used more bread pills, drops of coloured water, and powdered hickory ashes than all other medicines put together." The introduction of the double-blind trial resulted from the recognition of the power of the placebo effect and the importance of separating it from any really therapeutic benefit of a new drug being tested. However, there is less acknowledgement that the effect is as much due to the personality and competence of the prescriber and the subject's perception of him or her as to any expectation of the drug's potency. In the same way any consultation, examination or other intervention, whether or not psychologically directed, is commonly accompanied by a placebo effect which may be reinforced by the prescription of a drug.

Bargen's diplococcal serum [54] was a clear example of the personality of the prescriber being the effective agent and not the prescription. Between 1920 and 1923 at the Mayo Clinic the mortality for UC was 17%, but between 1924 and 1926 for patients treated by Bargen the rate fell to 3.5% [54], a figure never bettered in any series published since. Clinicians all over the USA and Europe clamoured for the serum, but in their hands it failed. Bargen himself was the therapeutic agent. His compassion for these notoriously difficult patients and paternal approach was probably the reason.

Another example is the reported remission of UC in a patient eating 2 lbs (0.9 kg) of raw pig's runners (intestines) per day [55]. The patient relapsed when the treatment stopped and remitted again after restarting. Two pharmaceutical companies then marketed dessicated pig's ileum, but trial results were equivocal. Soon the treatment was found to be no more effective than other remedies then in use [56]. Between 1934 and 1937 injections of histidine were claimed [57, 58] to promote remission in cases of DU. However, Barry and Florey [59] considered the response to be psychologically based. Gill later showed that injections of normal saline were just as effective as histidine.

Wolf [60] reported the effect of a placebo on gastric acid secretion in a group of medical students. When administered by one doctor, acid secretion rose, but when given by a second doctor it fell, thereby demonstrating that it was the investigator and the students' perception of the person who administered the placebo, that mattered. This lesson about the importance of what a stimulus means to a subject has yet to be learned by psychophysiologists using tests such as mental arithmetic, pain, discordant sound, etc. Lastly, Hambling [61] reported that a female graduate's diastolic pressure was always up around 110–120 mmHg when taken by a female doctor, but normal when taken by a male doctor. When Hambling took her blood pressure while simultaneously discussing her mother, from whose possessiveness she was trying to free herself, the diastolic levels were 96 mmHg and 105 mmHg, falling again to 80 mmHg when talking about general topics.

Readers wishing to discover more about the placebo effect should look at several references [62–65] and Taylor's [12] interpretation of the placebo as a *transitional object*.

2.10 Conversion Hysteria Versus Psychosomatic Disorder: Diagnosis

First, conversion hysteria is now rare in Western societies, whereas it was common in the early part of the century. It is still common in Third World cultures and in people living near the frontier where face-saving remains important. Reasons were discussed by Paulley [56]. Second, demonstrable pathology is absent in hysteria whereas in psychosomatic disorders physical changes may be evident macroscopically, or demonstrable by special radiological or other techniques, e.g. transient vascular spasm and dilatation in migraine or bowel spasm in IBS.

Third, in many hysterical presentations tell-tale physical signs enable a distinction to be made. For example, the pupillary light reflex is always present in hysterical blindness, contraction of antagonist as well as agonist muscles can usually be detected in hysterical limb paralysis, and hysterical sciatic pain with straight leg raising restricted to a few degrees can be shown to be exaggerated or to have no organic basis when the patient is able to sit up on request.

However, these clues are of less help, when pain presents without obvious physical signs, such as headache or some abdominal pains. It is here that the busy clinician has to depend on the way the history is presented and on non-verbal communication. In conversion hysteria there is always a degree of belle indifférence or of affect inappropriate to the symptom. Patients with psychosomatic disorders such as migrainous/vascular headache or IBS display anxiety and distress appropriate to their symptom. Exceptionally, they may use hyperbole, but that usually occurs when they have been told that nothing is wrong, and they feel they have to shout to be heard. The danger here is that the more vivid the descriptions of their pain become, the more likely they will be dismissed incorrectly as hysterics.

Another diagnostic clue is that patients with psychosomatic headache or abdominal pains usually continue to work even if they have to take a half day off to vomit. Hysterics tend to speak of their inability to work with a bland smile. A previous history of travel sickness, of migraine in first-degree relatives, or of syndrome shifts from other psychosomatic afflictions common in uptight, tense people such as PMT, apthous ulcers, proctalgia fugax, neckache, backache and PID is also valuable as a diagnostic pointer.

In H.E.P.'s experience conversion hysterics also tend to flutter their eyelids while giving their history.

Some people believe that a test dose of ergotamine will differentiate migrainous/vascular headache from conversion hysteria. It rarely helps.

References

1. Christie M, Mellett PG (1986) The psychosomatic approach: contemporary practice of whole person medicine. Wiley, Chichester
2. Creed F, Pfeffer JM (1985) Medicine and psychiatry: a practical approach. Pitman, London
3. Lipowski ZJ (1977) Psychosomatic medicine in the seventies. Am J Psychiatry 134:233–244
4. Graham DT (1979) What place in medicine for psychosomatic medicine? Psychosom Med 41:357–367
5. Halliday JL (1938) The rising incidence of psychosomatic illness. Br Med J 2:11–14

6. Engel BT (1986) Psychosomatic medicine, behavioural medicine, just plain medicine. Psychosom Med 48:466–479
7. Dunbar F (1943) Psychosomatic diagnosis. Hoeber, New York
8. Alexander F (1950) Psychosomatic medicine. Norton, New York
9. Alexander F, French TM, Pollock GH (1968) Psychosomatic specificity. University of Chicago, Press, Chicago
10. Ring FO (1956) Testing the validity of personality profiles in psychosomatic illness. Am J Psychiatry 113:1075–1080
11. Weiner H (1986) Die Geschichte der psychosomatischen Medizin und das Leib-Seele-Problem in der Medizin. Psychother Psychosom Med Psychol 36:361–391
12. Taylor CJ (1987) Psychosomatic medicine and contemporary psychoanalysis. International University Press, Madison (Stress and health series, No 3)
13. Bastiaans J (1977) The implications of the specificity concept for the treatment of psychosomatic patients. Psychother Psychosom 28:285–293
14. Kimball CP (1982) The concept of behavioural specificity. Psychother Psychosom 38:32–38
15. Klein M (1952) Some theoretical conclusions regarding the emotional life of the infant. In: Isacics S, Riviére J (eds) Developments in psychoanalysis. Hogarth, London
16. Winnicott, DW (1953) Transitional objects and transitional phenomena. Int J Psychoanal 34:89–97
17. Kohut H (1971) The analysis of the self. International University Press, New York
18. Mirsky IA (1958) Physiologic, psychologic and social determinants in the aetiology of duodenal ulcer. Am J Dig Dis 3:285–314
19. Bowlby J (1969, 1973) Attachment and loss, vol 1; separation, vol 2. Basic, New York
20. Hofer M (1984) Relationships as regulators: a psychobiologic perspective of bereavement. Psychosom Med 45:183–197
21. Grace J, Graham DT (1952) Relationship of specific attitudes and emotions to certain bodily diseases. Psychosom Med 14:243–251
22. Graham DT, Lumsby RM, Benjamin LS et al. (1962) Specific attitudes in initial interviews with patients having different "psychosomatic" diseases. Psychosom Med 24:257–265
23. Day G (1951) The psychosomatic approach to pulmonary tuberculosis. Lancet 1:1025–1028
24. Kissen DM (1958) Emotional factors in pulmonary tuberculosis. Tavistock, London
25. Halliday JL (1948) Psychosocial medicine; a study of the sick society. Norton, New York
26. Groen J, Bastiaans J, Van der Valk JM (1957) Psychosomatic aspects of syndrome shift and syndrome suppression. In: Booij J (ed) Psychosomatics. Elsevier, Amsterdam, pp 35–39
27. Kissen DM (1963) Significance of syndrome shift and late syndrome association in psychosomatic medicine. J Nerv Ment Dis 136:34–42
28. Wretmark G (1953) The psychosomatic theory of pathogenesis of the peptic ulcer individual. Acta Psychiatr Neurologica Scand [Suppl] 84:1–83
29. Sjöbring H (1923) Hysteric insufficiency and its constitutional basis. Acta Med Scand 59:387–405
30. Ruesch J (1948) The infantile personality: the care problem of psychosomatic medicine. Psychosom Med 10:134–144
31. Marty P, de M'Uzan M (1963) La pensée opératoire. Rev Fr Psychoanal 27 [Suppl]:1345–1356
32. Sifnoes PE (1973) The prevalence of "alexithymic" characteristic in psychosomatic patients. Psychother Psychosom 22:255–262
33. Nemiah JC (1973) Psychology and psychosomatic illness: reflections on theory and research methodology. Psychother Psychosom 22:106–111
34. Lipsitt DR (1973) Psychodynamic considerations of hypochondriasis. Psychother Psychosom 23:132–141
35. Parsons T (1951) The social system. Free Press, New York
36. Mechanic D (1968) Medical sociology. Free Press, New York

37. Pilowsky I (1967) Dimensions of hypochondriasis. Br J Psychiatry 113:89–93
38. Pilowsky I (1969) Abnormal illness behaviour. Br J Med Psychol 42:347–351
39. Mayou R (1986) Illness behaviour in cardiac patients. In: Lacey JH, Shergion D (eds) Proceedings of the 15th. European conference on psychosomatic research. Libby, London, pp 111–114
40. American Psychiatric Society (1980) Diagnostic and statistical manual of mental disorders, 3rd edn. American Psychiatric Society, Washington, DC
41. Monson RA, Smith GR (1983) Somatization in primary care. N Eng J Med 308:1464–1465
42. Katon W (1984) Panic disorder and somatization. Review of 55 cases. Am J Med 77:101–108
43. Escobar JI, Burnam MS, Karno M et al. (1987) Somatization in the community. Arch Gen Psychiatry 44:713–718
44. de Leon T, Saiz-Ruis J, Chinchilla A, Morales P (1987) Why do some patients somatize. Acta Psychiatr Scand 76:203–209
45. White PD, Hahn RC (1929) The symptoms of sighing in cardiovascular diagnosis. Am J Med Sci 177:179–188
46. Weiss E, English OS (1949) Psychosomatic medicine. Saunders, Philadelphia
47. Lum LC (1975) Hyperventilation: the tip of the iceberg. J Psychosom Res 19:375–383
48. Mayou R, Bryant B (1987) The quality of life after coronary artery surgery. Q J Med 62:239–248
49. Creed F (1981) Life events and appendicectomy. Lancet 1:1381–1365
50. Armstrong D (1986) Illness behaviour revisited. Proceedings of the 15th Conference on psychosomatic research. Libby, London, pp 111–114
51. Austen J (1972) Emma. Oxford University Press, Oxford
52. Kurland AN (1957) Drug placebo: its psychodynamic and conditional reflex action. Behav Sci 2:101–110
53. Brody H (1982) The lie that heals: the ethics of giving placebos. Ann Intern Med 97:112–118
54. Bargen JA (1928) Changing conceptions of chronic ulcerative colitis. JAMA 91:1176–1181
55. Gill AM (1945) Intestinal mucosa in ulcerative colitis. Lancet 2:202–204
56. Gill AM (1946) Ulcerative colitis treated with intestinal mucosa. Proc Soc Med 30:517
57. Bulmer E (1934) The histidine treatment of peptic ulcer. Lancet 2:1276–1278
58. Wingfield A (1936) Histidine treatment of peptic ulcer. Br Med J 1:1156–1158
59. Barry HC, Florey HW (1936) Histidine treatment of peptic ulcer. Lancet 2:728–734
60. Wolf S (1982) Psychosocial forces and neural mechanisms in disease: defining the question and collecting the evidence. John Hopkins Med J 150:95–100
61. Hambling J (1959) Essential hypertension. In: The nature of stress disorder. Conference of the Society for Psychosomatic Research 1958. Hutchinson, London, pp 17–39
62. Brody H (1982) The lie that heals: the ethics of giving placebos. Ann Intern Med 97:112–118
63. Knowles JB, Lucas CJ (1960) Experimental studies of the placebo response. J Ment Sci 106:231–240
64. Park LC, Covi L (1965) Non blind placebo trial. Arch Gen Psychiatry 12:336–345
65. Goulston K (1972) Drug usage in the irritable colon. Med J Aust 1:1126–1131
66. Paulley JW (1975) Cultural influences on the incidence and pattern of disease. Psychother Psychosom 26:2–11

3 Psychosomatic Disorders: Who Should Treat Them?

If one person is to provide management he or she should have sufficient clinical training and experience to be able to look after a patient's somatic condition as well as its underlying psychological basis. The few essential psychodynamic mechanisms to be understood are listed in Chap. 4. The doctor/therapist must also be prepared to modify the type of management according to the disorder being treated as described in the clinical chapters.

If two or more people are involved, their shared skills and experience should not be less than that of the single practitioner already mentioned, and they must understand each other's methods and meet regularly to coordinate therapy. Such cooperation has to be closer than is usually the case when patients are managed by several people in hospital or general practice. The reason, as Winnicott pointed out [1], is psychosomatic patients' inclination to split their care givers ("scatter of responsible agents"), reflected in the split in their own emotional expression between psyche and soma. If doctors do not take account of this, patients play one therapist/caregiver off against another to their own detriment and the frustration of all involved.

Thomae in Heidelberg [2] by arranging frequent meetings of all caregivers involved in the treatment of AN provided an ideal model of "the team". Trust and understanding forged between clinician and psychiatrist for the duration of an agreed piece of research seldom endure beyond the termination of the work, or extend to colleagues. One reason for this is that research workers are usually young and soon move to other posts.

The liaison developed by Treadgold and Wolff and their colleagues at University College Hospital, London, and many of the clinical consultants is another example. This began as a cooperative teaching exercise for students doing their clerkships or dresserships, but in the case of some of the clinicians it developed into shared clinical responsibility with the psychiatrist/psychotherapist. However, newly appointed staff on both sides are likely to have other interests and ideas, and then such arrangements break down.

3.1 A Need for Greater Clinical Exposure

Until psychiatrists, including liaison psychiatrists, are asked by clinicians to participate in the management of large numbers of the numerous psychosomatoses listed in this book, and are willing to take them on personally or under supervision, they will be just as handicapped as surgeons whose experience of a particular operation remains in single figures. Hambling (personal communication) was a consultant psychiatrist for 11 years before being asked to see his first case of UC.

M. D. Enoch (personal communication), after successfully treating children with this disorder at a district hospital, says that since moving to a teaching hospital 12 years ago he has not been asked to treat a single case. Indeed, psychiatrists who have conducted the psychological management of more than the odd case of hypertension, RA or oesophageal spasm are rare. Reasons for such low referral rates and how this may be changed have been suggested previously [3, 4] and they will be discussed in the final chapter.

3.2 Why Clinicians Gave Up Referring Classical Psychosomatoses

The following quotation partly explains why psychiatrists are not being asked to see enough psychosomatic disorders:

> A point of constant friction was our own reluctance to take over a considerable number of patients with classical psychosomatoses, as for instance peptic ulcer or ulcerative colitis for psychotherapy. Our clinical colleagues were disappointed and angry with us when we refused to treat these patients. On the other hand we did not want to paralyse our task trying to fulfil the very time consuming therapeutic demands. We, in turn, blamed our colleagues for not trying hard enough themselves to acquire the necessary skill so they could offer on their own at least a minimum of supervised psychotherapy to these patients [5]. (From the medical-psychiatric unit at Ulm.)

It follows that there is a need for many more liaison psychiatrists with sufficient experience to treat the range of disorders covered in this book, but because of the logistical difficulties mentioned and the number of patients involved, they will be unable to cope with but a fraction of them. Therefore, more physicians and general practitioners must learn to combine this work with their standard medical care, and contrary to current thinking this can be done in most cases without additional expenditure of time.

3.3 The Team

We have already stressed how psychological management is jeopardised by the tendency of patients with psychosomatic disorders to split and scatter their various care givers and will do so again in the clinical chapters with special references to Crohn's disease, asthma MS, etc. To counter this behaviour, whether in hospital or in general practice, care givers involved need to meet informally at a fixed time at least once a week. Half an hour is enough, and a cup of coffee or tea helps. In hospital medical and nursing staff are always involved, and depending on the nature of the case, a physiotherapist (asthma and hyperventilation), a dietitian (AN) and a medical social worker or occupational therapist as well.

  In the district hospitals at which most of these patients are treated – there being as yet few psychosomatic hospitals or hospitals with special units – effective psychosomatic management depends on the physician in charge of the patient passing on to the ward sister (head nurse) and staff nurse an understanding of the essential psychodynamics and *typical* emotional susceptibilities of the patients being treated. Only in this way is it possible for young nurses and doctors to avoid damaging pitfalls, e.g. in asthma, Crohn's disease or colitis.

3.3.1 Weekly Nurses' Meeting

Compulsory attendance of junior nurses and doctors at a weekly meeting led by the senior doctor or his deputy provides a valuable forum for learning about psychological management. Nurses ask questions about patients in their care, the responsible junior doctor answers, and open discussion follows. Invariably, nurses want to know about patients with whom they have problems in management; many of these have psychosomatic disorders. The meeting should be timed for a maximum attendance and least inconvenience to staff and patients. Half to three-quarters of an hour is enough and a 12.30 p.m. start seems to suit most people.

What has been said also applies to general practice, especially if more than one partner is involved in caring for a patient. Health visitors, district nurses, receptionists and physiotherapists should be included.

3.3.2 Combined Hospital and General Practitioner Care

Logistically this is the most difficult form of team work to arrange. It is nevertheless one of the most important. Occasionally, it is possible for members of the two teams to meet, but this is rare. For this reason scrupulous attention should be given to prompt and full exchange of information either by letter or telephone. Because such a situation is as yet seldom achieved, and its importance not understood, the chances for disastrous "splitting" and manipulation by psychosomatic patients remains very great.

"Team": Misuse of the Term. All too often departmental heads, social and nursing administrators use the term *team* as a smoke screen for doing nothing. It sounds good and looks good in a prospectus. For teams to be really effective, arrangements must be made for their members to meet informally, and talkative seniors likely to inhibit free discussion should keep out of the way.

3.4 Support Groups

It has been found that many care givers involved with people physically or psychologically very ill need the support of their peers. This applies as much to nurses and doctors in ICUs as to medical departments combining general management with psychological management of disorders covered in this book. Our experience of busy district hospitals has shown that the type of unit meetings and nurses' meetings we have described, also function fairly well as support groups. In hospitals or departments specially designed and staffed for the management of psychosomatic disorders, which are as yet very few, such group activity will be more intense, more sophisticated and, it is hoped, more therapeutic.

3.5 Couple Therapy

In some psychosomatic disorders management is facilitated by seeing the patient with a spouse, fiancé(e) or partner. This is often so in UC, Crohn's disease, MS, and for some cases of hyperventilation and disease phobias. The reader is referred to case reports in the relevant clinical chapters for examples. However, there are some disorders in which couple therapy is usually contraindicated; asthma is one of them, and the reasons are given in Chap. 7.

3.6 Group Therapy

Patients with certain disorders reap advantages through treatment in small groups, for example migraine, asthma and diabetes. An extension of this approach to MS has yet to be tried but would seem to offer promise.

3.7 Reassurance

For general practitioners "reassurance" is usually the first step in the psychological management of physical symptoms which are causing overt or covert anxiety. For it to be effective calls for the full history, examination and possibly limited investigations as described in Chap. 5. However, if such patients return a few weeks later, or their file is thick with previous attendances, the doctor should realise that further reassurance alone will not be enough. Yet many experienced doctors continue to refer patients to one specialist after another with the remark: "I feel sure that all she needs is *reassurance*" that she does not have heart disease, cancer, MS, brain tumour, AIDS etc.! If this book helps doctors to recognise that such patients require psychological management such as that described for hyperventilation and the IBS phobias, and that they are often the best qualified people to do it, it will have achieved something. This is because many such patients refuse to see a psychiatrist, or if so persuaded, soon "deskill" him by producing new somatic symptoms which they know are usually beyond his competence to assess. When this happens, another round of specialist referrals follows with increased introspection until some doctor is found who is competent to manage psyche and soma simultaneously.

Lastly, many true psychosomatoses, by Halliday's and our own definition, respond rather readily to psychological management or brief psychotherapy, just as Dunbar pointed out. Patients with behavioural disorders such as alcoholism or obesity know what they are doing and are more resistant to treatment. Because in the psychosomatoses the link mechanisms are always internal and unconscious, the therapist is provided with the powerful therapeutic tool of bringing them into consciousness. Many patients with psychosomatic disorders who have responded to psychological management say that the first important step was when they became *aware* that their emotional feelings were causing their somatic dysfunction or disease. Only after that are they ready to accept the need to change ingrained coping mechanisms by means of psychological management/psychotherapy.

References

1. Winnicott DW (1966) Psychosomatic illness in its positive and negative aspects. Int J Psychoanal 47:510–516
2. Thomae H (1963) Some psychoanalytic observations on anorexia nervosa. Br J Med Psychol 36:239–248
3. Graham DT (1979) What place in medicine for psychosomatic medicine? Psychosom Med 41:357–367
4. Paulley JW (1986) Psychosomatic medicine: a forward look. In: Lacey TH, Sturgeon D (eds) Proceedings of the 15th European conference on psychosomatic research. Libby, London
5. Karstens R (1973) Psychosomatic medicine 1V. Difficulties of integration. Psychother Psychosom 22:196–199

4 Psychodynamic Concepts and Mechanisms

Doctors early in their careers sometimes doubt whether their understanding of psychodynamic concepts is sufficient for them to undertake psychological management. A reason for this is that psychodynamic concepts have been expressed in language as foreign to them as their own specialist jargon is to most psychotherapists. Another reason is that until recently psychoanalysts, tired of ill-informed criticism and cheap jibes, sought the age-old defence of forming associations/societies ("gangs") requiring "initiation ceremonies" (training analysis). Soon, only initiates were regarded as competent to do psychotherapeutic work, and by implication others' attempts would fail, or the patient or client would be damaged. Yet Freud himself, without prior instruction or initiation, managed well enough, but admitted it would have been helpful had he known about transference earlier than he did. It was 10 years before he appreciated the value of working through it in therapy.

Can Psychosomatic Patients Be Harmed by Lack of Knowledge of Such Concepts? Most psychosomatic patients' psychological defences are so strong that their sensitive inner cores are well protected against even the most clumsy interviewing. However, patients with UC, MS, asthma, hypertension, post-MI and AI disease are prone to dangerous exacerbations when they are very ill, if *any* doctor who has been seeing them frequently does not realise when a transference has developed. The risk of this happening is greater if the doctor is not consciously carrying out psychological work, because otherwise he or she would be more likely to be aware of it. Something as apparently innocent as going on holiday without warning his patient, losing his temper without apologising, or passing the patient on to a colleague or a junior without explanation (interpreted by the patient as rejection) commonly provokes relapse. Engel [1] described how in UC *interruption* of the doctor-patient relationship was likely to cause setbacks. We describe comparable responses to doctors by asthmatics and by colitics.

The number of necessary psychodynamic concepts and mechanisms for a doctor wishing to pursue psychological management for psychosomatic disorders are relatively few; transference is the most important. To summarise, it is not the pursuit of psychological management which is hazardous, but what a doctor does *unwittingly* in dealings with sensitive and vulnerable patients. For the reader wishing to look further, the following books are recommended: Sandler et al. [2] and Wolff et al. [3].

4.1 Transference

From the many descriptions of transference we have selected three: first that by Bloomfield [4] who was also writing for students and young doctors:

We transfer feelings and attitudes developed in our early life experience on to people in the present. Since the earliest patterns of response are generally developed in relation to parents or parent substitutes, we are most likely to transfer feelings about these first authority figures on to anyone else in a position of authority, whom we encounter subsequently. Thus teachers, employers, therapists, doctors, priests, politicians or supervisors ... attract feelings which were originally evoked by significant people in our childhood.

Secondly, we quote Greenson [5]:

Transference is the experiencing of feelings, drives, attitudes, fantasies and defences towards a person in the present, which are inappropriate to that person, and are a repetition, or displacement, of reactions originating in regard to significant persons of early childhood. For a reaction to be considered transference it must have two characteristics ... it must be a repetition of the past and be inappropriate to the present.

And lastly, Bloomfield again [4] on the difficulties the concept poses for students and young doctors.

The concept of transference ... is often difficult for students in their early twenties to comprehend ... especially when a patient might be nearer their own parents' age ... They often cannot quite grasp that their particular patient could experience feelings of love, hatred, jealousy or fear towards *them* when these feelings are not the direct result of interactions which have occurred between them.

In all forms of dynamic psychotherapy, because of the length and frequency of sessions and how they are conducted, transference inevitably develops. Indeed, such therapies fail or are fraught with difficulty if the transference is not interpreted and worked through.

In standard general or hospital practice some patients who are seen frequently over a long period also develop a transference to their doctors, with feelings of dependence or even love. These often engender *inappropriate* parental or brotherly feelings on the part of the clinician *(countertransference)*. The hazard of sexual arousal in the doctor-patient relationship is so well-known that it is unnecessary to dwell on it here, but unconscious transference and countertransference are usually involved.

4.1.1 Hazards of Parent-Child Transference

Most adults when severely ill regress towards childlike dependence. Nurses and doctors encourage this because of their psychological need to be regarded as caring "Mums" and "Dads", which is often thought to be an unconscious motive for their choice of profession. However, children grow up, and patients get better. Both may then tire of the dependent role and begin to question the parent or doctor and refuse to do as they are told. If patients' questions are ignored, or they are treated like naughty children, they feel rejected or dominated. Negative transference may then become manifest when they return, complaining that they are no better for the treatment, or the operation has done them no good. They may want to indicate that they are not as ready for independence as the doctor thinks they are; alternatively, the doctor may be seen as the oppressive or possessive parent if the patient is not allowed to go when ready (transcript in Chap. 7). Equally, the doctor who is idealised as the "good father" is condemned to fail in that role. Patients, like children, are also expected by some doctors (parents) to be grateful, and suggestions that their treatment has been no good are then often resented. Doctors who lack this appreciation of parent-child psychodynamics are vulnerable; and the tendency of traditional medical teaching is to train them to remain aloof from their patients' emotions.

In transference a doctor may stand for any of the patient's key figures, irrespective of sex. For example, if the patient's mother was authoritarian and the doctor has a parade-ground voice, the patient may begin to respond as to the mother's strident commands. This is described in the management of asthma (Chap. 7), as those patients often play their doctors into a domineering role. Equally, asthmatics are prone to test their doctors' and nurses' tolerance to the utmost by their challenging or cheeky behaviour. In this way they court the very rejection which they so much dislike.

To summarise, in transference a doctor may stand for any significant figure in the patient's life, and in countertransference the patient may stand for any key figure in the doctor's life. Doctors who do not recognise when a positive transference has developed, are likely to meet some of the problems we have outlined, but failure to recognise a significant intrusion of countertransference into the relationship with the patient is likely to be more serious and jeopardise the outcome unless it is correctly identified and interpreted.

Negative transference is a term applied to a patient's dissatisfaction with the doctor, either from feeling disappointed after initial expectations to be cured, or from the doctor's manipulative behaviour, or because the doctor is acting like an oppressive parent. It may take the form of belittling the doctor/therapist, or in non-cooperation. It is essential for the doctor not collude with the patient (Alan, Chap. 7), but to interpret the transference reactions instead.

4.2 Ambivalence

Ambivalence is a term now so commonly used in ordinary conversation that explanation may be unnecessary. It originates from feeling two ways about an important figure, usually from childhood, i.e. love for a parent or sibling at the same time tinged with feelings of anger, envy and hatred. Love and hate are opposite sides of the same coin, so that normally the more intense feeling of hate is only aroused by those we love, or have loved. When hate is contained in an unconscious way it is a common cause of psychoneurotic or psychosomatic illness. The psychopathology of many psychosomatic disorders is based on unrecognised and unresolved ambivalent (two-way) feelings. In the clincial chapters we refer to it repeatedly and illustrate it which case histories. Effective psychological management depends on helping such patients bring these feelings into consciousness so that they can gradually accept them, together with repressed feelings of love.

Of course, many people who are not ill have ambivalent feelings for some close relatives. Illness for them may only arise when unresolved feelings are reactivated by some new event, such as the illness or death of the relevant figure(s), or someone who stands in their place.

4.3 "Identifying With"

Identifying is involved when someone experiences the feelings of another as if they were his or her own. It amounts to far more than empathy, i.e. the capacity to feel *with* another person, and the defence of *identification-introjection* should not be confused with it.

Identifying with another person is the most relevant psychodynamic in some psychosomatic disorders such as MS and UC. In both, separation from mother or surrogates in infancy is never achieved, or at best only partially (see separation-engulfment in MS in Chap. 9 and UC in Chap. 6). So close are these patients to their key figures that they sometimes say: "It is as if we are the same person." For example, in patients with MS, identifying with something happening to a person close to them, such as death or divorce, is experienced *as if the same thing were happening to themselves,* causing feelings of shock, panic, horror or emptiness (the giving-up response) which precede the demyelinating episode by hours or at the most a few days.

4.4 Defences

These are psychological mechanisms one or more of which everyone uses, including, of course, doctors and their patients. They include repression, denial, projection, rationalisation and splitting.

1. *Repression* is the keeping of certain disturbing feelings, usually dating from childhood, from reaching consciousness. Psychological management for many psychosomatic disorders will be ineffective until such feelings are *brought into consciousness* and find their emotional expression, often for the first time in the therapeutic relationship. The following analogy is a useful facilitation in explaining this to patients: "It is like having an enemy in a dark room; you cannot fight him because you do not know where he is. It is only when you can see him that you can fight him."
2. *Denial* is perhaps the most common defence used by psychosomatic patients and part of their shared "poverty of emotional expression" (see Sect. 2.6). Before treatment, some psychosomatic patients not only deny that they ever express anger, but also that they ever *feel* it, e.g. in UC and in the transcript of R.P. who states that his childhood was happy and his parents never quarrelled!
3. *Splitting* is regarded as a childlike defence of categorising everything into good and bad, especially people. In psychosomatic medicine it is particularly relevant

when patients play one "good" care giver off against another "bad" care giver, usually a replay of what happened with their parents. This applies to doctors in the same practice, or a GP versus a hospital specialist, a nurse versus a doctor, dietitians, physiotherapists, etc. and vice versa. Winnicott [6] pointed to this tendency of psychosomatic patients and described it as "scattering of responsible agents". Although such patients choose to express their emotions through soma, they may at times switch to psyche if they are deprived of the somatic outlet too suddenly, as for example by removal of a target organ such as stomach, colon or uterus by operation, or in asthma when insensitive psychological interpretations are made prematurely which may lead to the wheezing being replaced by florid anxiety or depression in a few hours. These are sometimes termed "flights" into somatic or psychological illness.

4. *Rationalisation* occurs when patients explain their feelings to themselves so reasonably that they do not have to be felt. Psychosomatic patients use this defence a great deal.

5. *Projection* means using other people to express and contain one's own feelings. Aggression or depression too dangerous to express oneself may be dealt with in this way.

6. *Resistance* was originally applied to the attitude of patients in psychoanalysis who could or would not cooperate in free association, presentation of dreams, etc. Ruesch [7] pointed out that this was true for most psychosomatic patients, and the reason why orthodox psychotherapy was suitable for but a few of them. Sandler, Dare and Holder [2] observed that the phenomenon of resistance was also common to therapies other than psychotherapy, including treatment by drugs, i.e. "non-compliance".

7. *Non-Compliance* is said to have been coined by health administrators and sociologists when asked to examine the waste of resources by patients, or because of overprescribing. Doctors unfortunately now use it in a punitive sense instead of looking for the reasons for such behaviour. One reason is some doctors' failure to listen, while another is negative transference, which we have discussed. We feel "non-compliance" is a term which should be discarded. Patients are people, not pawns, and some drugs are dangerous [8].

4.5 When Illness Is Gainful

Illness is clearly gainful in compensation neurosis. However, Groddeck's observation [9] that "the doctor is a threat to that part of the patient which wishes to remain ill" is likely to be less acceptable to young doctors fresh from medical school than a few years later when they will all have encountered such people. Recognition of this form of resistance may make all the difference between success or failure in some patients who do not make progress. Such cases may only resume progress towards health if the doctor points out that, although consciously they wish to be better, unconscious factors may be holding them back, and one of these is that the doctor may seem bent on depriving them of the only emotional outlet that they know. Frank acknowledgement by doctors of being the patient's servant and that the pace and extent of change is *not* in their control but in the patient's, often frees long periods of frustrating deadlock.

Not infrequently failure to return to health despite standard treatment is due to unresolved guilty feelings concerning the loss or alienation of a key figure(s). Here the martyrdom and punishment of a crippling disease such as RA, or recurrent fear of death, as in the phobias, are felt to be easier to bear by these patients than facing their feelings of guilt.

4.6 Stages of Personality Development

Personality development was described by Freud but greatly clarified by Erikson [10]. An understanding of this is particularly relevant to the psychological management of disorders such as MS and UC where failure to separate emotionally from early key figures or surrogates is the basis of the giving-up response to separation-engulfment threats experienced by these vulnerable people. We have summarised important aspects with examples in the section on MS (Chap. 9). They have also been set out clearly by Wolff, Knaus and Bräutigam [3], and illustrated with a light touch by Skynner and Cleese [11].

References

1. Engel GL (1958) Studies of ulcerative colitis V. Am J Dig Dis 3:315–337
2. Sandler J, Dare C, Holder A (1973) The patient and the analyst. Maresfield Reprints, London
3. Bräutigam W, Knauss W, Wolff HH (eds) (1985) First steps in psychotherapy. Springer, Berlin Heidelberg New York
4. Bloomfield I, (1985) The process of supervision: transference and counter-transference. In: Bräutigam W, Knauss W, Wolff HH (eds) First steps in psychotherapy. Springer, Berlin Heidelberg New York, p 55
5. Greenson RR (1965) The working alliance and the transference neurosis. Psychoanal Quarterly 34:155–181
6. Winnicott, DW (1966) Psychosomatic illness in its positive and negative aspects. Int J Psychoanal 47:510–516
7. Ruesch J (1948) The infantile personality: the core problem for psychosomatic medicine. Psychosom Med 10:134–144
8. Paulley JW (1979) Psychological resistance to treatment. Br Med J:23–24
9. Groddeck G (1977) The meaning of illness. Hogarth, London
10. Erikson E (1965) Childhood and society. Penguin, Hamondsworth
11. Skynner R, Cleese J (1983) Families, and how to survive them. Methuen, London

5 Interviews

5.1 The First Interview

5.1.1 The Appointment

Success may depend on events before a patient reaches the consulting room, for example on a secretary or receptionist's attitude. Some of them, like doctors' wives of the past, see themselves as protectors, but in so doing they may frustrate and irritate patients. The importance of secretaries was well put by Rosenow [1]:

> People generally do not sue doctors who are warm and friendly .... They sue the fellows in the biggest and coldest and most unfriendly centers – particularly the men who have rather snappy nurses (secretaries) who take the telephone calls and tell them "He can't see you – he doesn't work Thursdays."

The following dialogue is an example of a well-handled appointment.

P[1]:   Hello. Please can I make an appointment to see Dr. X?
S/R[2]: Of course, but I am very sorry that the earliest I can offer you is Wednesday, 21st October, at 9 a.m.
P: But that's rather longer than I want to wait – it is rather urgent.
S/R: The doctor is rather busy; can you give me a little more detail?
P: It's a headache, and I wonder if it is anything serious.
S/R: I will call you back. The doctor reserves a few short slots in which to fit your kind of problem; if so, it will probably be Friday evening. Can you manage that?
P: Yes, thank you very much. Goodbye.
S/R: Goodbye.

Any doctor can recognise open hostility but must also be able to sense silent hostility, one reason for which may be a secretary's tactlessness. It must be remembered that secretaries are often young and while good with most patients, may be less tolerant of aggressive, bossy people. If the doctor is aware of this, the situation can yet be retrieved by casting a general sort of "fly": "I hope you haven't had too much difficulty in getting here." This is the kind of facilitating remark that enables the patient to let off steam about almost anybody or anything, from his or her spouse who thinks it is a waste of time and money, to traffic and parking, as well as the idea possibly received from the secretary that the doctor's time is in shorter supply than their own!

---

[1] P = Patient.
[2] S/R = Secretary/Receptionist.

The more tense or hostile the patient at the beginning of the interview, the more important it is for the doctor to be friendly and welcoming, however irritated he or she may feel. All patients are entitled to good manners, such as a doctor standing up when a patient enters, or shaking hands and a quiet invitation to sit down. At follow-up interviews these civilities are usually less important, but many doctors overlook them at the crucial first interview to their cost when the history may take almost as long as getting blood out of a stone, and the patient does the opposite of everything requested during physical examination. Not all unrelaxed abdominal muscles are due to cold hands!

However, other causes for patients' hostility are more common. Among these are learned responses to excessively authoritarian key figures in childhood, commonly reinforced by subsequent experience of other authoritarian figures such as school teachers, policemen, employers, and in the present context doctors and nurses themselves. The last group may not see themselves as authoritarian, but because "they do things to you, make you take pills and tell you what to eat and what not to eat," they may appear to be, and as one patient said: "They control you, or try to." For such patients the doctor or nurse stands for the bossy parent and unconsciously evokes a bridling, hostile response acquired in childhood. Many patients' hostility arises from guilt and fear that retribution may have caught up with them, that they have a fatal affliction such as a brain tumour, cancer or venereal disease. Phobia for tuberculosis, once so common, has now vanished; tuberculosis is now no good to phobic patients because they know they are unlikely to die of it. Instead, there are new phobias, notably for leukaemia, AIDS and MS. The symptoms of the latter, paraesthesia and blurred vision, are nowadays described in detail on TV and in the newspapers, and they are sensations most people experience at some time or another for quite benign reasons, for example hyperventilation.

5.1.2 The Setting

Ideally, the room should be quiet enough for the patient and the doctor to converse without having to raise their voices; any voices heard from outside at all should be so muffled as to be unintelligible. Otherwise, the patient will feel that what he says may be equally audible outside and that will not only restrict the value of the initial interview but may lead him to seek privacy with another doctor. It is remarkable how many experienced doctors still have to learn the importance of privacy. Some delude themselves that because they are not psychiatrists they do not have to. They are wrong, and a nurse or a secretary in the room while a patient is giving a history to a physician or surgeon is equally unacceptable. Health service clinics are particularly deficient in these requirements, and administrators and architects need to be made much more aware of them.

Arrangement of Desk, Chairs, Lighting and Decor. Some doctors go in for very imposing desks and sit behind them in a chair resembling a throne. One may speculate what leads them to do this, but whatever it is, it does not help a patient already feeling "one down" to someone they see misguidedly as a kind of scientific wizard (Fig. 1). The lighting should be arranged in such a way that the patient is not

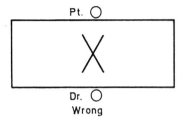
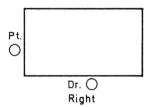

Fig. 1

dazzled or reminded of a "third degree" interrogation. The doctor in private practice will depend on personal taste, but in health service units it derives more from the whims of administrators and others and can be unnecessarily bleak. It is best to avoid garish or discordant tones. Pictures help, but frightening or lurid scenes are better avoided. The aim should be tranquillity but not treacle!

5.1.3 The Doctor's Appearance

It has been fashionable of late for some doctors to ape school teachers, social workers and some psychologists and be ostentatiously casual, i.e. jeans and no tie. The intention is to make patients feel more comfortable and communication easier. But just as an untidy waiting room may create an impression of carelessness, so dressing too casually may sow seeds of doubt of a doctor's competence, particularly among the majority of patients, who are past middle age. Some formality of dress is therefore desirable, but it may be counterproductive unless accompanied by friendliness, good manners and a display of professional ability. So, whereas some psychologists, for reasons of their own, have distanced themselves from the medical model and feel they gain by merging with their clients, doctors wishing to engage in competent psychosomatic management must be mindful that they have to straddle the two horses "soma" and "psyche" like a circus performer without falling off. Whereas in a hospital clinic the traditional white coat may convey clinical competence and thereby be useful in meeting the patients' initial expectation that their somatic complaints will be dealt with efficiently, it is likely to be counterproductive if continuing sessions for psychological management or psychotherapy are advised and agreed. At that stage the white coat can be seen by the patient, and sometimes unconsciously used by the doctor, as part of an impenetrable armour. However, doctors who manage to be warm and approachable *despite* wearing a white coat not only dent their starchy public image but find it no handicap. Hippocrates summed it up well when he advised doctors in their dealings with patients to aim at moderation.

So far we have been discussing the trappings attendant upon the first interview. None are as decisive as the interview itself, yet each can contribute to, or militate against, success.

5.1.4 Taking the History

All doctors develop their own method of taking a medical history. Our task is to stress points of special importance when dealing with a patient with a psychosomatic disorder. However, as the diagnosis is unknown in most cases when the patient is first seen, it is best to regard every patient as potentially suffering from a disorder with a major psychosomatic determinant – the majority.

GPs may feel the need to concentrate on a strictly organic medical history and examination when they see a patient for the first time and depend on "hunches" based on such things as non-verbal communication (see p. 40) as to whether they offer a longer appointment to obtain the biographical anamnesis.

Voice, Size and Manner. Doctors who do not have a quiet voice should try to lower it. Loud or strident voices set some peoples' teeth on edge, especially if it awakens childhood experiences. Fairly or not, people with loud staccato voices remind sensitive people of authoritarian figures, such as school bullies, some school teachers, policemen or sergeant majors.

Large doctors should try to appear smaller in relation to the patient. This is particularly important while interviewing asthmatics. If the interview is at the bedside, the doctor should sit down and not stand over the patient; in a consulting room one of us has been known to sit in the waste paper basket or on a low stool.

The doctor's manner should be empathetic and relaxed, thereby encouraging the patient to talk. Initial questions should be open ended: "Tell me about yourself."; "Can you describe the pain?"; "How does it compare with pain you have had before, like toothache or cramp?" Direct questions requiring "Yes" or "No" answers should be deferred until the end of the interview, such as: "Do you smoke"; "Do you get breathless?"; "Do you get pains in the chest?"; "Do you open your bowels regularly?"

The Importance of a Full History and Clinical Examination. Every patient must feel confident that the doctor has listened attentively to the complaints and that he or she has had a thorough clinical examination followed by sufficient, but not too many investigations. Psychosomatically orientated doctors should aim at being better than average as clinicians and not worse, or their patients will not give them the trust that is so essential when asked to consider a possible relationship between their disease and their emotions.

5.1.5 Biographical Anamnesis

This full and extended history of the patients' life, childhood, adolescence, adulthood, relationships with parents, grandparents, siblings, children, in-laws, close friends, neighbours, work mates, as well as hopes, ambitions, achievements, frustrations, sensitivity, ability to express emotions especially anger, etc. is essential if a doctor feels the patient needs psychological management or psychotherapy, but it can be gathered gradually. Dunbar [2] and Groen [3] have considered the anamnesis to be the most important investigative procedure for psychosomatic disorders, and

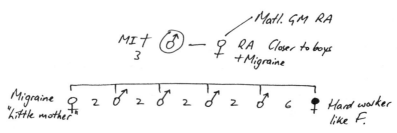

Fig. 2. Family history, psychosomatically orientated

also the first step in long-term psychological management, being in itself psychothe-rapeutic. Such a complete history is unlikely to be posible in general practice in a single interview. So what can health service practitioners do? Seeing a patient for the first time, many will find all the time taken up by the essential medical history and examination. However, depending on the suspected diagnosis, or on prior knowled-ge of the patients' family, or non-verbal "messages" from sighs, hesitations, wheezes, averted eyes, etc., the doctor can then decide whether it is necessary to give the patient more time by offering a special appointment, perhaps 15–30 min. If this time is added to the first attendance at the surgery, the time available is about the same as most physicians (internists) working in the health service are able to give to new patients referred to outpatient clinics. We have had many years' experience of working under this kind of time pressure as well as of private practice in which conditions, while optimal, are valuable as a yardstick against which physicians will be able to measure their health service performance.

Much information can be obtained in as little as 10–15 min, and it may be useful to continue the interview during physical examination. Many patients lower their psychological defences when lying undressed on a couch and readily admit things they had denied strongly as little as 5 min before in the consulting room.

The Extended Family History. One way of obtaining maximum information in the minimum amount of time is the extended family history, recording essential information with an occasional stroke of the pen on a family tree diagram with siblings and children declining in age from left to right (Fig. 2). The following transcript illustrates the use of the family tree diagram, showing how each piece of information is added, and it is offered as one way of recording information relevant to the management of psychosomatic patients, with retrieval at subsequent interviews made easy. The patient is a school teacher, unmarried, aged 23 years, presenting with migraine of 9 years' duration and a severe vascular headache and phobia for cerebral tumour for 2 years.

D[1]: Are you one of a large family?
P[2]: One of six.
D: Where do you come in it?
P: I am the youngest.

---

[1] D = Doctor.
[2] P = Patient.

D: By how many years?

P: Six

D: And your parents, are they well?

P: My mother has RA, my father died 3 years ago (stated without obvious emotion).

D: I am sorry to hear that (pause). Do any other relatives have RA or things like goitre or diabetes? [looking for hereditary disposition to AI diseases]

P: My mother's mother may have had RA but she died years before I was born. (Doctor makes mental note that mother's RA itself may have been precipitated by early loss)

D: Do any of the others have migraine?

P: One of my brothers, my sister and my mother when she was younger.

D: How many brothers and sisters do you have?

P: The eldest is a girl, the rest are boys apart from myself.

D: How many years between them?

P: Oh, short, not more than 2 years. (pause) I think I was an "after thought".

D: Were you told that?

P: No, but when I was quite small I heard my mum telling my aunt.

D: What did you feel?

P: I think I felt a bit different to the others, and a bit unwanted.

D: Your mother must have had her hands full? [facilitation]

P: Yes, she did.

D: Were you particularly close to your brothers or sister?

P: Very close to my sister, it was she who looked after me when I was small, she's more like a mother.

D: How about your brothers?

P: My youngest brother and I are close now, but when I was small we used to fight – he teased me.

D: Perhaps he was jealous having been Benjamin until you arrived?

P: Yes, I think that was the reason.

D: Tell me about your parents. Do you think you are more like your mother or father in temperament?

P: A bit of both, but more like my father.

D: In what way?

P: Both are hard workers, and although he was strict, he was a very warm person. My mother is sensitive but does not show her feelings – it is difficult to get close to her.

D: Did the boys feel the same?

P: Not the three eldest; she was not one to kiss and cuddle any of us, but she tended to spoil the boys with presents and treats. My sister felt this more than I did, because I had her, didn't I?

D: What was your father's trouble?

P: He died of a heart attack.

D: Any warning?

P: Not really, although he had been to his doctor with indigestion 2 weeks before (sadly?).

D: It is always distressing when these things happen without warning. You don't have time to say the things you might have if the illness had been longer. [psychological jargon "finishing one's business"] (Patient in tears.) You still feel it very much? (Doctor comforts patient either by getting up and putting an arm round her shoulders or putting a hand on her arm/hand but saying nothing except perhaps "Take your time".) [NB A doctor who behaves like an "embarrassed sphinx" will give the patient the impression of a lack of sensitivity; this may block further communication.] (As patient's emotion subsides) It seems your father is much in your thoughts?

P: He's always there, I adored my father.

D: I am sure you did, but sometimes the reason why people have difficulty in getting over the loss of people close to them is that they feel perhaps they could have done more, or were in some way feeling bad about it, or even responsible.

P: My father was rather possessive and didn't like my boyfriend, and I had a terrible row with him only a month before he died.

The cause of her tumour phobia is now apparent: guilt, fear of retribution and making reparation. For psychological management of pathological loss and mourning of this type see Chap. 10.

The date of onset of mother's RA should also be recorded. If it occurred many years before, it is likely to have been related to ambivalent feelings over the loss or alienation of a key figure such as her mother, father, or a surrogate such as a sibling or child, stillbirth or pet. If so, the RA will probably have worsened after her husband's death. Why the father had a MI may be thought to be academic but could be related to attitudes to work (type A, workaholic), and if some of these washed off on any of his children, that would be important to the GP. Apart from hereditary disposition, the basis of father's workaholic behaviour would have been set in his own childhood (Chap. 8, IHD and Chap. 6 DU).

In unravelling interpersonal relationships in the family it is necessary to ask whether siblings are married, have children, if they and their children are well and if not, what the trouble is, do they live near or far away? Do members meet or visit, where and when and if not, why? Christmas and other festivals are times when families meet, and infinite opportunities present for ultrasensitive members to take umbrage (see Chap. 6, UC and Crohn's disease, Chap. 9, MS).

However, interpersonal stress may not always be in the immediate family cirle; grandparents, close neighbours and friends may have to be included, and last but not least in-laws, or potential in-laws, if any. Colleagues, managers and foremen, if abrasive or dismissive, are provocative in a small minority of psychosomatic disorders, probably no more than 10%. Patients may greatly dislike such people but rarely hate or love them as they would someone in the family. (Interpersonal stress at work is more commonly seen in disorders such as migraine, hypertension and IHD than in IBD.)

The reader may be saying: "This is all very well, but can one possibly do all this in a limited time?" The answer is no, unless the time for the initial interview is not less than an hour; even then much will not emerge until later meetings. What has to be done initially is to obtain the basic extended family history as roughly outlined, which with practice can be done in 5 min, noting it down in abbreviated form, so that the doctor's whole visual and auditory attention can be given to the patient. All doctors develop their own method of note taking. The family tree format is merely one that we have found simple and time saving.

Is There Such a Thing as a Psychosomatically Directed Interview? The answer is yes, if the kind of consultation outlined is compared with the standard medical history. Does it differ then from a psychodynamically orientated initial interview for someone with a psychoneurosis? Yes, on two counts, first because the medical history and examination are included, and second because although there is common ground in the use of open-ended questions in exploring the patient's childhood, feelings and family polarities, and in the use of silence, patients with psychosomatic disorders pose a problem for doctors because of their shared "poverty of emotional expression" [4], "superstability" [5], "pensée opératoire" [6] and alexithymia [7] that psychoneurotic patients rarely display to the same extent. The doctor, therefore, has to adapt his or her approach to burrow under, or get round, the patient's defences. The methods are integral to effective management of PM disorders, varying from one disorder to another. These will be described in detail in the respective chapters. It is the concatenation of such evidence over hundreds, and not just tens, of cases that has taught psychosomatically orientated physicians the reality and value of *typicality* because only they have to deal with such numbers. Those who have disagreed, such as some psychoanalysts and many psychiatrists, have rarely had the same opportunities as clinicians to take on enough cases, because of insufficient referrals, or because their way of working was so time consuming.

Recent textbooks on psychosomatic medicine have neglected history taking, as they have also neglected guidance on psychological management or psychotherapy.

Dunbar [2] and Weiss and English [8] recognised the history as paramount in diagnosis over 40 years ago. Those wishing to learn more than can be conveyed in this book alone would do well to turn to both the sources mentioned, particularly sections on the psychosomatic history. Dunbar wrote:

> Gradually it became apparent that the usual psychiatric history as well as the usual medical history belonged to the either-or phase of medical practice ... That is, has this patient organic damage? If not, the practice ... was to tell him there was nothing wrong, or refer him to a psychiatrist. Such histories were essentially inadequate (p. 23) ... Personal data section (of the standard history) is useless unless it really gives personal data, and not just civic status, exercise, and addiction to tea, coffee or alcohol. (p. 32)

Yet half a century later that is still all the personal information the average medical history provides. On p. 54 Dunbar discusses:

> Degree and type of muscular tension ... the patient's muscle tension, his postural attitude, voice, gestures, and particularly their variations in relation to specific material under discussion were found revealing ... All patients are not tense in the same way ... generalised tension ... often escapes notice because of *their appearance of quiet control* ... furthermore they give great attention to correct external behaviour *(Superstability).* [Our italics.]

Dunbar also gives a transcript on pp. 58–72 of how an interview should be conducted, with open-ended questions, facilitations, observations and non-verbal communication. Today's students should be made aware of this mine of valuable information. Weiss and English [8] had this to say on history taking:

> One of our patients who had been through the mill of medical investigation recently remarked she was suffering from "testitis" ... If patients were allowed to talk more and were examined less, it would probably be a good thing for medicine as a whole (p. 74).

The introduction of the psychosomatic point of view does not require a different form of history taking; it only requires an awareness of the role that emotions play in illness, and consequently more emphasis on certain aspects of history taking. *Thus the history need not differ* in form but in substance (p. 75).

The essence of the psychosomatic approach in history taking is to give the patient sufficient time to tell his story (p. 76).

Weiss and English then discuss the problem that time appears to pose for the GP and came to the same conclusion as we did.

A third important book was written in 1948 by Halliday [9], sometimes known as the father of British psychosomatic medicine. His famous three questions should be engraved on every doctor's soul. They are:

Why did this man take ill?
Why did he take ill when he did?
Why did he take ill with what he did?

It is hoped that the quotations offered will encourage some to look at these sources which are as relevant today as when they were written, yet apparently ignored or deemed unfashionable by those who teach doctors and medical students.

5.1.6 Facilitations

It has long been recognised that patients with psychosomatic disorders "bottle up" their emotions, and this has frustrated psychotherapists using orthodox methods [4, 6, 7]. For this reason patients need to be helped first to recognise emotions, unconscious or heavily repressed, and then to be able to express them instead of denying them. Facilitations of this kind have been seen for good reason to be too directive and intrusive by orthodox psychotherapists working predominantly with psychoneurotic patients. However, unless doctors learn to use them discreetly in psychosomatic disorders, both patient and doctor will be frustrated by the lack of progress. At no time is this more important than at the first interview, because all forms of treatment, including psychological management, psychotherapy or even surgery depend on "holding" the patient long enough for it to be effective.

Therefore, some questions are necessary, but they should be open-ended or otherwise these heavily defended patients will reveal little of themselves. In helping the patient the doctor uses nods, smiles, encouraging grunts and giving total attention. There are many ways of saying "Mm"; some encourage the patient to go on, others may imply the doctor is bored or running short of time!

5.1.7 Hesitations and Qualifications

Doctors need to train their ears to pick up the slightest hesitation in replies to a quite ordinary question, like: "Do you sleep well?", e.g.P:"r – yes, thank you". Unless these are picked up, important opportunities are lost. The interviewer needs to say, "You seem a little uncertain."

P: Well, I haven't been sleeping quite as well as usual.
D: Why is that?
P: Since my wife started a job the youngest girl has been playing up.
or
D: Is your wife fit and well?
P: ..r – yes, thank you.
D: You seem a little unsure?
P: Well, she has an appointment to see a gynaecologist for bleeding, and there's a long wait.

Thus the hidden source of anxiety is revealed. Qualified answers should also be picked up in the same way:

D: Do you sleep well?
P: Oh, quite well, or fairly well.
D: What do you mean by that?
P: Well, I have been waking up a lot lately at about 5 a.m. and not getting off again.

The next question is obvious: "Can you tell me what you think about or whether there is anything on your mind?" Similarly, qualified answers such as "quite" or "fairly" as applied to the spouse's or children's health, behaviour, job satisfaction, etc. need following up. Even though the patient may try to assure the doctor that the hesitation or qualification was not significant, nine times out of ten it is highly significant.

5.1.8 Silences

Most people are uncomfortable if an individual falls silent, and doctors are no exception. Silence often conveys hostility. Doctors too often "jump in" prematurely to relieve their own feeling of tension. Silences of this sort are more likely in later interviews when a negative *transference* (see Chap. 4) may have developed. Subsequent progress in management/psychotherapy will be blocked until the cause has been identified and interpreted. Failure by the doctor to do so will increase negative transference and lead to more silences, and then the patient missing or coming late for appointments, the forerunner of dropping out altogether.

Such a policy on silences may be difficult to follow in a busy surgery or outpatient clinic, but even waiting a minute or two may achieve a great deal, or saying quietly: "I wonder what you are feeling" or "Can you tell me why you are silent?" For an example of a "silence" see the transcript involving asthma in Chap. 7.

5.1.9 "Tin-Opening" Questions

In the clinical sections of the book some questions will be suggested as appropriate to the disorder, e.g. migraine: "Can you sit still for long, doing nothing? How do you feel in a queue? Do you stand or walk up escalators? Can you leave dishes in the sink overnight?" or in the AI diseases: "Are any of the people you have lost much in your thoughts? Have you ever heard the expression: God doesn't pay his debts in money (gold)? If the answer to this last question is: "Yes", as it often is in people brought up in rural areas anywhere, the supplementary is "What do you think it means?" Similarly, there are appropriate "tin-openers" for colitis, IBS, DU, IHD, hypertension, etc.

5.1.10 Typicality

What has just been said clearly anticipates the whole question of *typicality* (old term *specificity*), not only of personality but also of *typically* provocative life situations which are discussed fully in Chap. 1.

Just as competent gardeners do not dig for potatoes in the rose garden, so psychosomatists need to know where to look, otherwise they will find roses and not potatoes, and dissatisfied patients may take off to herbalists or faith healers.

5.1.11 Non-verbal Communications

These include tense postures such as sitting on the edge of the chair, arms clasped high round the chest ("I am not letting you in" or "I am not letting much out"), vibrant voices or speaking between clenched teeth, to the more recognised ones of scratching or playing with a wedding ring or handkerchief. All these, as well as hostile coughs, gulping and expressive hand movements, etc. are channeled via the voluntary motor nervous system. Organs dependent for their innervation on the autonomic ("involuntary") nervous system may also "speak for the patient", e.g. borborygmi when a sensitive subject is being discussed, nasal congestion and sneezing, blushing of face and upper chest, particularly in women, palpitation and sweating.

Physical signs at examination may also tell much about a patient's state of mind: (a) oven burns on forearms = accident prone, angry, hurried, tired, careless; (b) dirty navels in women = prudish; (c) tidy pile of clothes = obsessional; (d) noisy undressers (men) whistling, humming = phobic (whistling in the dark); (f) quick undressers, "I am ready now, doctor" = obsessional; (g) patients looking out of windows and not listening are saying to themselves: "I know what I have got, even if he doesn't" =phobic; (h) cogwheel, irregular breathing on auscultation pointing to respiratory neurosis, hyperventilation; (i) adduction of legs in women while eliciting ankle reflexes suggests frigidity or sexual hang-up; (j) patients who sound their s's – "Yes'ssss" – between their teeth = suggests concealed feelings, especially noticed in UC; (k) little girl or childlike voices or expressions reflecting emotional immaturity, e.g. UC, Crohn's disease, MS (Chaps. 6 and 9).

5.2 Subsequent Appointments and Spacing of Interviews

For many psychosomatic disorders it will initially be the somatic part of the illness that determines how soon the patient needs to be seen again. This is particularly true for someone who has just had a severe attack of asthma, colitis, cardiac arrythmia, hypertension, RA, SLE, giant cell arteritis, MS, etc. If the somatic aspect is painful or uncomfortable but not dangerous, such as migraine, aphthous ulcers, IBS or musculoskeletal disorders, the need to see the patient soon is less pressing. This highlights once more the difference between psychosomatic management and standard medical or psychiatric management in that the psychosomatist has to listen and work at two levels, it is not either-or, soma or psyche, but both.

If doctors insist on seeing patients more often than necessary, they risk creating undesirable dependence in their patient, as well as using time they might be using more effectively elsewhere. On the other hand if they "cut *themselves* off suddenly" because the colitis, asthma, RA, etc. has remitted and no further prescriptions are necessary, they ignore the *transference* that may have developed, and may then be equated consciously or unconsciously with the neglectful, uncaring, rejecting parent. As we shall point out repeatedly, it is very often through transference that patients get better, although many doctors believe it due to the drugs, etc. that they have prescribed, just as mistakenly as did Bargen and Gill (quoted in Chap. 2). Doctors greatly underestimate their potency in this respect. Thus, any good which may have been done by doctors can be undone by then cutting themselves off peremptorily at the same time as their pills or injections. Instead, an appointment should be made in a month or two "to see how you are getting on". A patient may agree or say: "If I am O.K. could I phone you and cancel it?"

"Of course," should be the reply, "but if you do, we should arrange one final appointment in the next few months to discuss how we should leave things for the future." (See section on termination.)

Whereas in most cases spacing of interviews will be determined by the nature or severity of the somatic component, when continuing psychological management/ psychotherapy is felt to be the cornerstone of treatment, then the frequency of interviews and the duration form an important aspect of management.

In many psychosomatic disorders the necessary change in coping mechanisms and emotional attitude depends more on the passage of time than on intensity of treatment. This is in contrast to psychotherapy for the psychoneuroses, in which it has been traditional to require the patient to attend for an hour at least once a week over an agreed period of time, with tight boundaries. This view is quoted, not because we agree with all of it, but to assure readers that effective management for psychosomatic disorders can be achieved without such restrictions, and that the amount of time involved is quite modest by comparison. By allowing the patient to accept responsibility for deciding the dates of subsequent interviews, not only is dependency reduced, but emotional independence is encouraged. For the same reason face-to-face interviews take preference to the couch in the treatment of psychosomatic disorders. The exceptions are the few selected cases who after 1–2 years of directive therapies such as described in this book are then judged as suitable for full psychoanalysis. (See Chap. 2 for reasons why most psychosomatic patients are unsuitable for psychoanalysis and for the exceptions who are, read: Karush et al. [10] and Wittich [11].) Sufferers from disorders such as UC and MS display such childlike dependency and separation problems that psychological work at some depth is needed if they are to obtain even that small degree of emotional autonomy needed for their somatic presentation to remit, and to have a fair chance of staying in remission. Early on they should be given an estimate of how long a period of treatment will last, and the likely frequency of interviews. Experience has shown that in MS a minimum of 2 years is required with early interviews weekly or fortnightly, but soon being extending to monthly. By the 2 years three-monthly interviews may be enough. Patients are initially apprehensive if they feel the gap is too long but gain feelings of self-sufficiency when they succeed in setting longer spaces between interviews without mishap. In this way they test themselves and savour independence sometimes for the first time in their lives. Some patients with UC need psychological management at some depth, but many do not. The passage of time is more important than frequent interviews, and seeing relapses as stepping stones to emotional growth, not as unmitigated disasters. Patients with Crohn's disease need a minimum of 2 years, and the management of prolonged mourning and loss in AI diseases and phobias requires between 6 months and 2 years according to progress in its resolution.

5.2.1 Breaks in Care Continuity: Holidays

Doctors should warn patients whom they have been seeing frequently when they are going to be away. They seldom realise that transference may have been established, although they have not knowingly been doing psychological work. Where they have embarked upon the kind of psychological management or psychotherapy described in this book, not giving notice of their absence to their patients and the opportunity for them to express their feelings about it may put at risk any benefit from work already done. Patients with psychosomatic disorders not infrequently take ill when their doctor is away, and at the next consultation they may express feelings of anger and dissatisfaction that the doctor was not there when needed. In those psychosomatic disorders in which the inability to express anger is a "typical" personality trait, the doctor may be able to "use" the opportunity afforded, by accepting the patient's anger and with subtlety encourage it. Thereby the patient is helped to learn to express feelings openly to authority – the doctor standing for a parent.

A major cause of some patients' dissatisfaction with today's medicine is that they may see a different doctor each time they attend a surgery or outpatient clinic. This may not matter much for acute disabilities such as injury or minor infections, but it negates effective management of disorders with a major psychosomatic determinant. It is damaging for patients and bad for the doctor in terms of job satisfaction. Therefore, doctors who wish to pursue psychological management/psychotherapy must, as far as possible, ensure continuity of care from the first interview to termination.

5.2.2 Termination

It is evident that the longer the time over which a patient is seen, the greater the depth of the probable transference. Provided doctors remain constantly alert to this, and interpret during treatment sessions the implications of their patients' feelings towards them in the context of earlier or current feelings towards key figures, then termination, when it comes, will be less of a problem. It is wise to introduce the question of termination 6–12 months before it is due, and to raise it at almost every session. Only by so doing can very dependent patients express those feelings of anger and panic at being abandoned or rejected which have usually played such a large part in the psychopathogenesis of their disorder, and which hitherto they may have been unable to express because they were unaware of the relationship and largely unconscious of the feelings.

Where prolonged feelings of loss and mourning are involved in the psychopathogenesis, e.g. in RA, the AI disorders, the phobias and hypertension, resolution of the patients' feelings towards the doctor or therapist whom they are about to lose, is perhaps the most valuable part of the psychological management for this group of disorders. The patients are thereby enabled to work through their "unfinished business" with lost or alienated key figures with the doctor/therapist standing proxy for them in the transference (Chap. 4). (For examples of management of pathological mourning reactions see transcripts of patients with AI diseases in Chap. 10.)

In psychosomatic disorders "termination" for the most vulnerable patients must always include "an open door" with easy access to the doctor at the patient's request. Psychoanalysts of great experience of psychosomatic medicine support this view, e.g. in UC [10, 11], and it is typified by the card given to asthmatics on discharge from hospital (Chap. 7).

5.3 An Additional Note for General Practice

5.3.1 Confidentiality

GPs more often than hospital doctors meet their patients outside the professional setting, in the street, at a shop or on a committee. Because of this they may feel that such patients might be reluctant to discuss a possible emotional basis for a disorder. The difficulty cannot be ignored, but if *handled well* has been shown to be no hindrance [12]. The essential thing is for the doctor to be seen to be scrupulous about confidentiality, e.g. "I am not writing down what you are telling me, it's not going in the notes," and asking the patient's permission before anything is discussed with a spouse or third party. Doctors should avoid telling members of their own family that Mrs. X is ill and that they are looking after her. Mrs. X's surprise when she eventually meets the family and finds that they did not know she had been ill is soon passed on, and the doctor's reputation for discretion is enhanced. The setting and sound proofing of the consulting room is also important. Patients attending for special psychological management sessions should not be expected to run the gauntlet of a waiting room full of people who may know them. For a GP's own opinions on this, see [12]. Lastly, doctors who spend much time in pubs or golf club bars may not be trusted with confidences.

5.3.2 Certification

This is another problem particular to general practice, but the management of psychosomatic disorders should be little affected by it because although such patients may stay away from work when fearful about their symptoms, their records will show that hard work and competitiveness are much more characteristic of them than shirking. All doctors dislike being exploited, and young doctors are no exception. Bräutigam [12] describes this as follows,

> The doctor-patient relationship is clearly influenced by the fact that doctors (GPs) know they have authority and responsibility for their patient's social lives which they cannot avoid while at the same time they are financially dependent on their patients and are in danger of losing self-esteem if they give in to them.

We suggest that once doctors have identified such patients in their practice, they would by wise to reach a compromise and, rather than waste time and energy in argument with every case, decide sometimes to give in gracefully. They will soon realise that such patients are often the psychological or social cripples of society and if refused will only obtain what they need from another doctor or another social agency.

However, effective management of psychosomatic disorders requires doctors to distinquish as soon as possible between patients who are "lead swinging", malingering or have Münchausen's syndrome from those with psychosomatic disorders who can be helped. If they are in too much of a hurry or too dismissive, they will damage few in the first group but may lose the opportunity of helping the second group and at the same time the respect and trust which in a small community is so important.

References

1. Rosenow EC (1966) Residency in the clinical specialties (discussion). The ethical, legal and economic implications of the delegation of responsibility in a clinical teaching unit. Can Med Assol J 95:753
2. Dunbar F (1943) Psychosomatic diagnosis. Hoeber, New York
3. Groen JJ (1951) Emotional factors in the aetiology of internal diseases. J M Sinai Hosp NY 8:71–89
4. Ruesch J (1948) The infantile personality: the core problem of psychosomatic medicine. Psychosom Med 10:134–144
5. Sjöbring H (1923) Hysteric insufficiency and its constitutional basis. Acta Med Scand 59:387–405
6. Marty P, de M'Uzan (1963) La pensée opératoire. Rev Fr Psychoan 27 [Suppl]:1345–1356
7. Sifneos PE (1973) The prevalence of alexithymic characteristics in psychosomatic patients. Psychother Psychosom 22:253–262
8. Weiss E, English OS (1949) Psychosomatic medicine. Saunders, Philadelphia
9. Halliday JL (1948) Psycho-social medicine. Hyman, London
10. Karush A, Daniels GE, Glood C, O'Connor JF (1977) Psychotherapy in chronic ulcerative colitis. Saunders, Philadelphia
11. Wittich GH (1980) Discussion of "The role of conflicts in intestinal disease." 11th International conference on gastroenterology, Hamburg
12. Bräutigam W (1983) Psychotherapy in general practice. In: Bräutigam W, Knaus W, Wolff HH (eds) First steps in psychotherapy. Springer, Berlin Heidelberg New York, pp 100–147

6 Alimentary Tract

6.1 The Aphthoses

6.1.1 Aphthous Ulcer of the Mouth

Incidence. A common and painful affliction affecting as many as 20% [1] of people but in most only intermittently and with long remissions. Nevertheless, dental surgeons and GPs find the worst cases frustrating to treat. Cortisol pellets provide effective short-term relief but do not prevent another ulcer appearing in a few days in the most severely affected.

Aetiology. It has been reported as a complication of UC and coeliac disease, but with such a high general incidence of oral ulcers in the general community, the relationship cannot be strong. In 1976 a flat jejunal mucosa was reported in 20% of patients presenting with aphthous ulceration who had not previoulsy been recognised as having coeliac disease [2] and that a gluten-free diet brought satisfactory relief for the ulcers. However, Tyldesley [3] found the incidence of flat jejunal mucosa in aphthous ulceration to be much lower, at 6.2%. This is in agreement with our own findings. Other research [4] favours an immunological basis for aphthous ulcers with possible antigens ranging from virus and food to physical trauma. A sensitivity reaction involving mast cell discharge finds circumstantial support from the bleb reported by some observers to precede the ulcer, and from the beneficial effect of cortisone.

Personal Observations. Thirty years ago one of us (J.W.P) was impressed by similarities in the personalities and attitudes of these patients as well as by the fact that exacerbations occurred at times of emotional stress or pressure at work, and decided to carry out a trial of ACTH, which had just become available, and before cortisone could be prescribed. The value of ACTH and cortisone had already been established in other stress-related conditions in which histamine release was involved, e.g. glottic oedema. Two patients so treated with 20 units of ACTH per day remitted immediately and remained free of ulcers for 6 months, when they ceased to attend for follow-up. Clearly, the remission might have been due to placebo effect. Had not Gill (personal communication) found saline injections just as effective as the histidine advocated for DU (Chap. 2)? To test this, the next two cases of aphthous ulcers were given injections of 2 ml of subcutaneous saline daily. Both remitted, and remained in remission for 9 months, beyond which it was not felt justifiable to continue the trial. Whatever the instrinsic merits of ACTH or cortisone, the therapeutic effect of suggestion was evident. This led to a closer look at personality traits and attitudes and at whether particular forms of emotional stress were more common in these patients than in others. The conclusions reached at that time have been confirmed repeatedly by every patient with this condition ever since, a period of 25 years.

6.1.1.1 Psychopathogenesis

Patients with recurrent benign aphthous ulcers come from the same, uptight, industrious, perfectionistic subsection of the population which is also prone to migraine, IBS, dysmenorrhoea, PMT, urethral syndrome, back and neck ache, and intervertebral disc swelling, degeneration and prolapse. Syndrome shift between these disorders is common, as shown in cases in the relevant chapters, and aphthous ulcers and migraine share a familial incidence [5].

We are not alone in our view of these patients. Sircus et al. [1] in a study of 120 patients reported that 89% had a life pattern of conformity and good behaviour and that 35% showed obsessional features. Hard work, striving, neatness and orderliness were recognised in 71%. Unfavourable childhood experiences were present in 71%, and severe environmental or emotional stress preceded onset in 63%. In 9 cases the stress was the sudden unexpected death of a first-degree relative.

As early as 1898 Sibley [6] reported on three patients in an article entitled "Neurotic ulcers of the mouth". The first patient was described as "extremely active"; onset of her aphtha followed great domestic trouble, and her only significant remission over the next 23 years occurred after breaking a leg and enforced rest and convalescence in France away from her emotional problems. A second patient suffered from headaches, musculoskeletal pains and symptoms suggestive of hyperventilation. She had also had "climacteric hysteria" at the menopause. In her case the ulcers always corresponded to a more or less "trivial worry". The provocative stress in Sibley's last patient was reported to be money.

6.1.1.2 Psychological Management

We recommend the same approach as for migraine (Chap. 9) which involves helping the patients recognise ingrained intolerance of untidiness, unpunctuality or relaxation, all of which are equated with laziness. Management involves helping them to recognise their perfectionism and where it came from, parent or surrogate, i.e. inherited or learned or both, and offering a relaxation technique. They should be asked to say what they feel when they are inactive for more than a few minutes. The answer is usually: "I feel awful."

D: Why?
P: I don't know – I suppose I feel guilty. I am wasting my time.
D: Can you remember when you first felt that?
P: Well, my mother was always so busy.

Even at the first interview it is possible to help many such patients recognise for the first time the relationship of exacerbations of their symptoms to periods of increased tempo at work, either imposed by an employer or because someone is sick or on holiday, but more usually they impose it on themselves.

A Severe Case. The following case may be taken as representative. A woman of 63 who had had occasional aphthous ulcers in her teenage years presented with a recurrence of ulcers for 12 months. In middle life she had bad migraine for 4 years at a time of overwork and care of young children. There was unresolved mourning for a sibling and parent, and recent alienation from one of her children, a feature noted in several cases by us and also by Sircus et al. [1]. (Loss and immunological competence is discussed in Chap. 10.) She said she could not relax, was a "prize worrier", "paranoid about punctuality" and beset by high standards which she had acquired from her mother. She involved herself in every activity, in the garden, in business and in the community. A relaxation technique was advised, but at the time she said she found it too difficult. Yet at follow-up 5 years later, she said that the exercises she had learned had been a great help; she had practised them ever since when uptight and under pressure. She had remained virtually free of aphthous ulcers and had not had any need to see her physician or physiotherapist again. Her oral and palatal ulceration at onset had been as severe as in Behçet's disease and had caused her to lose 2 stones (12 kg) in weight. Because cortisol pellets had failed to relieve it, she was given IM injections of ACTH in a reducing dosage over 2 months. It was the only treatment she had had apart from psychological counselling and the relaxation exercises which at first she could not do.

6.1.2 Behçet's Syndrome

This was first described by Hulusi Behçet, a Turkish professor of dermatology, in 1937 ("a tri-symptomatic complex with hypopyous iridocyclitis, oral aphthous lesions and genital ulcerations") [102]. While a latent virus infection of a type somewhat similar to herpes simplex has not been excluded, interest of late has shifted to an immunological determinant, and consequently to some types of emotional stress acting through it. A systematic study of psychosomatic aspects was recently carried out by Professor Koptagel-Ilal and her associates [7] at a multidisciplinary Behçet's clinic in Istanbul. The work was done in cooperation with immunologists, ophthalmologists and dermatologists. Some 55 patients with Behçet's disease (30 male and 25 female) were involved. Of these 94.5% had experienced stressful life situations prior to onset, namely socioeconomic stresses or family conflicts. As in other psychosomatic disorders, a "poverty of emotional expression" was noted by the interviewers and their assessment of the patients' emotional stress was greater than the patients' own perception of it. Expression and handling of emotions were highly repressed. A Rorschach test revealed "highly pathological characteristics not permitting a free expression of emotions and establishment of social environmental contacts which had led on to ... aggressive drives which again had to be suppressed, leading to conflict situations and increase in psychic tension."

Incidence. Behçet's syndrome is relatively uncommon in Western Europe and in the USA compared with the high incidence in Turkey, Israel and Japan.

Psychopathogenesis. While the Turkish series quoted offers no data on the value of psychotherapy, it does provide indications of the type of psychological management likely to be effective, and the findings are very much in keeping with personal experience of three patients seen over 34 years, all of whom suffered familial conflicts with threatened loss or withdrawal of key figures. The personality and life situations are close to those already described in aphthous ulcers but associated with the added factor of loss and alienation.

The first patient was 18 at onset and her follow-up now extends over 34 years. After a stormy first 5 years necessitating high systemic corticosteroid dosage, she married and escaped the severe family dissension; at the same time, she found enough emotional space in which to grow up. As she moved away a few months after onset, these follow-up details are secondhand. The second patient, himself the product of an unhappy marriage, had already had 5 years oral and genital ulceration following a traumatic divorce; he developed intestinal symptoms and then a catastrophic haemorrhage from a large pharyngeal ulcer with complications which led to his death. When first seen he was already too ill for effective psychological work to be done. The third case history is instructive as it is the only one on which psychotherapeutic intervention was possible and carried through to termination. This woman of 22 with two children, a boy of 3 and a girl of 1, had married at 18. Oral aphthous ulcers had occurred occasionally since childhood, as had severe migraine. Her mother, a sister and her son had also had aphthous ulcers. Both parents were tidy, and she described her mother as firm. "I was not ever close to her." Her parents quarrelled, and her father left when she was 16. She had always been closer to him, and she was the only family member who continued to see him despite her mother's disapproval. Lately, she had felt only able to talk to him in generalities and on the telephone. Her mother started to cohabit with a man, and her disapproval of the daughter's contact with her father increased because she feared that if he heard about the new relationship, he would stop paying her an allowance. The patient's husband had been illegitimate, his first marriage had ended in divorce, and he had been violent to his first wife. When they married, the patient had told him that if he were violent with her, she would leave. The marriage was initially happy although the children arrived sooner than she would have wished. Her husband then became increasingly jealous, not allowing her to go out without him, and she felt as if she were "in a cage." Severe palatal and vulval ulcers had developed 7 months prior to first consultation at a time when tensions between them had escalated. "I can't argue; I stay quiet; he walks out; I can't win." Because she had been initially under the care of a venereologist, her husband had become even more suspicious of her and she of him. The first interview took place just after the patient received venereal clearance. She felt she could not go on with the marriage. Her husband had become even more jealous because she had played cards with one of the male patients in the hospital. Treatment involved a combination of prednisone, immunosuppressive and psychological management. It was suggested that while there might be no alternative to a separation, it might be worthwhile hearing her husband's point of view before reaching such a decision. It was also suggested that her husband's jealousy, intolerable as it was, probably stemmed from lack of love in his childhood, and for this reason his wife and children counted "double", i.e. were so important, representing the love he had not had or had not been able to find until his second marriage. His constant fear was that he would lose it, hence his jealousy and suspicion. It was also suggested to the patient that her own feelings for men were unconsciously ambivalent. Had not her father, whom she had loved, deserted her and left her to the ministrations of a mother who favoured her sister and her brother? The brother had been indulged and would fly off into tantrums if he did not get what he wanted. She acknowledged that some of her unexpressed anger with her husband's behaviour might relate to her own childhood experience. At the end of the interview the patient was asked whether her husband would come to a joint interview, and a date and time were offered in 7 days.

The patient was seen alone 15 min before that interview and said she had told her husband some of the things discussed the previous week, and that this released such a flood of feelings on both sides that they were still talking 5 h later. She thought that they had already resolved most of their problems, and she no longer wished to leave him. The joint session was straightforward with the couple talking a lot and with a great deal of eye contact, and only an occasional need for interpretation of unconscious activity being required. The husband turned out to be very caring, but frightened and suspicious. By helping him to feel what his wife felt when he did not trust her, progress was made. The patient's large and painful ulcers had healed within a month and were still in remission at the last follow-up, 2 years after the treatment started. She was then on prednisone 5 mg twice a day and azathioprine 50 mg twice a day. Psychotherapeutic interviews, four in total, ceased by mutual agreement with the patient after 5 months, but with the therapist's door being "left open" with easy access by the patient if she felt the need. At the last interview she said she had recently been screaming at her 6-year-old son. This was worrying her, particularly as he had started bed wetting, and she felt her own response was out of proportion to his misdemeanours. In the manner of a fisherman casting a hopeful fly, it was suggested that what might be annoying her was the boy's typically male behaviour. Had she not had reasons in her childhood for feeling two ways about males? She replied, "That's true, my son is exactly like my brother to look at, and he behaves in just the same way by pretending to be stupid and having tantrums ..."

6.2 Sjögren's Syndrome/Sicca Syndrome/Keratoconjunctivitis Sicca

An AI disorder, 50% of cases having a positive rheumatoid factor. Patients with the condition may have already had, or may develop, other AI disorders such as SLE or thyroiditis. The gastrointestinal presentation is dryness of the mouth, sometimes leading to soreness and difficulty in swallowing dry food for lack of saliva.

Parotid, submandibular or sublingual glands are usually enlarged and palpable. In the severe case repeated opening and closing the mouth produces an audible sticky sound because the saliva is so viscid. It may also be visible in elastic strands as the mouth opens.

Dryness and pricking of the eyes is as common a presentation as dry mouth. Other presentations are cough and bronchitis, dry skin and dry vulva, all due to reduced secretions, and polyarthritis and malaise. Strokes and other CNS manifestations may also occur [8]. For a recent review of diagnosis and treatment see [9] and on psychological management, Chap. 10 (Mrs. K. G. and Mrs. N. I.).

This brief outline of the clinical aspects has been included because the disorder is common but often overlooked in people past middle age, usually women.

Because many of them have unresolved mourning and loss, their symptoms are too often attributed to depression. Some are depressed as a result of a prolonged mourning reaction, but in many depression is enhanced because they feel unwell as a result of their systemic disorder and its troublesome somatic aspects.

6.3 Nervous Dysphagia/Oesophageal Spasm and Aerophagy

Early studies [10] suggested that the provocative life situation in this disorder was an inability "to swallow" some provocative emotional problem. We agree that this is often so, but point out that accepting or "swallowing" certain life stresses is common to many psychosomatic disorders, notably UC, asthma, MI and hypertension. Our experience, coupled with other sparse reports, suggests that there are recurrent similarities in provocative life situations and that the rage, which the sufferer experiences as a result, is conscious, as is recognition of their need to control it. Yet they are *unconscious* of the act of swallowing air and overbreathing associated with that control. By contrast, in disorders such as UC, Crohn's disease and MS not only is aggression and anger denied, but the link between psyche and soma involves involuntary mechanisms such as the psycho-neuro-immune or autonomic nervous systems rather than the voluntary motor nervous system as in pharyngeal spasm, aerophagy and overbreathing.

This unconscious habit of air swallowing is so common among the general population that it is difficult to regard it as other than a temporary exaggeration of the normal fight or flight response of deep breathing, and it rarely leads to medical consultation. The habit is apparent to doctors during medical interviews, or on examination when the patient's thyroid cartilage is seen to be bobbing up and down. Such patients may belch when something stressful is said or conveyed which they find it difficult to accept. It is then as revealing as an asthmatic's cough or wheeze, or of other people's sneezes or belly rumbles. Yet uncomplaining aerophagists unconsciously swallow air during much of their working or social day. For example, shy people may do it when they meet someone new or feel embarrassed at having to assert themselves ("stick their necks out") or meet someone in a position of authority and fear denigration. Indeed, any degree of anxiety may provoke it in sensitive individuals just as others will sweat, hyperventilate or palpitate.

Diagnosis. It must be emphasised that a psychosomatic basis for muscular irritability and spasm in the oesophagus depends as much on consideration of other causes as it does in the colon in IBS. For example, nocturnal oesophageal spasm may follow ingestion of too much pepper or garlic, etc. in people with a sensitivity, whereas concurrent swelling of the palate should point to an allergy. The commonest physical trigger is probably peptic oesophagitis.

6.4 The Splenic Flexure Syndrome

Excess gas in the stomach may lead patients to eructate persistently if they are able to relax the cardiac sphincter. Others who cannot belch or those who control the urge are now known to pass the air through their small intestines into the colon producing the classical splenic flexure syndrome and partial volvulus of the stomach (cup and spill deformity), or more commonly "gas" and anal flatulence.

Case management for the mildly affected involves explanation of the anatomical and psychological mechanisms and helping patients to become aware (conscious) of what they have been doing. They should be offered the help of a competent physiotherapist trained in teaching relaxation and relaxed abdominal breathing. This enables many of them not only to recognise when a situation or person makes them tense, but also gives them something they can do to reduce the tension. Most aerophagists are also hyperventilators (see Chap. 7).

6.5 Persistent Severe Disabling Aerophagy and/or Dysphagia

Such cases, fortunately rare, usually fail to respond to the superficial approach described and instead require psychotherapy or psychological management at greater depth. Philippopoulous [11] reported on three patients with fear of choking treated by psychodynamically based psychotherapy for 2 years followed by follow-up sessions every 2–3 months. There was almost complete remission of symptoms within 4 months of starting therapy and at follow-up 10, 9 and 8 years later all were in remission.

Klages reported an unmarried woman of 45 with aerophagy and borborygmi of 4 years' duration, which was so severe as to prevent her participating in social life or going to church. Radiography showed her stomach and colonic splenic flexure distended with gas. This case and those of Philippopoulous had the following features in common: (a) hostile-dependent relationship to a key figure or surrogate; (b) great conscious aggression, yet wholly controlled; (c) relief of symptoms by helping them to relate their feelings to their physical symptoms, and to be able to express those feelings and ultimately to accept them.

All four patients were unmarried at the outset of symptoms, as was the following patient.

An only child was referred at the age of 13 with attacks of hyperventilation and habit cough. Her first attack occurred after a nightmare in which horses were galloping towards her as she lay on the ground. She awoke panting for breath. An Oedipal and pubertal problem was suspected as a basis for her panics, and psychotherapy was advised in addition to re-education in breathing. The parents declined the advice, and she was taken to a psychiatrist who put her on psychotropic drugs. She continued to take the whole range of such drugs under the supervision of various psychiatrists for the next 18 years. During that period she had also seen physicians, paediatricians, behaviour therapists, and because she had developed idiopathic hirsutism, gynaecologists and endocrinologists.

She was referred again aged 31 because, despite these interventions, hyperventilation attacks had worsened, and because for 7 years she had suffered aerophagy and belching whenever she went out or met new people. It had become so severe that her social life had virtually ceased. It also affected her at night, and she was frightened of sleeping in case she should choke.

She said that drugs had not helped her and she wished to get off them, she also expressed a strong conscious wish to get better and lead a normal life and perhaps marry and have children. She agreed that she needed psychotherapy at some depth, and this was arranged with a trained psychotherapist. However, after the first consulation the latter's offer to try to help was declined by the patient, ostensibly because of the cost and probable duration of therapy, but the following comments made by the psychotherapist after seeing her seem relevant to the patient's refusal:

> The problem as regards psychotherapy ... is that she herself seems a long way from being able to accept that her difficulties have an emotional meaning ... She was unable to recall any recent dream to tell me (NB psychosomatic patients' failure to fantasise, free associate, present dreams [13]) ... She is unwilling to be spontaneous or "open with me", her anxieties are so completely somatised she is virtually inaccessible to me ... she would not acknowledge any hostility towards her mother (a chronic neurotic invalid) nor anxiety about her, and only a little concern about herself still living at home.

After a further 3-year round of consultations, including advice for group therapy, only to be told that this was not available, she returned with a new referral letter. Her symptoms had recently worsened after her father had been ill. One of us (J.W.P.) explained that as a physician with many hospital commitments, it would not be possible to offer the intensity and the depth of psychotherapy that she needed, but because so many approaches had been unsuccessful, he said he would try. She was seen 26 times over the next $2^1/_2$ years, an average of less than once per month, initially more frequently. Duration of interview was 30–60 min. Early on she was encouraged to decide for herself the gaps between appointments but was offered easy access at times of crisis such as her father's death 2 years after starting therapy, when she came the following morning.

Features included her admission that for as long as she could remember she had always found herself listening for her next breath, fearing it would fail. For this reason she particularly disliked cars, trains and noisy places where she could not hear it. During therapy it was felt that this may have originated in her traumatic birth and first few days of life. She had been 2 weeks premature, and labour was induced because her heart beat was becoming weak. The midwife told her mother to leave her lying down and not pick her up or feed her for 3 days. Mother said, "She did not sleep for ages, she just lay there with her eyes open and did not cry – she was a model baby." (Therapist's interpretation: "It sounds as though you were frightened of dying even then.") Apart from not sleeping well for 6 months and suffering from wind (?aerophagy), she developed normally and was walking at 15 months. Her mother lost her own mother when the patient was 4 months old and left home to look after her father in his house until the patient was 4 years old. This created family tensions. When the patient was aged 9 her mother developed depression after which she would not go out unless accompanied by her husband or the patient. This agoraphobic symptom never resolved. Because of it the patient from early teenage years began taking her mother's place at functions which her father had to attend (Oedipal problem). She resented mother's helplessness and despite being conscious of her anger, never expressed it. She developed panic feelings of losing either parent and fears of what would happen if her father died. She did not think she could live with her mother because "she never does anything in the house or goes out, and you can never have a discussion with her, she walks off."

The following comments by the patient at various interviews tell their own tale.

P: I am afraid to make mistakes, I feel self conscious.
D: Perhaps you create your own isolation?
P: (Tears) I do but I don't know what to do about it.
D: Is the burp a way of saying something – a form of speech?
P: I have never been good to crying – if I get angry it's when all the symptoms come on.
D: Angry with your mother? But you don't show it do you?
P: (Belches, burps loudly) I want to be liked by people. I don't get angry. (outwardly) [Tears and expressed fears about parents dying].
   My throat feels constricted if I eat anything and I feel breathless.
   I get frustrated if I don't let my feelings out.
   I fear being alone – it's always bad at night, it stops me sleeping, the gasping for breath and choking.
   I want to do things, but I am always in conflict.

After 12 months the patient recalled a disturbing episode with sexual content when she was 8 which involved a boy at school who got into trouble as a result. She presented a repetitive fantasy of herself being told off by a teacher. After this catharsis and that of other material relating to her Oedipal ambivalence, she acknowledged she had always pulled away from boyfriends, and her hyperventilation, choking and aerophagy gradually lessened.

Then she said, "I can't use tampons – I tighten up, I can't get them in." This problem was resolved with the help of an empathetic gynaecologist. After 18 months of therapy including membership in a migraine group, she began to go out more.

D: You seem to be shaking the shackles off?
P: I am now, but I am still not grown up.

I have a feeling I was taken in a car somewhere when I was 3 years old and told that I would be left if I was naughty.

I had a nightmare of a wall of water breaking over top of me.

D: A possible birth memory?

P: They (parents) won't let me cope while they are alive.

After the initial shock of her father's death and accepting the problem of undertaking some responsibility for her mother, she also recognised that this also involved being responsible for herself and her future, something she realised she would have found difficult to do while her father was alive.

At interview $2^1/_2$ years after starting therapy she did not belch (burp) once.

This case and those of Philippopoulous and Klages have some psychopathogenic features in common and suggest an overlap between psychopathogenesis and psychological management for oesophageal spasm, choking, aerophagy and in the above case severe hyperventilation as well.

While the basic, hostile, dependent relationship present in all these patients is also found in many other psychosomatic disorders, e.g. migraine, DU and hypertension, in the latter it is unconscious or barely conscious. However, in the case described and the others quoted, aggression was conscious, near the surface all the time, and had to be controlled by the use of muscles involved in swallowing and breathing via the voluntary motor nervous system.

Also significant in each case was that relief of the somatic symptom followed acceptance of the relationship of feelings to their symptoms and gradually being able to express those feelings verbally, first in therapy and then outside it.

6.6 Duodenal Ulcer

Reports of effective psychotherapy or psychological management for DU have been fewer than those on its psychopathogenesis. A decline in their number over the last 20 years in part reflects a falling incidence of the disease in most, but not all parts of the Western world [14, 15] but also the advent of more effective drugs, notably the H_2-receptor blockers. The fall in incidence began in 1945 in the southern United Kingdom and United States of America, in 1960 in the Federal Republic of Germany, but has been slower and later in Scotland, especially west central Scotland. The disease reached almost epidemic proportions between 1918 and 1939, and this led to a great deal of research just as in IHD today. Watkinson [16] recorded the cross association of the two disorders, as did an unpublished study by J.W.P. [17, 18], which showed it to be 20%–30%, and he suggested that a shared psychopathogenesis was a more likely link than diet or smoking. On that basis a comparable form of psychotherapy or psychological management might be appropriate for both diseases. However, regulation of gastric secretion as measured by serum pepsinogen levels has been found to be set at a higher than normal level from infancy and in part is genetically determined [19]. High acid secretion in medical students was also found to antedate clinical peptic ulcer and dyspepsia by 15 years [20, 21]. In other studies peaks of secretion have been shown to be related to *typical* life stresses and exacerbations of pain or the complications of perforation and haemorrhage associated with such peaks, subsiding during remissions [22]. Therefore, while psychotherapy has the potential to ameliorate, it cannot be expected to reduce acid and pepsin secretion to normal, especially nocturnal secretion.

The second factor against prolonged remission in DU, whether induced by drugs or psychotherapy, is the scarring at the site of the old ulcer, favouring relapses for reasons of ischaemia, or the thin covering of epithelium.

For the above reasons usefulness of psychological management in DU is limited to the following categories: (a) Young patients with short histories in whom scarring may be slight and damaging psychological attitudes and behaviour are less ingrained than in the older patient. (b) Patients with strongly expressed conscious motives to get off H_2-receptor blockers, e.g. fear of cancer, dislike of drug dependence. (c) Patients in whom despite effective H_2-receptor blockade, the ulcer remains unhealed on repeated endoscopy.

6.6.1 Prophylaxis for Duodenal Ulcer and Ischaemic Heart Disease

While preventative social medicine is not within the remit of this book, it is particularly relevant to these two disorders because of similarity in the "breeding ground" for their somatically damaging behaviour and attitudes set in the childhood of the sufferer. Effective psychological management requires an understanding of it. Davies and Wilson described the characteristic behaviour of DU patients in 1937 [23]:

> Peptic ulcer is common in the cities ... in the young and vigorous and those dynamic in outlook. The typical patient is a restless, active man of spare build ... of aggressive alertness and readiness to tackle any job or any problem (Citing Robinson [24]) They display enthusiasm for any project in hand and execute their tasks with zeal and sometimes with a degree of excitability.

Davies and Wilson compared their peptic ulcer group with hernia controls by Culpin scoring [25] and found: "The majority of ulcer patients differed from hernia patients in the degree to which tension is a constant characteristic and the ulcer patient was found first and foremost to be a worker." Davies and Wilson also found that the compulsive activity of the ulcer patient was sufficiently obvious to be a source of caustic or congratulatory comment by friends and relatives: of 75 male ulcer patients 40 were so classified against 9 of a corresponding group of 75 male hernia patients. In 25 women with ulcers the same characteristic was observed in 18 as against 5 of the hernia controls.

Mittelmann and Wolff [22] came to the same conclusion in 1942:

> The characteristic of assertive independence was outstanding in almost every instance ... superficial contact might lead to the conclusion that they were well adjusted ... but behind the facade of independence and self-sufficiency there was a background of longstanding insecurity accompanied by feelings of resentment and hostility ... Outstanding predisposing nurtural factors were the unhappy married life of the parents, separation or loss of father during the child's

development, early remarriage of the mother after separation from the father, feelings of the child being rejected by either or both parents or the foster mother [18]. Even superficial analysis made evident that the drive behind the hard work or sustained, relentless application to the pursuit of business and competitive effort was anxiety and insecurity ... The actuating motive – the desire "to achieve" at any cost, such a desire whipped into greater and greater intensity by mounting feelings of insecurity ... The insecure and anxious individual gains a degree of assurance by evolving a life style of being self-sufficient, independent; the "lone wolf" who, on the one hand, gains approval through extra effort, conscientiousness, perfectionism and meticulousness. While this is working, all might be well, but a change in life situation such as new responsibilities, courtship, marriage, criticism from without, is likely to challenge the patient's adequacy and he may then experience insecurity, anxiety and ulcer symptoms.

In 1959 Friedman and Rosenman [26] described what is now called "type A" behaviour in patients suffering from IHD:

1. An intense and sustained drive to achieve
2. Profound inclination and eagerness to compete
3. Persistent desire for recognition and advancement
4. Continuous involvement in multiple ... functions ... subject to deadlines
5. A propensity to accelerate execution of many physical and mental functions
6. Extraordinary mental and physical alertness

It will be evident that there is not substantial difference between type A behaviour in IHD and that described earlier in DU by Davies and Wilson and Mittelmann and Wolff [22, 23].

Likewise, in both disorders the underlying childhood insecurity, i.e. lack of overt love and esteem or even denigration [27–29], leads to this behaviour in an attempt to gain approval and esteem (love) from the working or social environment. IHD patients react in the same way as those patients with DU when described by relatives, friends and workmates [22, 23]. It has been estimated that 70% of IHD sufferers have type A personality. Apart from Zollinger Ellison cases and parathyroid adenomata all DU sufferers are type A, even though about 10% may not appear to be so at first sight because their show of hostile independence may lead them into trouble with employers, alcoholism and minor crime [30].

Much more research is still required to pinpoint social and environmental factors such as unemployment, broken marriages, one parent families or the lack of old-fashioned self-help and mutual support affecting the nurtural years of the child and adolescent, particularly in urbanised communities. Before measures are taken to ameliorate these things, we need to know much more or we may make them worse. For example, to put the blame on poverty or relative poverty [31] but ignore the basic problem of emotional deprivation, i.e. "emotional poverty", which thrives as well or better in affluent societies, would be foolish and even disastrous.

6.6.2 Psychological Management for Duodenal Ulcer and Ischaemic Heart Disease

The previous section on the *typicality* of early environmental influences in both disorders has been included because without understanding it any doctor or therapist trying to help such patients will be unnecessarily handicapped. Once again it is a question of a "gardener not digging for potatoes among the roses"; if the doctor does, he will waste the patients' and his own time.

The younger the patient, the greater the chance of helping him, first to understand the unconscious basis for the behaviour and then to express the anger and frustration felt in childhood, reacting as if by rote to certain cues and challenges. Many DU patients have been described as "willing horses". In fact they may be willing only consciously; subconsciously they are often not. Psychological management involves giving them the chance of saying "no". Prior to treatment they would have said "yes" because to say "no", as one patient said of his wealthy neighbour who was always borrowing his machines and returning them broken [30], would have led to being regarded as "awkward". "Awkward" in East Anglia means ill-tempered and therefore not highly regarded or loved. DU patients like to be liked and esteemed for the reasons already quoted.

6.6.3 Typicality of Double-Barrelled Stress

Onset or relapse of DU depends *typically* on the recurrence of typical forms of emotional stress in at least two areas of a *typically* vulnerable individual's environment simultaneously [27]. DU patients are likely to remain free of symptoms if they feel loved and highly regarded at home, even if their working and/or social environment is bleak and unrewarding. On the other hand, if employers think highly of them, pay them well, and promote them (see following note on foremen), they may remain well despite a carping spouse and children who tell them they are fools to overwork. It is then that the advent of a new unfriendly management, or threats of, or actual redundancy, leads to "double-barrelled stress" and often precipitates ulcer symptoms. Whereas in a previously tranquil domestic environment it may be the rebellion of a child or a parent coming to live in, and thereby diluting a spouse's attention, which is provocative.

Their community and social environment forms a third area in which these "willing horses" typically seek to gain the esteem (love) which from childhood onwards has been denied them. Thus, they make themselves useful by raising money for charity, running local flower shows, sitting on committees or parish/church councils, jobs most people try to avoid because of the envy, ingratitude and in-fighting which in the end seems to be inseparable from such activities. *Typically* ulcer sufferers relapse when their efforts are criticised or they are voted off such a committee or council and at the same time receive little sympathy from their family or colleagues at work.

Foremen. With the above in mind it should come as no surprise that foremen have been shown to have the highest incidence of DU in both the United Kingdom and the United States of America of all groups investigated [32, 33]. Not only do they select themselves for promotion by their diligence and willingness, but then more often than any other group they find themselves alienated from their old workmates and back in the "lone wolf" state. This sometimes leads them to undertake thankless jobs such as trade union secretary or welfare officer in an attempt to appease.

Patients who already have an ulcer and consult their doctor as to the wisdom of accepting promotion to foreman need help in reaching the decision with as much insight as possible into their unconscious, rather than their conscious motives for accepting or rejecting the offer.

In young, unmarried males with a short history it has proved useful to explore feelings about the kind of qualities important in a future wife. DU subjects tend to choose partners in the image of their undemonstrative mothers and/or fathers, who later when hurt by the patients' tendency always to put work first, distance themselves behind a facade of independence, and become critical and rejecting. DU patients need to be given insight into this; they do better with warmer, light-hearted wives whom they would initially ignore as flippant and not dependable.

For further case histories the reader is referred to [30].

6.6.4 Transcript

Mr. H. I. The following is from the second interview with a patient and his wife. The patient had had a DU intermittently for some years. When his DU was quiet there was syndrome shift to other psychosomatic disorders, migraine, costoclavicular compression and hyperventilation, but not more than one at the same time.

He was the eldest son of a hard working austere father who had suffered unemployment in the 1930s and was mean with praise and money. The patient's mother, kept short of both, had been unhappy and undemonstrative. This characterises the DU sufferer's childhood, and the transcript shows the response of striving behaviour and facade of independence now described as type A.

D: You said your father couldn't show you his approval and you had to keep trying very hard to try to get it?

P: That's it, he never came to my school and he never came to watch me in sports.

D: You had difficulty in pleasing him?

P: Yes, my wife can bear that out. W: Yes, we needed a hand with alterations in the house recently but when I asked him all he said was "Well I'll see and let you know." But there was no way that I would plead with him to come, so we took him a food parcel instead!

D: And what about the younger brothers, can he relate to them?

W: I don't think so.

D: So they don't get approval either?

W: No, but then I don't think they care. You see I think I notice it more because my family – the four of us – have been very close; until John came into our family, I don't think he fully understood family life.

D: You find her family very friendly?

P: Oh yes, their life is all about fun, and mother-in-law is absolutely the most wonderful person in the world.

D: Your own mother, could she kiss and cuddle you when you were little?

P: No, we didn't have that sort of relationship, from my point of view it was a protective relationship. My scholarship, young as I was, was an achievement, but it "blew out" because I had to take on things like paper rounds in the morning and evening to earn money, because whether father had it or not, he didn't give it to mother. It was a sort of a contributory relationship rather than one based on affection.

D: Yes?

P: I am sorry – I could not bear to see her hurt and father was hovering in the background between the two of us.

D: I suppose the Services must have had an influence on you?

P: It was the first time I was away from home, that didn't worry me, but I was always looking over my shoulder.

D: Did you get anything from the comradeship? Did you make good friends?

P: I think so while I was there, but there is always a little piece of me that I won't let go.

D: And perhaps you haven't even shown that piece of you to your wife?

P: Oh and I know why – (turning to wife) she's now hearing things she probably has not heard before.

D: But that may help her you see, as well as you.

P: I won't allow myself to be dented.

D: You said earlier that your father didn't like the idea of your marriage either.

P: No.

D: Why was he against it?

P: My father did not approve of what he saw of her family.

D: Perhaps he thought they were too flippant?

P: They had a tremendous life style, wonderful people, very happy.

D: Yes?

P: They would never have ulcers, the important thing is that life is about enjoyment for those people – he didn't like that, so when I came home I remember, and will remember until the day I die, telling him that we were going to get married.

D: Yes?

P: I had actually to tell him you know, that congratulations wouldn't come amiss.

D: Perhaps he had a puritanical background, being Welsh?

P: He is a very deep man, for instance when we visited as an engaged couple or later as a married couple, we would never sit on the same chair, because never in the whole of my life have I ever seen a gesture of affection such as a kiss or hug between him and my mother, therefore, you know we felt we had to sit on opposite sides of the room. After leaving the Services I began to realise what learning was all about, I had to recover some ground if I wanted to make something of myself. It was all about hard work and not being beaten – a pretty hard fight because I always felt somewhat vulnerable.

D: Yes?

P: When amongst people I know are brighter than me, for instance all the people in management on the same level are university graduates.

D: In a sense you have to try harder?

P: That's right, to maintain my position, it's all about being attentive and trying to stay with those guys.

W: That is why you can't take criticsm?

P: (Bridling a little) I don't see it that way, I am a perfectionist.

D: Perhaps the reason you don't like saying "No" when someone asks you to take something on is you don't like them thinking badly of you?

P: That's the size of it, yes.

D: So you are liable to be a bit of a "willing horse", people come to you and say "I suppose, John, you couldn't possibly manage to do this can you?"

P: And I say, "Oh yes, I can."

D: Do you know why you say "Yes" when you do not always want to?

P: I fear possible loss of people's respect.

D: You said at the first interview that you had always tried to protect your wife from certain things, and I said she might like to share some of those things. Perhaps you have doubted whether you could ask that of her – [to wife] are you aware of this?

W: Yes, very much so. We have been married 20 years – we like to protect each other, don't we? I don't think he means to shut me out but ...

D: Perhaps he has been protecting you like he did his mother?

P: Umph ... You're *right,* you're *right,* umph, you're *right!*

D: Maybe you can now release yourself a little from that earlier learned pattern of response and make a decision to do so irrespective of it?

P: Are you saying I have to unlearn and undo some of those reasons for problems I am wrapped up in?

D: Yes.

The patient and his wife were seen at intervals of a few months over a period of 2 years. The patient was able to relinquish some of his ingrained behaviour patterns, and communication and trust between the couple became evident with increased eye contact and speech, rather than for the therapist as in earlier interviews.

The patient's psychosomatic disorders settled, but 2 years later one of his daughters presented with obesity due to overeating when unhappy. She had found herself in conflict with her father's high standards and expectations for her school work. In the same way that he had been unable to please (be loved by) his father, she now found herself in the same position. It may be noted that her response of overeating, like with DU, was another manifestation of oral gratification in order to assuage her need for appreciation (love) which she felt her sister got without much effort.

6.7 Whipple's Disease (Intestinal Lipodystrophy)

We have been fortunate to have seen five patients with his rare disease, and yet many gastroenterologists of great distinction and experience have yet to see one.

The first two were reported in 1949 [34] and 1952 [35], and as the psychosomatic aspects were included in their histories they will not be referred to again except to say that the second patient was only the second recorded patient to survive and who received superficial psychotherpy in addition to chloramphenicol. At follow-up in 1959 his jejunal biopsy was normal [36]. Each of the subsequent patients had comparably severe emotional stress weeks or months prior to the onset of their disease and, as in the first two, suppression and denial of anger with key figures was prominent and additional to loss of other key figures. Each patient, as had the first two, showed a degree of dependence similar to that found in coeliac disease, Crohn's disease and UC and as in those disorders, sufferers feel hurt and brood instead of showing anger.

Incompetent immunological response [37, 38] is believed to be a major factor in the pathogenesis of Whipple's disease leading to proliferation of a bacterium, possibly a streptococcus in a protoplastic form [39], in the lamina propria of the jejunal mucosa. In some patients it may spread to the heart valves (endocarditis – it did in case 3) and to the joints, lymph nodes and brain by embolism.

For the effects of loss and mourning on the immune system the reader is referred to Chap. 10.

The reasons for including a condition as rare as Whipple's disease are (a) because of its exceptionally interesting pathogenesis, bacterial and immunological, a better understanding of which might well throw light onto other disorders such as Crohn's disease; (b) because of its combined psychopathogenesis comprising a mixture of the psychological *typicality* of IBD but also of loss and mourning; and (c) because patients not responding well to the penicillin antibiotics, now the accepted treatment for the condition, we think should also receive psychological management/ psychotherapy to help them express their feelings of anger and to work through their mourning reaction.

6.7.1 Case History

A first generation Greek-American's symptoms began a few months after his mother's death following a prolonged illness from cancer during which he, who had always been closest to her, had been the only one of the family to make regular hospital visits. Because he had a mentally handicapped brother at home, his father sent him back to Europe to find a bride, marry her and bring her back to look after father, brother and himself. His trouble set in when his wife had a baby which the brother resented and attacked physically. This led him, due to pressure from his wife, to tell his father that if his brother did not leave, they would. His father then abused him verbally "as a bad son" and would not allow it. Unfortunately, there was no opportunity to offer the psychotherapy he needed as he was seen on a fleeting visit to the USA. The diagnosis was confirmed on jejunal biopsy.

6.8 Coeliac Disease (Idiopathic Steatorrhoea)

One of us has found [40–42] that emotional stress is closely related in time to the onset of this disorder, whether in the infant or the adult, a finding supported by Prugh [43]. The discovery that a gluten-free diet, in general use since about 1953, brings remission in nearly all children and most adults has made psychological management/psychotherapy unnecessary except for the few adults who fail to respond or suffer the complication of jejunal erosions and ulceration. For a description of cases treated by psychological management before the introduction of gluten-free diet or by psychotherapy directed to the parents of coeliac children, see Paulley [42] and Prugh [43].

The reason why wheat gluten is so noxious to these people and not the rest of the population is still not understood. It has been suggested that the permeability of the jejunal mucosa [44] may be a factor allowing the large gliadin molecule to pass through the epithelium into the intercellular spaces where it may set up a sensitivity reaction, and that such permeability could be the result of stress-induced jejunitis comparable to ileitis in Crohn's disease, or colitis or mucous colitis in the colon. In favour of this is that the provocative life situation in both children and adults with coeliac disease is similar to that found in UC and Crohn's disease, and that the adults certainly share the same personality traits. Whether the children have these too is not possible to judge because they are usually too young to communicate verbally.

6.9 Appendicitis

In 1955 evidence was produced [45] that acute appendicitis should be considered a psychosomatic disorder. Binning [46], a school medical officer in Saskatoon, came to the same conclusion in a study of tonsillitis and appendicitis in school children for whom he was responsible. More recently a life events study with controls reported by Creed [47] has been confirmatory.

Both these studies showed that the provocative life situation in acute appendicitis was a short-term threat, such as an interview, examination, wedding or a coronation as in the case of Edward VII. In the 1955 article [45] it was suggested that lymphoid hyperplasia in the appendix as part of the *alarm reaction* might be instrumental, with parallels in acute appendicitis associated with measles and infectious mononucleosis.

A recent example was a man who said he had had a perforated appendix shortly after waking to find his wife in status asthmaticus, "the colour of a corpse and I thought she would die." However, she recovered, and he developed his appendicitis 3 weeks later. After her discharge from hospital he was at first in constant fear she would have another attack while he was working away from home. His wife had no further asthma, and his anxiety subsided, but he had *typically* lost his appendix on the way.

It will be evident that there is no place for psychological management in *genuine acute* appendicitis because of the suddenness of onset, but for those patients operated on in error and found to have normal "lily white" appendices, it is quite different. They are usually misdiagnosed cases of spastic colon (IBS) and need psychological management appropriate for the condition. It was these patients, as Creed pointed out, who remained symptomatic and psychologically unwell for as much as a year after their operations.

6.10 Crohn's Disease (Regional Enteritis)

It may be surprising to learn that the first reports of emotional stress in a close time relationship to the onset and relapses of this disease were made by surgeons [48, 49] – people whose usual image is that associated with practicality and technique. However, in view of the often distressing course of the disease followings surgery 30–40 years ago, and that so many patients were tragically young, it is not so surprising. Physicians did not have much to offer until the introduction of ACTH, cortisone and immunosuppressives in the 1950s and 1960s. Before that, it was usually surgeons who week after week and month after month treated these mainly young people and inevitably got to know their feelings, sensitivity, vulnerability and immaturity. The surgeon Eastcott summed it up well in 1958 [49] when he said they were regarded by other patients in the ward as "rather nice people" and as "peacemakers". It was not until the 1950s that it was recognised that surgery ought if possible to be avoided in the acute stage of disease as bowel wall oedema often led to leaking suture lines and consequent sepsis with a 5-year mortality rate as high as 20% in some centres.

6.10.1 Previous Reports

For a list of references to psychological factors in pathogenesis, 16 for and 4 against, see Paulley [50]. Additional to that list and in favour of the findings are Parfitt [51], Cohn et al. [52], McKegney et al. [53] and McMahon et al. [54].

Of the four investigations which were against the psychological determinant in Crohn's disease, three were flawed methodologically, either because of insufficient interviewing time – Crockett's [55] 16 patients were restricted to a one-hour psychiatric examination while Feldman et al.'s [56] interview arrangements with a team of three interviewers would have been doomed to failure in any psychosomatic disorder, but particularly so in Crohn's disease and UC because of the patients' extreme sensitivity and characteristic defence of denial. This was pointed out at the time [57–61]. Despite this, Feldman et al. [56] are usually quoted alone by critics to bolster their case against the psychosomatic determinant, yet they would to be first to condemn such unrepresentative selection of references in their own field.

6.10.2 Psychological Management

Grace [62] criticising Crockett's study stressed "the need for frequent interviews over a long period of time in order to gain the patient's confidence. Frequently, patients will not confide for many months." Ford et al. [63] were also critical:

> It should not be surprising if patients with the degree of rigidity, repression and guardedness noted in our study were to answer negatively to direct questions about emotional stress ... Our patients were seen extensively (and) ... had a much greater opportunity to talk spontaneously and reveal themselves.

Ford et al. [63] made additional points especially relevant to psychological management, gleaned from their study of 17 of the total of 20 unselected patients. For example:

> Tranquillizing drugs are of little or no value for the obsessively preoccupied patient ... Before these very guarded patients can allow themselves to talk freely, a relationship must be established ... Hurried rounds consisting of "Nothing is bothering you today, is there?", of course result in only one answer: "Nothing." ... Many can be helped by psychotherapy.

It is unfortunate that the authors were unable to carry out a long-term follow-up as their grasp of the *typicality* of the Crohn's personality profile and life situations was so sure. Insufficient interdepartmental cooperation may have been a factor, a problem we discussed in Chap. 3. Another perennial handicap is that research workers are usually young "birds of passage" only too aware of the truth of the axiom "publish or perish". Goldberg's [64] study could have yielded so much more had he been able to see his patients over a period of ten or more years, the minimal time needed to comprehend the natural history of a chronic disorder such as Crohn's disease with its relapses and remissions, appearing to be spontaneous but which are not.

The reader is advised to refer to the report by Reinhart and Succop [65] on 13 of a total of 17 children with regional enteritis referred to them for psychiatric evaluation and/or treatment in Pittsburg, 1941–1966. This study is one of the few published so far, which describes psychological management in sufficient detail to be a real help to anyone wishing personally to treat such a patient. They will be sure to find among these case reports a replica of the emotional problems faced by their own patient.

Experience of Management. Reinhart and Succop stress the same point made previously by Sullivan [66] in the comparable disorder UC about a frequent consequence of effective psychotherapy, namely "Loosening the ambivalent ties to the family poses a continual threat, as much or more, to the parents than to the child." Sullivan's patients (and also Murray's [67]) were often young adults in conflict with their parents' wishes over intended marriage (see transcripts Mrs. F. O. and Mrs. P. K.) We agree, but in most of the children or adolescents we have treated, it has been possible to bring one or both of the parents (or siblings) whose behaviour has been provocative into the therapeutic work in joint interviews. *These parents had no idea before this that their arguments, quarrels or shouting which they had considered normal could have any bearing on their child's disease.* Such recognition is usually critical to the patient's recovery. Empathy with, and not condemnation of, the aggressive parent or sibling is the key to their willingness to change.

"Pig-in-the-Middle". On other occasions psychotherapy enabled patients to see the relevance of the typical life stress of Crohn's disease, i.e. being "in-between" quarrelling factions, *typically* described by them as "pig-in-the-middle" (see transcripts Mrs. M. C., Mrs. F. O., Mrs. P. K. and Mr. S. Q.). They were then able to take some positive action to get out of it.

For example, a young man of 18 presented with a 2 year history. He was the youngest of four, and his elder siblings had all left home as soon as they were old enough, because of the quarrelling between the parents. This had dated from his mother's stroke years earlier when as a result of the brain damage she had become aggressive, frequently provoking a response from his father. Asked about recreations, football, darts, disco, etc., he said he never went out. Because of J.W.P.'s *prior knowledge* of the *typical* peacemaker role which these patients repeatedly get into, it was suggested that this patient did not go out because he feared his parents would injure or kill each other in his absence. He said this was true, but he had not until then connected his stomach trouble with his emotional dilemma. Two months later he returned in remission saying he was hardly ever at home and had joined the local club. Asked how he had been able to do this, he said he had told his parents what is illness was due to. After that, their attitude to each other improved and at last he felt it safe to leave them for a few hours.

Of the four case histories described by Grace [62] three involved classical "pig-in-the-middle" situations, first between parents and later with in-laws, between husband and children, husband and another woman, and in one case persistent differences between a paranoid father and the mother. These histories suggest the need for psychotherapy or adequate psychological management early in the disease, before too much gut is damaged. Feldman et al.'s [56a,b] criticism was that the study was retrospective. Nevertheless, the material could only have been obtained by the most sensitive, unhurried interviewing, in this instance a minimum of 14 h over a period of months. This is in contrast to Feldman's two free association type interviews in front of a team of four and the patient seen as much as possible by the team during the hospital stay. Teams of interviewers will get little from these patients, and it is not surprising that Feldman's results were negative.

A Follow-up Study. One of us published in 1959 [30], 1971 [44] and 1974 [68] a personal approach to psychological management in Crohn's disease, and the 1971 paper included a 1- to 18-year follow-up of 40 cases. Other reports of successful therapy have been given by Sperling [69] of one patient treated psychoanalytically and still well 3 years later, by Parfitt [51] of one case, and by Reinhart and Succop [65] of psychological management in liaison with paediatricians and surgeons of 13 children and adolescents. They found that the more severe the illness, the greater the arrest in psychological growth and of "continued symbiosis and failure to move away from parents to function autonomously". Chronic illness in children, because of their physical dependence, inevitably compounds any abnormal immaturity they may have. The same factor obstructs progress in the sister disease UC, and unless carefully handled, reinforces the dependence which is at the root of the disease. However, Reinhart and Succop were able to say in less severe cases of Crohn's disease: "There seemed more awareness and ability to cope with the anxiety around separation, a greater appreciation of the child's individual pattern of behaviour, and an easier disruption of the symbiotic state of the child in the family." Their article drew attention to the difficulty posed by shared clinical responsibility between two or even three departments. Of their 13 cases, only in the last was psychotherapy "carried to successful termination to his family's and our mutual satisfaction." Winnicott [70] referred to the "scatter of responsible agents" as a defence used by patients with psychosomatic disorders. It applies especially to Crohn's disease because of the unconscious predilection to return time and again to the in-between position. Nowhere are such opportunities of "splitting" better than between the doctors responsible but jealous for their own discipline and denigratory of others. Until all clinicians understand this psychodynamic it will be better for patients with Crohn's disease if their physical and psychological management is in the hands of one doctor sufficiently competent in both fields. Such a doctor could theoretically be a surgeon, GP or psychiatrist, but the problem is that Crohn's disease is not common enough for one GP to gain the sufficiency of skills necessary in *physical* management, nor to date is it usual for psychiatrists in their training to have acquired *enough* of such skills to enable them to undertake full clinical responsibility either.

Two cases quoted in a 1959 article [42] are worth mentioning. Psychological management over a period of 3 years with interviews every 1–6 months enabled the first man to leave home and eventually the district. At 10 years he was reported to be still in remission. The second patient, dwarfed by the malabsorption caused by uncontrolled jejunal disease, remitted with treatment and continued to grow in height until she was 24. She also grew emotionally, first doing the things she would have done in her 'teens, with menarche at 19, then getting a job and finally marrying at 26. Sadly, she developed the recognised but rare complication of jejunal cancer at 33, and it was inoperable.

Five other cases were described in 1974 [68], which may be referred to as *typical.* Of the total series of 141 cases, a further three have been selected to illustrate psychological management, followed by an edited transcript of another patient.

6.10.3 Case Histories and Transcript

Mrs. M. C., aged 21, ileocaecal disease found at laparotomy at another hospital in 1974, shortly after her wedding. Her GP's letter of referral 2 months later underlined the *typical* family tensions:

> Last March she married into a large family ... Her husband is one of 11 children, 9 of whom are already married. His father has never been to any of the children's weddings and his mother says of the father: "He isn't a husband – might as well live separately." The patient and her husband were forced to live initially with his family, and her symptoms started soon after landing herself in this inhospitable household.

In June 1974 having moved to their own home, she was asked if she thought she was sensitive. "Things upset me." Asked for an example, she said, "If I think have offended anyone – I don't like atmospheres, I try and clear them up." Her mother and brother were also sensitive and quiet, unlike her quarrelsome father, who in drink had caused rows for as long as she could remember and which she hated, the replay of which she met with her in-laws after her marriage.

At the second interview in July her husband said he had had a quarrel with his mother before the wedding and would not speak to her for 3–4 weeks. It was in this abrasive atmosphere that she (patient) spent the first days of married life, sleeping in the bedroom next to her mother-in-law who would shout: "Shut up and stop laughing."

The patient was seen for $1/2$–1 h at lengthening intervals, latterly annually until termination in 1982. There was no major relapse; a minor one occurred in 1975 when her husband thought he was in love with another woman and apparently expected her to tolerate this liaison. She felt very hurt but had found enough strength to say she would not accept it, and left. It is doubtful if she would have done this without the psychological help she had received. Her husband soon came to heel and left the other woman. She had loose stools and abdominal pain for 2 weeks after her father died of cancer in 1976. She then became pregnant but lost the baby at 2 months; despite disappointment and grief she was able to express it and did not relapse. She was soon pregnant again, and a baby girl was born in 1977. In 1978 there was trouble with a landlady, and she had a mild relapse lasting 2 months, but it remitted when she confronted the landlady after a therapeutic session.

In 1980 she said there had been no upsets for a long time; at one time she would never go anywhere on her own. "People say I have changed – I will now row with my sister Joan which I could never do before." She and her husband had decided to have another baby.

In 1982, still no relapses, mutual agreement to terminate. Address and telephone number given for access if in need.

Mrs. F. O., aged 21, onset of symptoms occurred in 1963, laparotomy carried out 3 months later, ileocaecal Crohn's disease diagnosed. Abdomen closed – referred to medical department.

At first interview, there was a large teddy bear in her bed. She said she would avoid quarrelling at any price and bottled up her feelings. Her Belgian father had left her Belgian mother when she was 3, and she was brought up by her mother who then remarried a British soldier and came to the UK when she was 6. Since then there had been constant tension between her stepfather and her mother because of his lower social status. They lived in a rather rough housing estate, and mother felt she had been deceived by him.

Exacerbation of emotional tension dated from February 1963 when the patient became engaged to be married. At this point, her stepfather, who had made a fuss of her when she was younger and had become jealous when she went out with boys, retired to a backroom every time the patient and fiancé came into the house. She said there was an atmosphere that "you could cut with a knife". There had been rows as to what dress should be worn at the wedding, stepfather refusing to get into ceremonial clothes. She had wanted to ask her Belgian father, of whom she was very fond, to the wedding. Stepfather announced that if he came, he would not attend himself.

A letter to her doctor in 1963 stated:

> The situation this girl has found herself in is classical for Crohn's disease – finding herself
> jammed as it were between warring parties and only wanting peace. After several sessions the
> girl has decided not to invite her Belgian father but instead to visit him with her husband as
> soon as possible after the wedding. The Crohn's disease is now quiet as a result of drugs and
> psychotherapy, but we have not seen the end of the trouble here. The girl is extremely
> immature and dependent, and the mother extremely dominating, and I am not sure of the
> quality of the future husband.

A daughter was born in 1964, a son in 1967 and a daughter in 1974.

She had two major relapses in 1970 and 1973, both requiring admission with subacute
obstruction and reactivity of Crohn's disease, despite the unchanged small maintenance dose of
prednisone and oxytetracycline.

The first relapse related to a visit of her Belgian family, in particular her stepsister, described
by the patient as "a little bitch, trying to get me to do things father would not approve, constantly
arguing with father. I certainly don't want them over again." The second relapse occurred when
friends tried to involve her and her husband in a wife-swapping circle.

Termination of interviews, by then only annual, was mutually agreed in 1975 with access if
required.

Mrs. P. K., aged 29, ileocaecal Crohn's disease diagnosed at laparotomy in July 1977. An only
child, married, with a son of 4 and a daughter of 2. First symptoms of right iliac fossa pains in
April 1977, but the disease had probably started earlier.

At interview December 1977, she said she had been frightened of her father in childhood. He
was

> remote, I was closer to mother ... I was very good as a child and never remember doing
> anything wrong, my mother tried to get me on her side and "cut my father out" by using me as
> an ally – I was always pig-in-the-middle ... Nowadays, my father tries to get me on his side
> against my grandmother, who lost her husband and now lives with my parents. My father will
> not talk to her ... My mother now also has pains and diarrhoea, and she is always between my
> father and grandmother.

Asked if she were sensitive, "Yes, to people's moods – what they are thinking." She said she could
get angry but only with her employers behaving unjustly to her husband or herself. She never lost
her temper with her parents, husband or in-laws. Her father-in-law was Polish and rigid and
strongly disapproved of his son's marriage; father-in-law and his wife were always quarrelling and
when she said she would leave, he threatened suicide. Visits to the in-laws were always fraught
because of the father's dislike of her and denigration of her husband.

One may wonder why she chose to go north to have her second child in her in-laws' house,
unless it was her predilection to get "in-between". There was trouble almost at once, and her own
mother had to come and take her and the baby home. She tried to go back but gave up after a week
because of rows between her intolerant, foul-mouthed, argumentative father-in-law and her
husband.

Following that, her husband took legal action against their joint employer for wrongful
dismissal, which he lost. She felt aggrieved because of the publicity and that it would reflect on her
own reputation and career. The husband, who shared with his father comparable problems with
authority, started smoking cannabis. Just prior to the onset of the patient's first symptoms, there
was a knock on the door, and the police entered with a warrant to search the garden for the
cannabis growing there. Again, there was a court case; she was now "in-between" her husband
and the authorities as well as her own disapproving parents and neighbours.

Seen over the next 5 years, usually with her husband, she did well. He began to grow up and started a successful business. He now understood her sensitivity and anticipated in-between situations. They discussed them or avoided them for the most part. One mild relapse occurred when her mother took the grandmother into the house against her father's wishes, and another when her husband bought a new van before selling the old one. As a result he spent all her housekeeping money, and she found herself between her husband and the trades' people wanting to be paid. Interviews were mutually terminated in 1983 with access if in need.

Summary. The patient was initially between her parents, then between her husband and his father, then between her father and her grandmother and finally between her husband and her disapproving parents, neighbours and employers when he went to court for growing cannabis. Management involved helping her to change her hitherto damaging coping mechanisms and enlisting her husband as a co-therapist, i.e. the value of couple therapy.

Mr. S. Q. (seen in 10 interviews over 18 months), an only child, aged 32, with Crohn's disease, was born while his aggressive father was away in the war, but after his return, the child was always in the middle between his parents and between his noisy father and the neighbours. He spent as much time as he could with a friendly farmer. In courtship he found himself between his mother and his girlfriend, and after marriage "pig-in-the-middle" between people at work, and then between his work and his wife. She became annoyed because she felt that she and the children were being neglected. At the time of presentation his father had broken his leg, and the patient had to visit him in hospital and met as usual his father's awkwardness and ingratitude.

First Outpatient Interview October 1984: Edited Transcript

D: What sort of temperament do you think you've got, I mean are you sensitive?

P: I'm afraid I do take things to heart a bit too much, it's the same as at work, I am involved in security. I think I take it too seriously.

D: If somebody annoys you, are you liable to flare up or get in an argument, or how do you respond?

P: Sometimes I get in an argument, but being supervisor you've got to take a bit – I mean you can't afford show-downs.

D: Do you think you take after your mother or father, I mean were they both quiet people, or was one of them fiery or argumentive?

P: They are both quiet really.

D: You mean there were no quarrels?

P: No, there was never any quarrel. (Note: *typical* denial in view of what he says later)

D: Is your wife liable to speak her mind? For example, she said what she thought of the holiday situation; didn't she?

P: Oh yes.

D: In a mild way?

P: She can be, yes.

D: Does it hurt you?

P: It does at times, but then our relationship is not as good as it could be.

D: Can you retaliate easily when she gets like this? I mean do you ever have a good up and downer with her?

P: Mm, not really, I usually go in the garden by myself, you know, I don't like arguments. I just let it slide by, nobody likes arguments.

D: Well, you don't, it doesn't sound as though she minds so much.

Seen with his wife not long after she said: "He would never argue," and added: "I am never comfortable when we visit his mother and father because they are always bickering." The patient then said, contrary to his earlier denial: "If I do anything for my father on his allotment, my

mother immediately wants to know why. If I do anything for her, my father wants to know why."
In August the patient visited his father every day in hospital, but since he had become ill his father
had not bothered to come, although he had been able to catch a train to his favourite pub several
miles away, which had annoyed the patient. During the next 14 months he was seen on eight
occasions, mostly with his wife; his improved physical condition occurred in step with
improvement in his ability to express his feelings both at home and at work.

10th Interview January 1976:

D: Weight today 12st. 1lb (77 kg), and when you came to see us when this began in October 1974
   you were 10st. 3lbs (65 kg)?

P: Yes.

D: So that's an improvement.

P: I've put on a lot.

D: How many motions are you getting now?

P: Mostly about one a day, on odd occasions twice.

D: Mm, and of course originally when you had this diarrhoea?

P: Mm, a dozen times a day.

D: You also had a little blood at times?

P: Yes.

D: Looking back on that time, what do you think was the most important factor in getting out of
   that particular hole?

P: Mm, well my home life never did a lot of good, I was sort of never at home.

D: Yes?

P: And I didn't realise that kind of thing could ...

D: Of course – your wife was a good soul, but she got a bit sharpish at times?

P: Yes, yes.

D: And there was trouble with your father too?

P: Yes.

D: Not an easy chap to deal with?

P: No.

D: Do you remember the rows when you were a child?

P: Yes.

D: I remember you describing to me some of the rows which were offensive to you.

P: Yes, at times he used to go off and upset the neighbours and other people, you know, trying to
   be on top you might say – the girl next door used to aggravate him – that one landed up in
   court, that did.

D: Yes, that caused a lot of trouble?

P: That caused a lot of trouble with the neighbours all round, it wasn't a very nice thing to live
   with.

D: If he was shouting about the place, stirring things up, what did you do?

P: Well at times didn't know what to do really – but would get caught up in the arguments, you
   know neighbours throwing words at me same as they done to him ...

D: Mm, which you didn't deserve?

P: No, you had to put up with it, I suppose you didn't fight back, you took it in.

D: But maybe fighting and rows were things that you chose to avoid?

P: Yes, I never liked getting in any of them, I suppose at times if one had gone in and stirred them
   up and got it over with, it might have been better.

The patient remained in remission until termination of treatment in 1982.

6.10.4 Summary

1. It is necessary to help these patients to become aware of the close temporal relationship between what they feel and experience emotionally and the onset and relapse of their disease.
2. To begin with, as in UC, their *typically* dependent needs should be met and manipulative behaviour accepted.
3. Once the acute episode or threat to life has receded, the patients need to be helped to forego some of that earlier dependence on their physician or therapist, which is initially so therapeutic. This phase of management, if not sensitively handled, may promote relapse [74].

   Physicians and gastroenterologists often fall unwittingly into the trap by fostering continued dependence through insisting on measures necessitating frequent outpatient supervision. We recommend gradually attenuating the link between patient and physician to the vanishing point but never to sever it totally. Hospital patients should have free access to clinics without having to make an appointment. To begin with they need fixed appointments according to their clinical or emotional state. Later, they will come when a particular emotional situation threatens *before* their Crohn's disease relapses – a genuine therapeutic "gain". Thus far, their psychotherapeutic management does not differ from UC.
4. However, the patient with Crohn's disease, while sharing an extreme aversion to a strife-ridden environment with a patient with UC, differs in adopting the active role of peacemaker, whereas the UC patient usually walks away. Patients with Crohn's disease *typically* find themselves sandwiched between two bickering parents, or parent and sibling, or two siblings, or a spouse and a neighbour. Refusing to come down on one side or the other for fear of incurring the wrath of either, the patient unconsciously perpetuates the conflict and pays the penalty of so many peacemakers of being denounced by both parties.

These patients' predilection to continue the same pattern of behaviour and to reconstruct comparable abrasive situations at work, in their marriages and in their children's marriages necessitates long-term psychological management and repeated interpretation. By these means patients gradually become aware of old, damaging coping mechanisms and develop new ones.

With a substantial post-operative 5-year relapse rate psychological management is as strongly indicated after ressection as before it. Patients are all too often returned home without such help, and therefore are as vulnerable to the same abrasive environment as they were before operation.

Resistance to sensible psychological management of Crohn's disease has grown rather than diminished over the years, which is a pity. As long ago as 1958 the third edition of Harrison's textbook of medicine [71] stated that "accumulating clinical evidence strongly suggests that it is a psychosomatic disorder. Emotionally, the patients are and have been frustrated for one reason or another. Unsatisfactory patient-parent relationships often exist. Emotional storms and upheavals precede the onset of the disease and the occurrence of relapses. Most of the patients are very intelligent and are less dependent and more mentally mature than those with UC." Subsequent editions of the book have omitted this important passage.

6.11 Ulcerative Colitis

Many articles and one book have appeared since Murray's [67] initial report while still a medical student in 1930. The book, entitled *Psychotherapy in Chronic Ulcerative Colitis,* was published in 1977 [72] and can be recommended for its appraisal of the limited place for psychoanalysis in the treatment for the majority of UC patients and for its comprehensive review of the literature. Karush et al. found intense symbiotic needs for dependency in two-thirds of the patients. Other publications which contain useful advice on psychological management of UC are Sullivan [66] and Groen [73], and Engel [74] with both of whom we are in close accord [30, 75–77]. *The Human Colon* [93] is also essential reading.

The hypothesis about pathogenesis of UC advanced in that book is still the most likely, and is in accord with our own research on emotion and colonic motility [75].

Between 1946 and 1949 in a clinical study of 173 cases of UC J.W.P. reported:

The usual methods of history taking were found to be of little value. It was necessary to develop a new approach. A thorough search of the patient's background had to be made, and at first one's technique was clumsy. Colitis patients may be ready talkers about their symptoms but they are "dumb" about their emotional feelings [75, see also 13, 78–80]. After 6 months I began to be impressed by a similarity of history and personality in many instances [*Typicality* of life events and *typicality* of behaviour and personality] ... The following groups of features were constantly appearing, whereas in the controls they were generally absent or only a few were present in any one person ... They were excessively dependent, parent-controlled people, usually maternally controlled ... They were never outwardly aggressive though often querulous. Anger is apparently not felt by them in the usual way, instead only a dull prolonged resentment ... They are excessively sensitive and brood for months over real or imagined wrongs or insults [with hindsight perceived for imagined would be more accurate] ... The men are rather effeminate, and fastidiousness and neatness are commonly found in both sexes ... They tend to self-righteousness, smugness ... and have a poorly developed sense of humour. They are generally described as model children.

This old report shows that the conclusions on typicality of personality and of life situations reached 35 years ago are the same now as then, after confirmation by a further 2000 patients. What may have changed has been the effectiveness of psychological management, thanks to learning from patients, trying different strategies, such as couple therapy, and assessing the results as measured by relapses and remissions over many years.

6.11.1 Psychological Management

Predisposing Cultural and Childhood Influences. Doctors and/or therapists will waste time and suffer unnecessary frustration unless they employ the short cuts afforded by prior appreciation of UC patients' sensitivity, emotional immaturity and extreme dependence on key figures, the result of childhood experience, and cultural factors such as race, religion and social class. Matriarchal dominance in strict Jewish families and the patriarchal equivalent in strict, non-conformist sects [75, 81] are likely to inhibit development towards emotional independence in some members of a sibship. Both religious groups mentioned have been shown to carry a 2–3 times higher than anticipated incidence of UC [81, 82]. Whether a particular child will conform or rebel depends both on inherited tendencies towards obsessionality, docility, timidity, aggressivity, etc., and subsequent parental, cultural and environmental pressures.

Background to Aversion to Quarrelling. The extreme aversion of UC patients to speak their mind stems from two different childhood backgrounds. The one is rather "cosy", as in some strict religious sects "with never an angry word, where all is peace and light", at least on the surface; the other background is of quarrelling, bickering parents, and memories of hiding in the garden shed and blocking the ears to avoid the terrifying shouting of a drunken father coming home. Children brought up in that environment were sensitized first hand to the threat that quarrels posed to their security, and from then on, as do all UC patients, they avoid quarrels at any price. The "cosy" background fails to equip the children with the ability to cope with the hurly-burly of normal life, and they fail to learn that parents and siblings can argue even to the point of shouting, but can then make it up. Patients with UC are so sensitive to atmospheres that they know at once when they walk into a room if there has been argument.

Other Causes of Sensitivity. An only child is particularly exposed, perhaps also babies born near the menopause or when the gap in time from the preceding sibling is wide. Death of a child can result in excessive parental concern for the next born, while early rearing problems commonly lead to over-concern reinforced by conscious or unconscious guilt. Extreme fearfulness of illness, doctors, dentists, bad news, even thunderstorms, may be passed on to the more vulnerable child, while emotional deprivation in a parent's childhood is a common cause of a parent clinging to one or more of their own children. Such parents may freely admit that they found their first happiness in the love of a spouse or children and therefore cling to them. Put another way, they "feed" on them emotionally. To treat UC effectively doctors have to understand this extreme sensitivity which originates in childhood backgrounds like those described.

Engel [74] emphasised that the basic problem of UC patients was in separating emotionally from a key figure (usually mother and subsequent surrogates).

One gains the impression that the patient lives through a key figure (e.g. mother) and that the key figure lives through the patient ... [He stressed the implication of this for physicians] ... It is also a general experience that the patients who develop a "dependent" relationship, whether or not it is consciously planned by the physician, do better than patients who do not. Once a relationship has been established, it is unusual for the patient to relinquish it and still remain in good health. Any interruption of the doctor-patient relationship, especially early in the relationship, is likely to be accompanied by some relapse of symptoms.

The First Interview. Engel agrees that doctors treating patients with UC will be helped by a prior understanding of the personality traits and of childhood and nurtural influences.

> Knowledge of the psychologic processes ... provides us with important aids in the treatment of the patients ... the way the physician relates to and behaves with his ulcerative colitis patient, may result in harm as well as help ... psychologic understanding ... is far from an academic matter.

First, patients must feel that they have had a full hearing of their symptoms and a full examination which must include sigmoidoscopy. An essential part of the history in UC as in other psychosomatic disorders is the extended family history including positions in the family, births, deaths, illnesses, similarities and dissimilarities of sibling and parents, and polarities between them and with the patient. After that, enquiry should be pursued as to what the in-laws or neighbours are like and whether relationships are friendly or tense. For example, who visits whom at festivals, or spends holidays together, and who does not and why (see transcript Mr. S. P.).

Sensitivity: Ways of Extracting What Patients Feel. With the foreknowledge about UC patients' extreme sensitivity to quarrels and shouting, it is necessary to establish the truth of this with each patient, using open-ended questions such as: What kind of a temperament have you got? The answer may be anything from "I am quiet", "I am happy-go-lucky", "Nothing worries me" to a frank admission of being "easily hurt". If the answer has been unhelpful, it is useful to ask: Do you think you are a sensitive person? The answer in 90% will be "Yes", and the supplementary question is obviously: In what way? or Can you explain what you mean? UC patients often hesitate at this point but may say that things can upset them.
D: What sort of things?
P: Well, things that people say.
The supplementary question should again be, What sort of things? Can you give me an example of anything that happened recently? As often as not with facilitating grunts or smiles and remarks such as, "There's plenty of time – think for a bit", the patient will tell the doctor the provocation of the current attack.

However, if the patient "clams up" having admitted sensitivity but cannot give an example, it is necessary to put the question: How do you deal with quarrelsome or awkward people, not so much at work but neighbours or your own family or friends? The answer invariably is "I do not like quarrelling – I prefer to walk away – they can get on with it."
D: But don't you ever feel like saying something or feel angry?
P: I don't feel anything, I just ignore it.
D: You don't even feel a little hurt or put out? (facilitation)
P: Well (reluctantly) perhaps just a little. (Even this may be denied until two or three interviews later, perhaps with the prompting of a spouse, who may say, "You know you haven't visited your sister since she made that remark at Christmas," or "You didn't say anything all the way home, and every time I have mentioned it you said you didn't want to talk about it." The spouse may receive a look, but the shell has been cracked.)

If the early open-ended questions betray some insight by the patient, the following "tin-opener" is worth asking: Would you be surprised if I were to suggest that this trouble might have an emotional basis in part related to your sensitivity? Experience has shown that about 50% will say that they would not be surprised. When asked to provide their reason and an example, given encouragement and suitable silence by the doctor, the patient often comes up with the precise incident which had provoked the attack, thereby saving a great deal of therapeutic time.

A Therapeutic Essential. Having established an empathetic relationship on the lines mentioned, effective psychological management then depends on uncovering, if possible at the first interview, or not later than the second or third, the precipitating insult, which may have been verbal or a situational threat. For example, the unilaterally declared intention by a bossy, aggressive relative to visit the patient for Easter or the summer holidays. One of us recalls such a patient whose sister had been converted to a strict religious sect and who proposed to convert the patient too! Being *typically* colitic, the latter could not bring herself to say "no" for fear of the sister's aggression.

If the interview is unproductive with such a denial as: "Nothing has upset me, Doctor, of course I would tell you if it had," other means can be employed. It is useful to explain to the patient that problems that provoke UC are often so trivial that they may feel ashamed of mentioning them. It may help to tell patients that what may be petty to an outsider can be vexing to someone as sensitive as they are. To prime the pump at this point, doctors or therapists can call on their own actual experience of previous cases or the published experience of others. It is also useful to ask the patient: How would you have felt or reacted had you been in that situation? In this way UC patients often reveal their true feelings; and as with the Thematic Apperception Test (TAT) it is a technique that can penetrate the alexithymic defence in a way that other methods and tests fail to do [83].

The Importance of Festivals and Holidays. Special note should be taken of the onset or relapse of UC close in time to Christmas, New Year, Easter, Whitsun or summer holiday period. At these times families meet, and the opportunities for tensions, snide remarks and umbrage to be taken by the sensitive "no-boo-to-a-goose" UC patient are numerous. When the time relationship is close, the doctor should ask how the patient spent the festive days or summer holiday (see transcript Mr. S. P.). Equally unwelcome are further invitations from relatives or friends after a previously traumatic holiday which may prove to be provocative because the patient fears refusal will cause a rift.

Births, Deaths and Marriages. Lindemann reported [84] that loss by death or alienation or a threatened loss as by illness of a key figure was the most common provocative stress in the psychopathogenesis of UC. Most authors since then have accepted this view but without convincing evidence. Sometimes numbers are too small, e.g. 12 out of 18 [72]. However, whereas pathological and prolonged mourning is the provocative stress in RA and other AI diseases [85], in UC it has rarely been so in our experience. It may sometimes *appear* to be so, e.g. when a very immature and dependent UC patient loses his or her prop either by death or withdrawal and when their ego resources prove to be inadequate to cope with the ordinary problems of living alone. They then relapse into childish, sulking resentment when relatives or friends are unable or not prepared to assuage their great dependency needs. Lindemann's cases 2 and 3 appear to have been examples of this when brothers acting as protective surrogate parents were drafted into the army. In neither case are we told about the relationship with parents or other siblings; in case 1, a nurse in whom UC developed 4 days after the death of her father whom she had nursed through his terminal illness, we are not told what her mother was doing at that time, or what she felt about the mother delegating to her "all the errands and decisions concerned with the funeral", or what she felt when told she might "hurt her mother by making her nervously upset". We have found that when death appears to be related closely in time to onset, there are usually events surrounding the death which are responsible, e.g. ill-chosen remarks at the funeral, allegations of neglect by relatives, the theft of trinkets, disputed wills, unwelcome remarriages, etc.

In one instance, a patient's doctor requested consultation because he felt that the death of the patient's daughter 6 months earlier had precipitated UC; however, the real cause became apparent when she revealed that her son-in-law had remarried and that the new wife was not kind to the grandchildren and restricted her access to them. Her problem was not one of unresolved mourning but of smouldering resentment against the new wife which she had to bottle up if she wished to continue to see her grandchildren at all.

Births, like deaths, offer endless opportunities for parents or in-laws to interfere; in the following instance a first-born baby much wanted by the father at a conscious level suddenly posed a threat. Seen in a relapse of UC and a week after the birth, his wife's nodding head revealed the cause when it was suggested that babies can be fun but also competitors. While bathing the baby her husband came in from work and wanted his tea. She called from the bathroom: "It's in the oven." She said she could see he was offended and was quiet for several days, i.e. sulking and resentful. Immediate remission of UC followed ventilation of his feelings and being made aware of their relationship to his relapse.

When alienation of a parent, sibling or in-law precipitates UC because some trivial event is perceived by the patient as an insult, it is feelings of smouldering resentment rather than loss which dominate the patient's thoughts for months or years. The offending relative will often try to make amends, but the patient will prefer to sulk.

For example, a sister asked a patient's daughter to be her bridesmaid and then put her off for someone else. The patient broke off all contact although the sister only lived in the next road. "What do you do if you meet in the street or in a shop?" she was asked, "I look the other way or go out." Hostilities were thus maintained by the patient for 5 years, during which time her bowel continued to bleed.

The Value of Couple Therapy. Personal experience over the past 15 years has shown couple therapy to be more effective than seeing the patient alone, and this is also true for Crohn's disease and MS. In contrast it is usually contraindicated in asthma (see Chap. 7) and has no important place in the management of disorders such as migraine or IBS.

It has been our experience that young doctors find listening to, and asking about, patients' feelings embarrassing even on a one-to-one basis, but to discuss them when a spouse or fiancé(e) is present who may be very emotionally involved is even more threatening. Young doctors and students who are still close in time to their own dependency and separation problems tend to find a couple's disharmony as too much like similar rifts, actual or fantasied, in their own family or personal relationships. Thus, they may use the defence of not feeling it right to intrude, or of not wanting to be responsible for breaking up a marriage, thereby making the assumption that the voicing of feelings about an unstable relationship will worsen it, when in reality openness is often the beginning of mutual understanding and acceptance.

We advise doctors who recognise the value of couple therapy in the disorders mentioned but are wary of it, to seek a co-therapist, preferably someone versed in psychodynamics, such as a medical social worker, health visitor or counsellor. In this way they will soon learn enough for their fears to abate and then they will be able to manage such interviews on their own. That is not to say that two therapists are not better than one in seeing more of what is going on in couple or family work, but simply that it is rarely logistically possible in a busy surgery or outpatient department.

Much of the value in couple therapy is to allay or reduce the infantilising effect of overconcern of a partner arising from conscious or unsconscious feelings of responsibility. Feelings of guilt arise when anything more than trivial illness affects close relatives, and they are made worse by an inability to help. When the complaint is something invisible, such as headache, diarrhoea or rectal bleeding, which is not easy to talk about, patients feel how much easier it would be if they had something obvious like a broken leg. However, if they do not specify their symptoms, relatives are apt to be unsympathetic when they conceal their complaint and merely say they feel tired and unwell. This leads to tetchy remarks such as: "Why don't you go to the doctor and get some new pills?" In couple therapy it is useful to ask the partner what he or she feels about the patient's illness and "droopiness", and whether they feel frustrated by its chronicity and their inability to help. This permits expression of the overconcern often arising from guilt over feeling in some way responsible, rarely recognising that the patient's limited coping mechanisms had their origins in childhood, long before the couple had met. Acceptance of shared responsibility for the roles they unconsciously play each other into, e.g. a sulking, demanding child on the one hand and the rejecting and/or overpossessive parent on the other, is a paramount step in the therapeutic progress for both patient and spouse. After that it is usually possible to enlist the spouse or partner as a co-therapist. Once the latter understands that bottled up resentment can cause a bowel to bleed as easily as a face can blush, and that the stress may seem outwardly trivial, he or she can often anticipate and identify likely provocative stress before the patient does. In management we sometimes describe this as "defusing the bomb" or acting as a "lightning conductor".

For example: "I told her to stop worrying. That sister of hers is always upsetting people but when she insists on us going every weekend, my wife fears to refuse because her sister will tell the rest of the family that she has become standoffish since we married." Gradually the patient learns to feel emotions and then free to express them, first in the consulting room and then beyond it. That important step is greatly facilitated by the understanding and encouragement of a spouse as co-therapist – a very different role of the infantilising overconcern of "parent" before couple therapy began.

Psychosomatic Patients Split Therapists. The dangers of psychosomatic patients splitting their various therapists symbolically into psyche and soma, first described by Winnicott [70], has been dealt with in Chap. 4. This applies to GPs, physicians, surgeons, dietitians, nurses, not to mention homeopaths, herbalists and meditators. Because the somatic aspect of UC can be so life-threatening, unless the psychotherapist feels competent to deal with the physical aspects of a relapse, the chances are high that the patient will escape from psychotherapy into illness, perhaps to a surgical ward and colectomy. Equally, the surgeon or internist not practised in dealing with psychoneurotic or psychotic breakdown may be stampeded into admitting the patient to a mental hospital when the patient switches from colitis to mental illness.

Interrupted Therapy: A Disadvantage of Somatic Therapeutic Success. Psychotherapy for psychosomatic disorders including UC has to take into account that once the somatic component remits, the strongest motive for the patient to remain in therapy ceases. This necessitates an open door policy and easy access in the event of relapse. The longer a relapse persists, the longer it takes to achieve a remission. After initial therapy the emotional insult causing the relapse is usually within the patient's consciousness although almost instantly suppressed and denied. Reluctance to acknowledge it to the doctor, even though comparable acknowledgement had led to previous remission is understandable, despite the unpleasantness of the disease. Thus, the doctor or therapist learns to be grateful for small morsels, however irregularly offered. In a previous publication [75] this was described as seeing relapses not as disasters but as stepping stones to understanding and emotional growth. Daniels [72, pp 105–111] expressed this very clearly in case 2, with a follow-up over 47 years.

Management of the Severe Case. Initially, this should be gauged according to the gravity of the disease. For the acutely ill patient every infantile demand must be met or anticipated. Not to accede reinforces the patient's feeling of rejection by a key figure. Some doctors and nurses find querulous and demanding patients hard to tolerate, especially when they appear supine and apparently prefer to die despite all that medical science can offer. Failures to conceal their frustrations may prove lethal. Without an experienced ward sister (senior nurse) with a sixth sense who understands these patients' sensitivity and can convey this understanding to her staff, the management of severe UC will always be unnecessarily hazardous. It is better, therefore, to treat these patients as far as possible as outpatients. Even with the best management wards can be abrasive places, with verbal attack from other patients being particularly damaging for these vulnerable people. It has been claimed that psychotherapy in the acute stage is dangerous. We think this is so only if the therapist is insensitive, remote or makes interpretations prematurely. On the other hand we recall many patients who continued to deteriorate until given an opportunity to talk in privacy out of the ward along the lines already described, and who then immediately recovered.

The Importance of the Team. Detrimental scattering or splitting of care givers, so damaging in UC and Crohn's disease, can only be managed effectively by a team approach, with all members having sufficient understanding of the psychodynamics of the patient's manipulation to avoid falling for it. We have discussed how this can be done in Chap. 4.

Syndrome Shift. Either spontaneously or as a result of treatment, including surgery, there may be a shift to another syndrome. A shift to schizophrenia can occur, but it is rare in practice. Personal examples of a shift to another psychosomatic disorder in which the spectrum of personality traits is closest to that met in UC, e.g. MS number 11 currently [77], and a neurologist, Arnason, made a similar observation [86]. Both disorders share the same extreme emotional immaturity and hopelessness in the face of separation threats. However, threat of engulfment, which is a feature in MS, is not so important in UC. The shared obsessionality and fastidiousness explains why many UC patients also suffer from migraine at times. Syndrome shift to psychosomatic disorders such as asthma and hypertension, in which the *typical* attitudes and traits are different to those in UC, are rare.

Follow-up Studies. There have been all too few follow-up studies, one reason being that since the advent of effective agents such as ACTH or corticosteroids it is rarely justifiable in the severe or moderately severe case to depend on psychological management alone. In consequence, remission cannot be claimed for one or the other form of treatment. For follow-up studies on psychological management alone, see [87–89]. However, in patients with mild or moderate colitis seen in outpatient clinics, it is quite justifiable to depend on psychological management alone, particularly when the precipitating insult has been uncovered at the first interview and if emotional factors have been acknowledged. The transcript of Mr. S. P. was just such a case. The reader is referred to previous publications [89, 76, 30] for a variety of case histories.

6.11.2 Transcripts and Case History

Mrs. I. K., aged 30, looked and sounded ill and resentful at her first interview in 1976.

D: What do you feel when you get eight motions a day?

P: Very tired and very tender ...

D: You had a bit of inflammation of the lower bowel in 1971. Have you lost any weight with these troubles?

P: Well, I have actually.

D: How much have you lost?

P: 12 lbs (5 kg).

D: Do you think anything makes this troubles worse?

P: I think emotional stress makes it worse.

D: It does, does it?

P: Yes.

D: What sort of temperament have you got?

P: Mm ... I'm very calm, but sort of trying to analyse myself I realise that probably I keep everything inside me. (Gesture, places hand on upper abdomen.) It might be the cause of me getting this illness.

D: Do you find people who get awkward easy to manage? How do you feel with them?

P: I always keep my temper, always, although I am extremely angry inside.

D: Perhaps you don't like quarrels?

P: No, I don't

D: Did your parents quarrel or bicker at all much?

P: Yes, I can remember quite a few arguments with my parents.

D: Did you argue with your father, or tell him off?

P: Once, yes, he was very annoyed. (Puts her hands to her throat in a throttling gesture.)

D: Did he hit you?

P: Yes.

D: You didn't like that? Did he frighten you?

P: Yes, I remember I didn't like my father very much – after that ...
We had a cottage in the country in 1970

D: Perhaps that was when you took ill, was it?

P: That was the time when it started, yes. I remember one particular incident that upset me during this period. Other than that, I think it may have even been started off when my husband used to go to the pub with the next door neighbour's husband, you see, on a Saturday night, and when he came back a bit later on he said they had been invited to a party, a sort of golfing party thing, but he didn't tell me. It was downright deceit and it upset me terribly, and well, that was the first time.

D: I should think you felt rather hurt about that? (facilitation)

P: I was.

D: Were you able to express it to him?

P: Oh yes, he realised I was upset because I was crying.

D: I understand you were crying, but did you tell him how angry you were?

P: Well, I think he knew.

D: I think he knew all right.

P: I think he knew that he had hurt me.

D: I understand that, but you were actually feeling very angry. (facilitation)

P: Yes, I was, well, I *suppose* I was angry.

D: Were you able to express it to him? I am just questioning whether you were actually able to express the anger to him? (facilitation)

P: Oh no, I cried, that's all. That's the kind of thing he does that hurts me. He is *so* sorry, he *so* sympathetic with me that I *never* actually throw the kitchen sink at him.

D: Does he "defuse" you?

P: Yes.

D: Yes, I understand very clearly. Well, that's why you've got the bowel trouble all right.

Note: (a) *typicality* of childhood and (b) *typical* inability to express, supine response to aggression, brooding and hurt feelings instead.

Four interviews and 1 year later: Appearance happy, smiling, attractive, self-confident.

P: I did go over 9 st. once (56 kg). I'm back into keeping my own weight.

D: I see.

P: Well, I suppose I keep all my feelings inside me instead of letting fly at times, and this has probably helped me a lot.

D: You weren't fully aware before I saw you that that tendency you had could cause your bowel trouble?

P: Because I'm not really a very violent person. (Excuses herself by laughing.) I think I've broken the front door glass, the window, and dented rather badly a teapot since I last saw you.

D: Very good! (Doctor shakes hands to reward patient for a change in coping mechanism.) I hope it was the teapot that was thrown at your husband?

P: Yes – it was full. (Laughs.)

D: Did he catch it?

P: No, we were thinking about getting a new one and I said, "No, we must keep that to remind us."

D: That's very good. Do you think he is happier with you as you are? I expect he finds you less moody.

P: Most definitely.

D: At one time I said you didn't beam your message loud and clear. I remember you said, "I wasn't beaming it at all." How many bowel actions are you getting at the moment?

P: One, occasionally two.

Patient returned a year later in mild relapse again, related to her husband's attitude. On threatening to leave him he apologised, and the colitis remitted.

Mr. S. P., aged 34; neatly dressed, unemotional, precise man. *First interview*

P: Going to the toilet – sitting down – blood – the beginning of 1975.

D: January about?

P: Yes.

D: What sort of temperament do you think you've got?

P: Calm. I don't like arguing for the sake of arguing if it's something unimportant then you know, perhaps I will agree, just to keep the peace.

D: Wife's people?

P: They live in L. Her stepfather is very docile, her mother is very strong-willed, and I find it difficult to get along with her, but I don't make it obvious. I just go along with her and keep the peace. We both went up there this Christmas, and because of this trouble I was having, I was, you know, absolute waste of time my being there, you know – fed up – so I, so we both came back on the Friday – we were going to stay until Sunday.

D: Can you tell me what it is about her that gets under your skin?

P: Well, she's so dominant and tries to organise everybody's life. I'll give you an example. My wife's sister said, "As you are coming up at Christmas, come and stay with us and everything will be all right, it'll be nice to see you". That sentence had hardly finished when mother-in-law pipes up and says, "Ah, well you won't come up with an empty car, will you? How about you bringing L. and J. up as well? Now that's the sort of thing she jumped right in and said, she did two things, one, she presupposed that I wanted to take two people along, and the second thing was that she hadn't even asked L. and J. whether they wanted to come for their first Christmas to L. You know, this is the sort of thing she does which really annoys me. My wife and I were going to go up there and stay with my sister-in-law, and we thought everything was OK and then sister-in-law telephoned my wife and said there's all sort of trouble up here about who you are going to stay with, and my sister-in-law thought to keep the peace and keep everybody happy, we had better go and stay with mother-in-law.

D: You didn't want to?

P: We didn't want to, but we did it.

D: This kind of experience you describe and the thoughts going through your mind, coming up to Christmas could have made you very resentful, if you like, angry inside is another way of putting it, do you know what I mean?

P: Yes, I think that's possible.

Typically avoiding arguments and feeling resentful instead, *typicality* of stress when families meet at Christmas, Easter, etc.

Three months later, with wife:

D: How many bowel actions now?

P: One a day average

D: It is conceivable that you may get another patch of trouble, particularly when you go to L. (Laughter; wife's comments inaudible.) I don't think you probably had associated in your mind the trouble up there, certainly the blow-up at Christmas?

P: I think really, until we first spoke about it, no one had related that to me as a sign of some sort of stress, and therefore, obviously, I hadn't got anything to think about. I just thought it was something physical, but obviously if it did re-occur, then I would just sit down and think what's happened in the last 2 months – so that ...

D: That's right, that's right, and talk with your wife because she might be able to spot it before you could.

P: Yes, thanks very much.

NB Therapeutic effect of "awareness".

Another example of the importance of visits and festivals was a man who seemed surprised when his wife pointed out in an interview that his bowel always started to bleed 3 days before dreaded visits to his mother in another part of the country.

Case History. The following case illustrates the value of short-term psychological intervention, the importance of *typicality* of childhood background leading to inadequate coping with strife and also the *typicality* of life situations. A married man of 42 with proctocolitis for 3 years was referred by a gastroenterologist because relapses occurred every Christmas or at times of stress despite standard drug treatment. His sensitivity to quarrels dated from childhood when there had been constant tension between his mother who had a fierce temper and his adopted sister whom he recalls being stiff with rage in her high chair, and because his father who was a Roman Catholic had been despised by his kin for marrying outside the faith. Christmas had always been a time of strain between the families because of religion and injured feelings over presents and cards. The patient had been much hurt by his paternal uncles's behaviour at his father's funeral and their subsequent neglect of his widowed mother. As a result he refused to have anything more to do with them. Proctocolitis started some months after this insult, but as he no longer had anything to do with his paternal uncles it seemed unlikely that they were accounting for his disease persisting 3 years later.

For this reason the direction of the interview was switched to his feelings about his wife and her family. Once again there had been a long history of tension between his wife's parents, of such severity that his wife had left home as soon as possible. Mother-in-law had developed a manic depressive psychosis after the death of her son in a traffic accident, and the patient had found himself "adopted" in his place, whereas his wife had been rejected from her birth, which took place shortly after her brother's death. The patient's wife had never been able to cope with her mother when she was manic, and because the patient could do no wrong he became the unwilling recipient of his wife's anger and frustration; such tensions were also invariably worse at Christmas time when the families were together.

After three joint interviews with the couple, the patient's colitis remitted and remained in remission. He later stopped his drugs and felt that he no longer needed to attend the GI clinic, or for further psychological management, but as usual he was offered open access in the event of relapse. He said that prior to being seen he had not related his colitis to his emotional tensions, and because his wife was also now able to appreciate this, they were communicating their frustrations in a more mature way. As a result he was taking less umbrage at being "put on the spot" (ambushed) either by his wife or by his mother-in-law.

6.11.3 Summary

Salient points are as follows:

1. An understanding of the predisposing cultural and childhood influences leading to *typicality* (specificity) of personality traits is essential.
2. As in all psychosomatic disorders the patients must feel that the organic aspect of the history has had a full hearing and has been fully examined and investigated before being able to accept possible emotional links.

3. The precipitating emotional insult or life situation must be uncovered, if not at the first interview, then at the second or third. Joint interviews with spouse, partner or siblings can be facilitating and time saving.
4. Facilitation. Because of these patients' failure to express emotions, techniques of facilitation (Chap. 5) by the doctor are necessary. The doctor also needs to know the kind of threats to which these people are typically so vulnerable.
5. For some weeks or months the doctor must empathise with the patients, respond to their infantile needs and accept their behaviour, however manipulative.
6. Continuing management, psychotherapy and/or couple therapy. The aim is to help these patients to use their hitherto undeveloped ability to feel emotion, especially anger, and express it. An alternative to childish sulking is offered. Spouses or partners can be very useful as co-therapists once *their* overconcern and the patients' manipulations have been exposed and accepted. With the more adult communication which ensues, previous childlike responses become unnecessary.
7. As stated above, death or illness of a key figure is only provocative of UC when the patient's dependence makes even the normal problems of living abrasive. Much more often it is events arising *from* the death, which are provocative, such as contested wills, allegations by relatives at the funeral, early remarriage, etc.
8. Festivals and holidays are occasions for relatives to meet, and the opportunity for hurt feelings are notorious. When onset or relapse of UC is closely related to these events, detailed enquiry is called for of who went where, and who met whom, and will they go again next year.
9. When the somatic component remits, patients are reluctant to stay in therapy. An open door policy is required, and relapses should be seen as stepping stones to understanding and emotional growth rather than the disasters which many doctors usually regard them,
10. Unthinking remarks by other patients and young doctors make a hospital bed dangerous for these patients. For inpatient management it is necessary to train a team to understand these patients' sensitivity and vulnerability.

6.12 Irritable Bowel Syndrome

IBS is a common disorder accounting for 44% of referrals to gastroenterological clinics. Gastroenterologists of the greatest experience, such as Almy [90], speak of "wrestling with the irritable colon", but they are able to add: "While defeat is likely, both reward and enjoyment may be in store for the successful tactician." Kirsner [91], after 40 years of day-to-day involvement, says: "It is treatable and even curable, yet few GI tract illnesses are approached so awkwardly and so ineffectively." The nearest parallel in inept management which comes to mind are the number of cardiac invalids caused by the medical mishandling of effort syndrome, ectopic rhythms, innocent murmurs and hyperventilation in the 1914–1918 war and subsequently, despite the teachings of Mackenzie [103] and of White and Hahn [104] (Chap. 8).

Diagnosis. Throughout this book it has been assumed that diagnoses have been established before starting definitive psychological management. To have done otherwise would have left insufficient space for the main objective.

However, it should be stressed that the diagnosis of IBS, while reached by eliciting positive points in the history and on examination, including sigmoidoscopy, also depends on exclusion of organic causes. This is especially so when the history is *only* of diarrhoea or loose stools. IBS *may* still be the cause, but the chances of protozoal or bacterial infections, disaccharidase insufficiency, Crohn's disease, duodenal diverticulum, one of the malabsorption syndromes or malignancy are high and need exclusion. When the history is of intermittant constipation, with hard, "rabbity" stools coated with mucus, and some alternating diarrhoea, IBS is more likely, especially if left or right iliac fossa pain and tenderness is present, and if a rubbery, rope-like, descending colon or loaded caecum is palpable. Sigmoidoscopic appearances of dilated and injected vessels with normal surrounding mucosa also favour IBS, but where the mucosa is congested without the classical bogginess or contact bledding of UC, an infectious cause is likely, or chemical irritation by lactic acid resulting from disaccharidase insufficiency and/or free fatty acids in malabsorption states. The texture, colour and smell of the faeces can also be a useful pointer to malabsorption. Blood in the lumen or contact bleeding calls for barium studies and if these are unhelpful, colonoscopy.

Once again it is not a question of either or (psyche or soma); equal attention to both is needed and never more so than in IBS. Psychosomatically orientated clinicians should try to be as knowledgeable of its organic causes as their gastroenterological colleagues, and no less concerned about them.

6.12.1 Psychological Management

Having excluded the organic causes mentioned, it is our experience [92] that approximately 90% of cases have a *typically* provocative life situation of indecision or "fence-sitting". This, however, is usually overlooked because patients are rarely asked the right questions with suitable facilitations (see below and case histories). IBS patients with psychosomatic aetiology are always from the same group of tense, uptight people who from time to time suffer from migraine, vascular headache, aphthous oral ulcers, prolapsed intervertebral discs, neck and back ache, dysmenorrhoea or urethral syndrome. Doctors need to recognise that syndrome shift frequently occurs between these common afflictions, so that a single patient may have suffered three or four of them at different times. Because the section of the population who suffers intermittently from these disorders, including IBS, is so large (10%–20%), there is no justification for it to be regarded as more neurotic, more anxious or more depressed than the mean. Otherwise it would be difficult to explain why 13% of apparently normal people have had IBS but have never consulted a doctor about it [96]. The same point applies equally to migraine, aphthous ulcers, etc. Where they do differ from the mean is in being more uptight and possessing some obsessional characteristics. Thus in approximately 90% of psychosomatically based IBS there is a combination of a *typical* life situation and a patient with a *typical* personality. In some cases the *typically* provocative situation does not occur until middle life (for example see last Transcript).

"Fence-Sitting" – The Typical Life Situation. Support for the relevance of fence-sitting is to be found in the literature. Weiss and English [10] described a classical case in a

young woman undecided whether to jump into a career or into marriage (a common conflict today). It was suggested to the patient in question that she should try to make up her mind. When seen a month later her bowel symptoms were much improved, and she said she had given up the idea of marriage and had decided to pursue her career.

Grace, Wolf and Wolff [93] mentioned conflict and indecision as provocative factors in disturbed colonic function, and Wolf recently confirmed this in a personal communication. To some "conflict" means primarily a battle or clash of interests between people, whereas psychotherapists usually mean conscious or unconscious emotional conflict. In IBS the fence-sitting is usually conscious, although the origin for indecisiveness is unconscious. The following case illustrates this.

A young unmarried woman of 24 and the youngest of her sibship had lived at home since she had left school and worked in her father's office. She liked the work and knew it was important to her father that she continue, but as she matured from child to adult she had become increasingly infuriated that her father did not recognise this; he remained dictatorial and took her for granted. She was in conflict in both senses of the word. However, battle with her father was unvoiced for reasons in her unconscious, while the conflict of indecision as to whether she should pack up and leave was conscious and was the basic cause of her IBS. With the type of facilitation already mentioned of suggesting that the usual cause of symptoms such as her's was a fence-sitting life situation, followed by a few examples, she told her story. After being encouraged to resolve it one way or the other, she returned 3 months later symptom free. She said she had made the decision to tell her father what she felt, and to her surprise he had accepted it and from then on began asking her and not telling her to do things.

The following question is recommended to uncover fence-sitting: Do you think you are a person who finds it easy to make up your mind, not just buying things but over bigger issues such as changing jobs, moving house, emigrating or having a baby? After the reply ask: Has anything like that been happening lately? Almost invariably it has, e.g. a woman is to be married and wants children but knows her fiancé does not. She knows she should settle it before marriage but avoids it, fearing he will leave her. A woman with a 15-year liaison is nearing middle age but knows the man will not marry her and that she should leave him and puts it off. A business man after entering a partnership finds his position intolerable; he has either to assert his rights or leave at considerable financial loss. A woman has moved house because of her children's education but is unsettled because of her isolation and hankers after moving again. Resolution of the dilemma is followed by remission of symptoms; the clinician's task is to help identify the dilemma and encourage decision-making instead of fence-sitting.

Other examples are quoted in the case histories and transcripts.

Cancer Phobia. Most of the remaining cases of IBS (approx. 10%) in which organic causes mentioned at the onset have been excluded, are phobic, usually fearing cancer or leukaemia, etc. as the cause of their symptoms. It is important to identify them early if their neurosis is not to be fed by a multitude of costly investigations. Instead, appropriate treatment is called for. They will usually deny their fear at first, but remarks at the end of a careful explanation such as: "But there must be something more than spasm to cause all this, doctor" belie their denial, or it may be hostile and bored inattention during the examination, e.g. looking out of the window, humming, etc., which can be interpreted as "He's wasting his time, I know what I've got even if he doesn't." Such patients have problems of guilt, usually related to pathological mourning or loss of key figures for whom they have had conscious or unconscious ambivalent feelings. They fear retribution and the need for reparation and require psychotherapy to help them resolve it.

Emotional Diarrhoea. Although it may masquerade as IBS, emotional diarrhoea is rather rare, and it also needs a sophisticated psychotherapeutic approach. Such patients' apprehension is so great that they fear leaving their house unless there are accessible lavatories every 100 m on their route, and in many the disorder is secondary to underlying agoraphobia; just like infants and young animals, they void their bowels in panic. They invariably hyperventilate (Chap. 7), and treatment should combine re-education in breathing with psychotherapy for their phobia.

6.12.2 Case Histories and Transcripts

The following three case histories illustrate the intractability of such cases with standard treatment and the technique of management needed. The first patient unfortunately dropped out of therapy after initial improvement and for reasons which are instructive. The second case on the other hand responded dramatically, and the third case after six sessions spread over 2 years.

Mrs. B. L., aged 48, had had cancer phobia superimposed on the pain and bowel symptoms of intermittent IBS for 2 years. Major problems of indecision were affecting this tense, house-proud secretary. These included moving to another part or the country, which she did not want to do, but was necessary if her husband was to obtain promotion. He was restless and applying for jobs. Another point of indecision was whether she should have a confrontation with her only child, a teenager who had been a problem since infancy and was now in rebellion. The origin of the phobia was unresolved ambivalent feelings for her father who had died when she was a baby, and then for her mother who had been dead for 10 years. "When my mother died I was bitter about it (pointedly). You see she went into hospital with one diagnosis but in fact had another [cancer]. I felt I had not done enough and felt guilty." Always frightened of the dark and being alone, she had slept in the same room as her mother up to the time of her marriage. She felt she could never get so close to her as she would have wished and resented the fact that other girls at school had fathers and she did not. Following an interview she had a hyperventilation attack. The patient said she was convinced that her stomach pains must be "more than spasm" that there must be something there". Unfortunately, after progress in the resolution of her unresolved mourning and the hyperventilation attack, she persuaded her husband to support her view that "something nasty had been missed" and spent the next years seeing specialists and having every possible investigation for her symptoms with negative results.

Mrs. L. T., aged 30, was referred because she was convinced that her IBS symptoms of 6 years duration were due to cancer. Her mother had had an abdominoperineal resection, and the patient had been anticipating and dreading her own death because of her ambivalent feelings for which she felt she would have to pay with her own life. The youngest by 8 years, she had been told by her mother that she was "a mistake". She had unresolved mourning and guilt feelings for her father who died when she was 4, leaving her defenceless against her mother.

She had memories from the age of 4 of her mother giving her enemata and making her hold them, of her mother's anger at her enuresis, and going on and on at her until she implored her to hit her instead, of mother whispering in her ear when they were out, "Just wait until we get home", of mother's repeated threats to kill herself and of running for protection to her aunts up the road only to be forbidden to do so ever again because of her mother's jealousy. Astonishingly, this sanction was still in force at the time of the consultation. That interview enabled her to pour out her feelings of guilt and fears of retribution, and she went home and talked with her husband for 5 h. The following day she visited her friendly aunts and said she would "be damned to her mother". She remitted and remained in remission after 5 years of ill health which had distanced her from her husband and children. She was now able to accept her feelings of guilt, particularly after talking with her aunts, resumed her life as wife and mother and was still well at follow-up.

Mrs. M. N., a married Dutch woman, aged 65, with IBS, and cancer phobia was subjected to daily pressure by telephone and letter to return to Holland, about which she had strong reservations. Her sister inferred that she was neglecting the family and that she had also neglected her mother who had died 6 years before. The patient was the oldest and had always been exploited by her sickly mother and younger siblings, yet it was the youngest sister who was mother's favourite and spoilt. Even after working for the Resistance in the war and spending 2 years in a labour camp, she was told she should not have left her mother. "My poor mother had everything wrong – I had to look after her – while it was my sister who was sent to a nice school". The patient's fence-sitting began after her mother's death and with her sister's increasing pressure for "little mother" to return. At the same time her own long-standing guilt over her ambivalence to her mother and guilt over leaving her began to take their toll. Her first recorded phobic symptoms were cardiac, i.e. hyperventilation in 1977. When she was seen in 1979 with IBS she said, "I convinced myself I had cancer." She also feared she would be punished for her badness by losing her husband who had tuberculosis.

Two years and six therapeutic interviews after the first attendance she was symptom-free, although her husband was not well. Holland was no longer worrying her, and her mother was rarely in her thoughts instead of daily as when first seen.

6.12.2.1 Other Views on Psychological Management

Kirsner [90] said,

> Avoid any implication that IBS is imaginary ... maintain a kindly professional interest ... arrange regular visits ... and remain alert for any new symptoms ... but do nothing to decrease confidence.

As Almy [89] so rightly said,

> Clinical strategy calls for open-ended questions, a relaxed manner, sensitivity to non-verbal cues, and a readiness to re-explore and amend a supposedly complete history ... closely resembling the manner of the office based psychiatrists ... It is helpful to begin this social history at the first encounter.

Two Outcome Studies of Psychotherapy. Without special psychological training, Hislop [94] employed a form of brief psychotherapy (average 2.2 h) incorporating the basic tenets of psychodynamic theory aimed at resolution of the somatic complaint together with development of increasing insight and responsibility. Of 60 consecutive IBS patients so treated, 52 responded to a self-assessment questionnaire 20–30 months after completion of treatment, and of these only 22% had failed to obtain some relief. Svedlund and Sjödin [95] divided 101 IBS patients with at least 1 year of complaint into a control group treated by the usual medical means, and a second group treated similarly with the addition of psychotherapy 1 h per week for 10 sessions. The criteria of improvement were scored by independent raters at 3 months and then at follow-up at 12 months. Both groups improved mentally and somatically, but the group receiving psychotherapy had improved at 3 months; after 12 months this group had continued to improve while the control group showed some deterioration.

The following four transcripts of edited videotape of first and second outpatient interviews further illustrate how to uncover fence-sitting life situations and the benefit to patients and clinicians of this therapeutic short cut. Readers will appreciate that in the unedited interview the fence-sitting question comes only after 15–30 min.

Male lawyer, Not obviously tense, disarming smile, appearance and attitude rather precise; IBS for 12 months.

D: What are the motions like? Do you have any diarrhoea or loose stools?

P: No, the motions are very hard and comparable with rabbit pellets, and it is then that the slime is there – when I have what I call "normal motions" the slime is not there at all.

D: You are in the legal business?

P: That's right.

D: Well now, what I find is that some people who get this trouble either get themselves into positions where they find decisions difficult to take or they get themselves in a fence-sitting situation, or on the horns of a dilemma.

P: Yes, I suppose I have, about 15 months ago my chief officer did mention there would perhaps be some redundancies within the department, and since my particular job was suffering under the government cutbacks, I might be subject to redundancy.
   At the same time I was approached by a private firm of solicitors who said they would like my services, and you can perhaps appreciate my problem in that I hadn't been made redundant, and I might not be, but on the other hand, there was a job going in private practice and the future for that perhaps could be equally as bleak.

D: How long ago did they come forward with this offer?

P: The offer came about this time last year.
   Seen after a few months his symptoms had remitted after deciding to stay in his job. However, in a relapse 12 months later he revealed that he was once again undecided.

D: Are the private people still badgering you?

P: No, they are not any longer, but that position is still open to me.

D: Do you ever get a hankering for it?

P: Yes.

D: You do?

P: (Laughing) When things get bad I constantly feel I want to chuck it up and move to this firm. I know, I think, that I won't, but you know how it is – you get fed up from time to time.

D: Oh yes.

P: You think: "I'll get out, I'll move," but next day you change your mind again.

Female secretary aged 24, tense initially; IBS for 4 months.

D: Show me exactly where you get the pain?

P: Just here is where it swells up sometimes. (Points to left iliac fossa)

D: Do you ever get diarrhoea?

P: No, no.

D: It's usually more constipation?

P: Yes.

D: I mean, is it so bad sometimes that you have a job to clear the bowels?

P: Hm, yes, I'd say yes, yes.

D: The present attack has lasted about 4 months?

P: Hm.

D: Do you ever get into situations where you can't make your mind up about things, or else you are undecided as to whether to take up another job or move somewhere else, or get engaged to somebody or not get engaged? Do you find these decisions easy to take?

P: No, I can never make decicions. A few months ago I was seriously thinking about leaving and about moving, but I was very depressed at the time as well.

D: What sort of things were affecting you in balancing the decision at the time?

P: When I was depressed? Well, there were problems with my love life and I was a bit fed up with my job, and my immediate reaction was, "I want to get out, I want to get away." There was another girl there, and she wanted to go out with him.

D: When did you actually finally make up your mind to stay and bury the hatchet with your boyfriend?

P: It all happened gradually, and things are now a lot better than they have been for months and months previous to the big break-up.

D: You say you are not good at making decisions. Have you found in the past at times that you tend "to sit on the fence" a bit?

P: Yes, I can never make decisions, never. If I see something I like in a shop, I know I like it, but I need someone else to come along and say well, shall I get it or not, I just need them to say either yes or no. I know what I want but I can never decide whether to do it or not.

Three months later:

D: Have you had the same amount of pain, and you were also getting a bit constipated weren't you before?

P: Yes, that's right, it's alright now.

D: Has that eased up?

P: Yes.

D: When did all that begin to improve do you think?

P: I don't know – about the time I came here I suppose.

D: As I said, you may get a recurrence at times when things are a bit difficult and perhaps particularly when you can't make up your mind one way or another because that's often how it goes.

P: Yes, I know.

D: You know?

P: Yes, yes.

D: You know deep inside that's so?

P: Oh no, it's just that I never know what I want to do.

D: Yes. (Patient laughs).

Female school secretary, aged 30, tense, sitting on edge of chair, appeared younger than her age.

P: The lump in the stomach and the side pain.

D: Show me. Yes, I see, a sort of lump in the side feeling. Does the stomach ever get distended or blown up?

P: Yes, it does swell out here.

D: Are you one of a large family?

P: No, I'm an only child.

D: Did you have pain with your periods in your 'teens?

P: Yes.

D: You remember it then?

P: Yes, because I had to go to the doctor about it then.

D: Sometimes people have this kind of complaint that you have, who are undecided about some things in their lives, indecision, sitting on the fence if you like – do I change a job or don't I, or do I emigrate or don't I, do I get married or don't I, these kind of questions. Do you think you have problems of decision-making?

P: Well, funnily enough, it more or less started at the time when I met somebody who I thought was married who had a child in the school. Since I found out he was divorced and we started becoming friends, it started off and then I thought it was just – since you mention it – it was more or less from then, I thought people might raise their eyebrows slightly, I don't know, I'm always rather worried about what people think.

D: I understand that. And then the decision whether to go on seeing him or not seeing him, do you think that was a problem for you?

P: I suppose it was really.

D: Do you think you are a person who finds it easy to make up your mind about things?

P: Not really. (Laughs) I keep putting things off.

Three months later:

D: When have you seen these rather hard motions with slime on – have you had that again?

P: That's normal now.

D: The other thing was that you were a bit undecided about advancing that relationship which we talked about, do you remember?

P: Yes, that's just continuing as a friendly relationship – we see each other from time to time.

D: But it's pretty platonic?

P: Yes, you know.

D: So you are not really – ?

P: Not bothered about it now I've sorted it out – you said to make the decision one way or the other, no, and to let it go and carry on as it was progressing.

D: So you're quite happy about that? But before that I think perhaps you were feeling that you ought to put a stop to it?

P: Yes, for various reasons, but I've sorted them all out.

D: I'm glad you did that.

Female school cook, aged 50, cheerful, sensible woman; IBS for 12 months.

D: Can you show me where it was again?

P: In here, and low down there (points to abdomen) and very constipated.

D: Pains, left side, and then you pass rather hard, rabbity stools?

P: Yes, yes.

D: And sometimes you think there might be some slime?

P: Yes.

D: Sometimes people who get this sort of complaint have a little difficulty in making up their minds on certain things. I mean what I am saying is that you probably might have difficulty in deciding whether you were going to say give up work or change your job.

P: Yes, yes.

D: Move house?

P: Yes, well, this is it. I find that my job gets on top of me, and I did say to Dr. S. you know, I kept saying, it's getting a bit much, shall I give it up, you know. But then on the other hand, too much time on your hands is not good for you sometimes, I think.

D: People probably depend on you quite a bit, and they might find it difficult to replace you immediately? (facilitation)

P: Well, this is it, this is it.

D: Is it?

P: Yes, I think so.

D: Do you feel you might let someone down? I mean –

P: My assistant, my assistant cook –

D: Ah, it would be her your have in mind?

P: Yes, definitely.

D: What does your husband think about it? Does he think you ought to give it up?

P: Oh yes, he says, give it up, give it up, that's his answer, but I think I would miss seeing the children start with.

D: So that's another thing, you'd miss the children?

P: Yes.

D: Your mother, do you see much of her?

P: Well, I try and see her because she's seventy-five, but she knows I'm working.

D: Does she think you should give it up?

P: I think so, I think she would like me to give it up, but then I think, well, if I give it up, she'll expect me to be round there looking after her all the time and that's it, you see.

D: That's right, so you won't have a little alibi, will you?

P: No, no.

D: So we could say there are certain pressures on you from various directions. When I find people who have this trouble, I say to them "Look, I can't solve the problem, only you can solve it." (Patient acknowledges.) If you can resolve the problem one way or the other, you may well find your stomach gives you some peace. When it is unresolved, it tends to keep niggling away.

Five weeks later, all investigations negative:

P: Well, I don't seem to get so much pain now. I have more or less made up my mind that I am going to have to give it (job) up I think and look for something else.

D: When do you think you are going to be able to come to it?

P: I hope soon. Now's the time to do it, I have been sort of thinking about it a long while, as you say, I'm one of these people who dither too much.

6.12.3 Summary

The patients described are representative of hundreds seen by one physician in a district hospital, outpatient clinic or private consulting rooms over many years. The majority accord poorly with the more pessimistic of the reports recently reviewed by Creed and Guthrie [96], as regards both chronicity and frequency of a prior history of psychiatric disorder. Only one, Mrs. B. L., fits the picture of illness behaviour or "the patient who does not get better". Even she might have done so if she could have been held in psychological management a little longer. Her own, and her husband's manipulative behaviour prevented this, but flitting from one doctor to another is not peculiar to IBS; it is common in many disorders including musculoskeletal pain, MS, hyperventilation, etc. None of the patients mentioned briefly in the text, or who speak for themselves in the transcripts, had suffered a chronic psychiatric disorder. All were at work and had been for years. However, all were tense, uptight, conscientious people, who had had major problems of decision at the time of onset of IBS; their symptoms persisted until the problem resolved spontaneously (second transcript) or were helped to resolve it with the modest psychological aid described. One said she had been depressed at the time of onset, but it clearly did not amount to a psychiatric illness. Had she not felt depressed while her boyfriend's affection was being undermined by another woman, at the place the three of them all worked and being urged by friends not to run away, she might indeed have been judged as emotionally abnormal, Mrs. L. T. and Mrs. M. N. have been included to illustrate the psychopathology of the minority of IBS patients whose symptoms start as usual in a situation in which they feel torn and undecided, but because they also have had long-standing conscious or subconscious feelings of guilt about ambivalence for dead or alienated key figures, fear that their badness has caught up with them (retribution). It may be noted that both these patients, despite very traumatic childhoods, had substantial ego strength. Both responded to a modest amount of psychodynamically orientated management directed at enabling them to express their feelings of guilt and unresolved mourning with much emotional release. Patients in this category resist all forms of treatment until (a) their phobic feelings are diagnosed – they usually deny them at first – and (b) receive the form of psychological management or psychotherapy as outlined. This is quite within the competence of any GP or internist who is prepared to acquire it. Some psychiatrists have the skill but many do not and tend instead to prescribe anti-depressants, which are useless in this type of case.

Why then have so many reports about IBS been so gloomy? Part of the answer may be that these reports have tended to come from large university hospitals or gastroenterological units where these patients tend to be considered as uninteresting and too often passed from assistant to assistant at each attendance. After multiple investigations they are often told there is nothing wrong with them, without explanation of their abdominal pain or bloating, etc.; when in addition they are told that it is due to their nerves, they gain the impression that the doctors think they are imagining the symptoms. In such circumstances it is not surprising that these single-minded people who expect explanations of symptoms become more tense, hostile and increasingly introspective about there being "something seriously wrong" as doctors failing to understand what to do with them send them for investigation after investigation.

The lesson to follow is the wise advice of Almy and Kirsner [90, 91], and that an experienced doctor rather than a series of juniors should undertake the management throughout. As Hislop [94] and we have indicated, the psychological skills required to treat most cases are well within the competence of any GP or internist, although specialist psychotherapeutic help may be needed to treat the minority who start with phobic symptoms or who develop them as a result of inept medical management. For the majority, however, early referral to a psychiatrist is counterproductive because it is resented, being seen by the patients as inappropriate and dismissive.

6.13 Proctalgia Fugax

An intensely sharp fleeting pain in the rectum, usually but not always at night, was first described by Myrtle in 1883 [97]. It has been likened to the insertion of a red hot poker. Myrtle described the disorder as "purely neuritic in nature". From 1935–1958 several articles on the personality characteristics of patients with proctalgia described them as irritable, perfectionistic, meticulous, obsessional, tense and anxious and were summarised by Pilling et al. [98], who also reported similar findings in a series of 48 patients. We recall a paper presented by Ryle, himself a sufferer, to the Annual General Meeting of the British Society of Gastroenterologists [99] and the ensuing discussion during which various senior members of the society contributed their personal experiences. Remedies varied from manual dilatation of the anal sphincter to self-administered enemata. The meeting acknowledged tension and frustration as provocative and that doctors and nurses as a group were particularly prone.

The subset of society affected is the same uptight one whose members at various times have shifts of psychosomatic presentation from migraine and vascular headache to Menière's disease, aphthous ulcers, IBS, dysmenorrhoea, pseudo-cystitis, backache/neckache and intervertebral disc disorders. These shifts in our experience are attributable to changes in typically provocative life situations, e.g. in migraine it is the clock and sustained tension in reaching deadlines without lowering standards, or maintaining very high standards in adverse circumstances. In IBS it is typically indecision and fence-sitting over some major issue, whereas backache and disc prolapse may occur when the same individuals find themselves "in a struggle" either with someone in the domestic, social or working environment. Typically the individual would prefer to avoid head on conflict but disdains the easy way out. Such tension is usually conscious but before a psychosomatic type of interview rarely, it ever, associated by the sufferer with the somatic complaint. Other types of life stress may come to be identified as commonly provocative of other afflictions such as aphthous ulcers or pseudo-cystitis. Alternatively, genetic determinants may prove to be decisive in selecting to which of the above disorders an individual may be most prone.

At present the most effective psychological management of proctalgia fugax would appear to be the same as that described for migraine and aphthous ulcers. That is a relaxation technique learned individually or in a group and of a type suited to the patient's personality and acceptable to him or her. At the same time patients should be helped to become aware of being tense and of the personalities, events and situations which make them tense. At least two interviews are required for this, during which patients should be encouraged to explore possible temporal relationships of tension and uptightness to attacks of proctalgia fugax, to pinpoint what it is within themselves that subconsciously leads them to react in this way, and then to try to change such ingrained responses.

6.14 Chronic Relapsing Amoebic Dysentery

In such cases unsuspected proctocolitis has been found to render the bowel susceptible to invasion by *Entamoeba histolytica* [100, 101]. Recurrent courses of amoebicidal drugs fail to promote remission unless accompanied by psychological management as recommended in the section on UC and Crohn's disease.

6.15 Chronic Constipation

Chronic constipation and/or encopresis may be thought to warrant a place in this book, but apart from the costive form of IBS which has already been covered extensively, we do not regard chronic constipation or encopresis as genuinely psychosomatic. Instead, the factors involved are those such as insufficient activity, low fluid intake, inadequate care and diet (anorexics) especially in the elderly or psychotically depressed, or in younger patients due to a refusal to conform or laziness or not giving enough time at stool. The last and prudery were the cause in a mother of three who, before taking a job, had delayed defaecation until her children and husband had left the house. After starting work, she had been unable to get to the only lavatory before leaving the house as it was always occupied, and if she felt like going to stool at the office she held it in because she did not want to leave a smell. Psychosomatic and psychological management in her case would have been pointless; instead, advice to get up a quarter of an hour earlier before the rest of the family and take a book to read was all that was needed.

Children with encopresis come from disturbed families, but here again suppression of the defaecation reflex may be as much due to neglect or conscious refusal to cooperate as to the psychoanalytic concept of obsessional retentiveness or feelings of anal gratification.

References

1. Sircus W, Church R, Kellesher J (1957) Recurrent aphthous ulceration of the mouth. Q J Med 26:235–250
2. Ferguson R, Basu MK, Asquith P, Thompson RA, Cooke WT (1976) Jejunal mucosal abnormalities in patients with recurrent aphthous ulceration. Br Med J 1:11–13
3. Tyldesley WR (1981) Recurrent oral ulceration and coeliac disease. Br Dent J 151:81–83
4. Lehner T (1967) Autoimmunity and management of recurrent oral ulceration. Br Dent J 122:15–20
5. Wolff HG (1948) Headache and other head pains. Oxford University Press, Oxford
6. Sibley WK (1899) Neurotic ulcers of the mouth. Br Med J 1:900–901
7. Koptagel-Ilal G, Tuncer O, Enbiyaoglu G, Bayramoglu Z (1983) A psychosomatic investigation of Behçet's disease. Psychother Psychosom 40:263–271
8. Alexander EL, Provost TT, Alexander GE (1982) Neurologic complications of primary Sjögren's syndrome. Medicine (Baltimore) 61:247–257
9. Moutsopoulas HD (1980) Sjögren syndrome (Sicca syndrome). Current issues. Ann Intern Med 92:212–226
10. Weiss E, English OS (1949) Psychosomatic medicine. Saunders, Philadelphia
11. Philippopoulous GS (1975) Three cases of cardio-spasm treated successfully with psychotherapy. Psychother Psychosom 26:265–269
12. Klages (ca. 1970) Case report, available from author
13. Ruesch J (1948) The infantile personality. Psychosom Med 10:134–144
14. Susser M, Stein A (1962) Civilisation and peptic ulcer. Lancet 1:115–119
15. Pulvertaft CN (1968) Comments on the incidence and natural history of gastric and duodenal ulcer. Postgrad Med J 44:597–602
16. Watkinson G (1956, 1958) Relationship of chronic peptic ulcer to coronary sclerosis. Gastroenterologia 85:201–204; 89:292–301
17. Paulley JW (1979) Ulcers, heart disease, and Type-A behaviour. Lancet:1238
18. Paulley JW (1975) Cultural influences in the incidence and pattern of disease. Psychother Psychosom 26:2–11

19. Mirsky IA (1958) Physiologic, psychologic and social determinants in the aetiology of duodenal ulcer. Am J Dig Dis 3:285–314

20. Lee Lander FP, Maclagan NF (1934) 100 histamine test meals on normal students. Lancet 2:1210–1213

21. Doll R, Avery-Jones F, Maclagan NR (1949) Gastric secretion and subsequent dyspepsia. Lancet 2:984–985

22. Mittelmann B, Wolff HG (1942) The emotions and duodenal functions. Experimental studies on patients with gastritis, duodenitis and peptic ulcer. Psychosom Med 4:5–243

23. Davies DT, Wilson ATM (1937) Observation on the life history of chronic peptic ulcer. Lancet 2:1353–1360

24. Robinson SC (1935) On aetiology of peptic ulcer: analysis of 70 patients. Am J Dig Dis Nutr 2:333–343

25. Culpin M (1935) Temperament and digestive disorder. Br Med J 2:102–106

26. Friedman M, Rosenman BH (1959) Association of specific overt behaviour pattern with blood and cardiovascular findings. JAMA 169:1286–1296

27. Groen JJ (1964) Psychosomatic research: a collection of papers. Pergama, Oxford

28. Van der Valk JM, Groen JJ (1967) Personality structure and conflict situations in patients with myocardial infarct. J Psychosom Res 11:41–46

29. Arlow JA (1945) Identification mechanisms in coronary occlusions. Psychosom Med 7:195–209

30. Paulley JW (1959) Stress and the gut. Br J Clin Pract 13:314–320

31. Paulley JW (1981) Inequality, health and the small community. Lancet 2:205

32. Doll R, Jones FA (1951) Occupational factors in the aetiology of gastric and duodenal ulcer. HMSO, London. (MRC Special Report no 276)

33. Dunn JP, Cobb S (1962) Frequency of peptic ulcer among executives, craftsmen and foremen. J Occup Med 4:343–348

34. Avery Jones F, Paulley JW (1949) Intestinal lipodystrophy. Lancet 1:214–217

35. Paulley JW (1952) A case of Whipple's disease (intestinal lipodystrophy). Gastroenterology 22:128–133

36. Paulley JW (1964) Whipple's disease. Acta Gastroenterol Belg 27:159

37. Maxwell JD, Ferguson A, McKay AM, Irvine RC, Watson RC (1968) Whipple's disease. Lancet 1:880–889

38. Martin FF, Vilseek L, Dobbins WO (1972) Immunological alterations in patients with treated Whipple's disease. Gastroenterology 63:6–18

39. Charache P, Bayless TM, Shelley WM (1966) Atypical bacteria in Whipple's disease. Trans Assoc Am Physicians 79:399–408

40. Paulley JW (1949) Chronic diarrhoe. Proc Soc Med 42:241–24

41. Paulley JW (1954) Observations on the aetiology of idiopathic steatorrhoea. Br Med J 2:1318–1321

42. Paulley JW (1959) Emotion and personality in the aetiology of steatorrhoea. Am J Dig Dis 4:352–360

43. Prugh DG (1951) A preliminary report on the role of emotional factors in idiopathic coeliac disease. Psychosom Med 13:220–241

44. Paulley JW (1971) Determinants of adult celiac disease. N Engl J Med 284:916

45. Paulley JW (1955) Psychosomatic factors in the aetiology of acute appendicitis. Arch Middx Hosp 5:35–41

46. Binning G (1950) The influence of perturbations of childhood life on the occurrence of appendectomy. Can Med Assoc J 63:461–467

47. Creed G (1981) Life events and appendicectomy. Lancet 1:1381–1385

48. Blackburn G, Hadfield G, Hunt AH (1939) Regional ileitis. St. Barts Hosp Rep 72:181–224

49. Eastcott HGG (1958) Regional ileitis: personality pattern and cause of the disorder. Society for Psychosomatic Research, Meeting. October 1958, University College London

50. Paulley JW (1971) Crohn's disease: treatment by corticosteroids, antibiotic and psychotherapy. Psychother Psychosom 19:11–117

51. Parfitt HL (1967) Psychiatric aspects of regional enteritis. Can Med Assoc J 97:807–811

52. Cohn EM, Ledermann II, Shore E (1970) Regional enteritis and its relation to emotional disorders. Am J Gastroenterol 64:378–387

53. McKegney FP, Gordon RO, Levine SM (1970) Psychosomatic comparison of patients with ulcerative colitis and Crohn's disease. Psychosom Med 32:153–166

54. McMahon AW, Schmitt P, Patterson JF, Rothman E (1973) Personality differences between inflammatory bowel disease patients and their healthy siblings. Psychosom Med 35:91–93

55. Crockett RW (1952) Psychiatric findings in Crohn's disease. Lancet 1:946–949

56a. Feldman F, Cantor D, Soll S, Bachrach W (1967) Psychiatric study of a consecutive series of 19 patients with regional ileitis. Br Med J 4:711–714

56b. Feldman F, Cantor D, Soll S, Bachrach W (1967) Psychiatric study of a consecutive series of 34 patients with ulcerative colitis. Br Med J 3:14–17

57. West R (1967) Psychological factors and ulcerative colitis. Br Med J 2:56

58. Engel GL (1967) Psychological factors and ulcerative colitis. Br Med J 2:56

59. Gainsborough H (1967) Psychological factors and ulcerative colitis. Br Med J 3:499

60. Paulley JW (1968) Emotion and ileitis. Br Med J 1:180

61. Brown D (1968) Emotion and ileitis. Br Med J 1:179–180

62. Grace WJ (1953) Life stress and regional ileitis. Gastroenterology 23:542–553

63. Ford CV, Glober GA, Castelnovo-Tedesco P (1969) A psychiatric study of patients with regional enteritis. JAMA 208:311–315

64. Goldberg D (1970) A psychiatric study of patients with disease of the small intestine. G 11:459–465

65. Reinhart JB, Succop RA (1968) Regional enteritis in paediatric patients: psychiatric aspects. J Am Acad. Child Psychiatry 71:252–281

66. Sullivan AJ (1936) Psychogenic factors in ulcerative colitis. Am J Dig Dis 2:651–656

67. Murray CD (1930) Psychogenic factors in the aetiology of ulcerative colitis and bloody diarrhoea. Am J Med Sci 180:239–248

68. Paulley JW (1974) Psychological management of Crohn's disease. Practitioner 213:59–64

69. Sperling M (1960) The psychoanalytic treatment of a case of regional ileitis. Int J Psychoanal 41:612–618

70. Winnicott DW (1966) Psychosomatic illness in its positive and negative aspects. Int J Psychoanal 47:510–516

71. Harrison TR (1958) Principles of internal medicine. McGraw Hill, New York

72. Karush A, Daniels GE, Flood C, O'Connor JF (1977) Psychotherapy in chronic ulcerative colitis. Saunders, Philadelphia

73. Groen JJ (1947) Psychogenesis and psychotherapy of ulcerative colitis. Psychosom Med 9:151–174

74. Engel GL (1958) Studies of ulcerative colitis V. Psychological aspects and their implications for treatment. Am J Dig Dis 3:315–317

75. Paulley JW (1950) Ulcerative colitis: a study of 173 cases. Gastroenterology 16:566–576

76. Paulley JW (1972) Psychosomatic and other aspects of ulcerative colitis in the aged. Mod Geriatrics 2:30–34

77. Paulley JW (1981) Pris en charge psychologique des malades atteints de colite ulcereuse. Med Hyg 39:269–273

78. Marty P, de M'Uzan M (1963) La pensée opératoire. Rev Fr Psychoanal 27 [Suppl]:1345–1356

79. Nemiah JC (1973) Psychology and psychosomatic illness: reflections on theory and research methodology. Psychother Psychosom 22:106–111
80. Sifneos PE (1973) The prevalence of "alexithymic" characteristic in psychosomatic patients. Psychother Psychsom 22:255–262
81. Paulley JW (1963) Ulcerative colitis. Br Med J 11:308
82. Acheson ED (1960) The distribution of ulcerative colitis and regional in US veterans with reference to the Jewish religion. Gut 1:291–293
83. Roubiçek J, Martonova F (1957) Psychopathology of ulcerative colitis. Cesk Psychiat 53:220–230
84. Lindemann E (1949) Modifications in the cause of ulcerative colitis in relationship to changes in life situations and reaction patterns. Proc Assoc Res Nerv Ment Dis 29:706–723
85. Paulley JW (1983) Pathological mourning: a key factor in the psychopathogenesis of autoimmune disorders. Psychother Psychosom 40:181–190
86. Arnason BHW (1975) Multiple sclerosis research. MRC Symposium. HMSO, London, pp 238
87. Groen J, Bastiaans J (1955) Studies on ulcerative colitis personality structure, emotional conflict situations and effects of psychotherapy. In: O'Neill D (ed) Modern trends in psychosomatic medicine. Butterworth, London, pp 102–125
88. Grace WJ, Pinskey RH, Wolf HG (1954) Treatment of ulcerative colitis. Gastroenterology 26:462–468
89. Paulley JW (1956) Psychotherapy in ulcerative colitis. Lancet 2:215–218
90. Almy TP (1978) Wrestling with the irritable colon. Med Clin North 62:203–210
91. Kirsner JB (1981) The irritable bowel syndrome. Arch Intern Med 141:635–639
92. Paulley JW (1984) The psychological management of the irritable colon. Hepatogastroenterology 31:53–54
93. Grace WJ, Wolf S, Wolff HH (1951) The human colon. Hoeber, New York
94. Hislop IG (1980) The effect of very brief psychotherapy on the irritable bowel syndrome. Med J Aust 2:620–622
95. Svedlund J, Sjödin I, Ottoson G, Datevall G (1983) Controlled study of psychotherapy in the irritable bowel syndrome. Lancet 2:589–592
96. Creed F, Guthrie E (1987) Psychological factors in the irritable bowel syndrome. Gut 28:1296–1318
97. Myrtle AS (1883) Some common afflictions of the anus often rejected by medical men and patients. Br Med J 1.1061
98. Pilling LF, Swenson WM, Hill JR (1965) The psychological aspects of proctalgia fugax. Dis Colon Rectum 8:372–376
99. Ryle JA (1948) Proctalgia fugax and discussion. Gastroenterologia 73:289–293
100. Paulley JW (1950) Amoebiasis and personality. Br Med J 2:525
101. Crede RH, Rosenbaum M, Ferris EB (1948) Amoebic colitis. Psychosom Med 10:223–229
102. Behçet H (1937) Über rezidivierende aphtöse, durch ein Virus verursachte Geschwüre, am Mund, am Auge und an der Genitalien. Dematol Wochenschr 105:1152
103. Mackenzie J (1913) Diseases of the heart, 3rd edn. Frowde
104. White PD, Hahn RC (1929) The symptom of sighing in cardiovascular diagnosis. Am J Sci 177:179–188

7 Respiratory Tract

7.1 Hyperventilation Syndrome

No one has done more than Lum [1, 5] in recent years to alert all clinicians to one of the most common disorders in medical practice, often undiagnosed because of its diverse manifestations. Masquerading as disorders of the heart, lungs, GI tract, CNS, eyes, ears, musculoskeletal system, or as psychoses or psychoneuroses, it beats as "greatest simulator" other claimants such as polyarteritis nodosa and carcinoma of the bronchus. This was acknowledged as far back as 1929 by White and Hahn [2], and had their report received the attention it deserved, not only could countless investigations have been avoided, but effective treatment made available.

Early psychosomatists such as Weiss and English [3] in their chapter "The effect of emotions on breathing" were clearly aware of the multiplicity of symptoms including chest pain, arrhythmias, hallucinations and depersonalised feelings. The two case histories they quote from 1934 and 1938 would be exceptional even today because the emotional as well as the physical aspects were recognised.

J. W. P.'s first understanding of the syndrome arose from the outpatient teaching of Evan Bedford in the 1930s. Bedford was a cardiologist of repute and a friend of Paul D. White, already mentioned. Bedford would ask, "What is your complaint?" The patient, usually a young male, replied: "I have got a pain over my heart." Bedford would ask: "Where is your heart?" Patient answered: "Here", pointing to the left submammary region. "No, it isn't," would come the reply. He would then continue the history and after careful examination reassure the patient that there was absolutely nothing wrong with his heart. This approach, although abrupt, was a great advance on the management of cases of "disorderly action of the heart" in the First World War when physicians still learning to use the modern stethoscope mistook ejection systolic bruits or ectopics in anxious men with tachycardia as evidence of heart disease and invalided them. By the Second World War the condition (then renamed *effort syndrome*) was widely recognised to be associated with hyperventilation. As a result cardiovascular casualties in the Second World War were 1/50 of those of the First [4]. Instead young home-sick recruits, frightened and chased by noisy NCO's, reporting sick with chest pain and fears of heart disease, were reassured. Later, they were sent on courses of graduated exercise in which they learned that their hearts would stand 20-mile route marches in full kit without mishap. Since the last war the early reports on the essential role of hyperventilation in cardiac and other manifestations of the syndrome have become accepted. For the sake of brevity the reader is referred to Lum [1, 5] as well as for key references and for the biochemistry of hypocapnia.

7.1.1 Psychological Management

The first essential is early diagnosis and effective treatment before multiple referrals and investigations have increased the patient's fears. Diagnosis depends on doctors improving their knowledge of the many presentations of the syndrome. Treatment requires competent physiotherapy to help the patient unlearn an ingrained habit of upper chest breathing and overfilling which, when it is suddenly augmented by emotional or physical stimuli, promotes an attack. As Lum has pointed out hypocarbia can be demonstrated in two-thirds of chronic hyperventilators between attacks, but in the remainder biochemistry is in the normal range. For them it is sudden drops below the baseline, which provoke attacks. Stimuli with a psychological content include claustrophobic threats such as small spaces, lifts, underground railways, crowded airless shops, or agoraphobic, i.e. anything beyond the security of the front door. Other phobias include spiders, heights, water, etc., but most common in our experience are unvoiced fears of a lethal disease, e.g. cancer, brain tumours, heart disease, leukaemia and recently, due to media publicity, MS and AIDS. It has already been noted that phobia for tuberculosis, once common, has become extinct because it now poses insufficient menace to fulfil a phobic individual's need for punishment and thereby make reparation for the conscious or unconscious guilt. Physical triggers of attacks for the persistent hyperventilator involve anything increasing depth of inspiration suddenly, such as going into a cold wind or even explosive laughter.

Some cases of hyperventilation syndrome can be brought into remission by re-education in breathing alone, but many fail to respond or soon relapse unless their underlying ambivalent feelings for dead, ill or alienated key figures or surrogates are identified and worked through as described in Chap. 10 by psychotherapy or effective psychological management. What is required for optimum handling of these cases, are a correct diagnosis and the acquisition of modest psychological skills.

7.1.1.1 A Need for Clinical Awareness

Increased dependence on sophisticated tests at the expense of physical examination is one cause of cases being missed.

Allergy. A much publicised case of a so-called total allergy syndrome in 1981 cost well-wishers thousands of pounds to send a woman to a special clinic in the USA. It was clear that she had in reality an undiagnosed hyperventilation syndrome [6]. An increasing number of people suffering from hyperventilation are being incorrectly diagnosed and treated for allergy at some cost.

Neurology. In this speciality less attention is usually paid to what is going on in the chest or cardiovascular system than in the CNS. Thus hyperventilating patients presenting with paraesthesiae, vertigo or attacks suggestive of epilepsy may be misdiagnosed.

Psychiatry. Hyperventilating patients commonly present with anxiety or feelings of unreality leading to fears that they are going mad, often too frightening for them to voice. Examination of the chest and cardiovascular system is just as necessary in this speciality as in neurology.

Rheumatology. Hyperventilation frequently presents with pains in the chest, shoulders and arms, and costoclavicular compression is almost as often due to the first rib being pushed up against the clavicle from habitual overfilling of the chest as to drooping of the shoulder girdle.

Gastroenterology. Aerophagists and sufferers from the splenic flexure syndrome or oesophageal spasm are essentially hyperventilation sufferers.

Otology. Many such patients are first referred to ENT surgeons for dizziness. Specialists in this field are usually quick in identifying a psychological basis but less often recognise the underlying hyperventilation.

Endocrinology. Glandular "deficiency" is often suspected by sufferers or their physicians to account for the symptom of "exhaustion" and are referred to endocrinologists. Recognition that many such patients are hyperventilating would save a great deal of money and effort currently spent on an increasing range of complex investigations.

Gynaecology. Many female hyperventilating patients between the ages of 30 and 60 think they are "menopausal" and are treated as such by GPs and gynaecologists.

Cardiology. Hyperventilation and the soldier posture are present in many patients after MI and relate to fear of a further attack. It is a common cause of the persistent ectopic's, failing to respond to drug intervention, which the CCU staff finds so worrying. If as much attention were paid to the recognition of hyperventilation as is currently given to anti-arrhythmic drugs and if it were treated by physiotherapy and helping patients to talk about their domestic and work problems, professional anxiety in CCU staff would lessen (see management of acute MI, Chap. 8).

The above list is by no means complete! For instance, in the USA in the 1950s hyperventilators were wrongly diagnosed as chronic brucellosis, whereas today thousands are being told incorrectly that they have myalgic encephalomyelitis (ME).

7.1.1.2 Other Reasons for Lack of Adequate Psychological Management

First and foremost, some doctors assume that their duty is done once they have excluded organic disease. Hyperventilator's symptoms tend to be seen as trivial because they are presumed to be due to "nerves" or be "all in the mind". This attitude has some of its roots among northern Europeans in the abhorrence of things emotional, but it is enhanced in the medical schools by medical scientists and teachers denigrating anything not organic or which cannot be measured. This leads to unnecessary feelings of impotence in dealing with disorders having a partial or total psychological basis. It follows that some students once they have graduated are dismissive and even punitive to such patients with the implication that they are wasting doctor's time or "putting it on". This may be apparent when an overtly hysterical female patient is admitted with florid tetany. Knowing grins are the order of the day with a comment such as "breathing into a paper bag cured her, her boyfriend has just left her, you see" and that is that. Rarely is an attempt made to find out what in her background may have made her so vulnerable to being abandoned or to uncover possible underlying guilt. Should she be referred to a psychiatrist this may be explored, but often treatment is restricted to a tranquilliser or an anti-depressant. Once again students and young doctors fail to learn because they see their seniors managing hyperventilation syndrome either physically *or* psychologically, i.e. soma *or* psyche, but rarely both at the same time.

7.1.2 Psychosomatic Management

Where diagnosis is not immediately apparent, as with witnessed tetany, it will depend upon a combination of clues in presentation and important physical signs. First, patients who have had one or two attacks are usually very frightened and seek urgent appointments. They or their relatives often browbeat their GP or the secretary to obtain priority. This should always be granted even if hyperventilation is suspected. The temptation to punish and make them wait is wrong as well as counterproductive: a common result is a night call! Secondly, all doctors *need a high suspicion index for hyperventilation on history taking.* The following "tin-opening" questions may provide valuable clues:

D: What did you feel like in these attacks?
P: Terrible, I felt I was passing out.
D: Do you ever feel you might not come round or even die?
P: (reluctantly) Yes, I suppose I do.
D: Have you ever felt that you cannot get enough air or get a deep enough breath?
P: Yes, often.
D: How long have you had these feelings and have you ever had them before? (invaluable in relating previous episodes to emotional crises).
   Have you had pins and needles in your hands or feet, or palpitations or cramp in your hands like this? (demonstrates the main d'accoucheur.)
P: (replies positively to one or more)
D: Do you ever have the feeling that you are not really there or in touch with things? [depersonalisation; many patients experience this but do not like to talk about it because they fear they are going mad]

Physical Signs. Upper chest breathing throughout the interview may be apparent, while during an examination the chest may be obviously overfilled, resembling a guardsman lying to attention. Hyperventilating patients tend to sigh a lot, and the doctor's ears should be attuned to this during interview or examination. Likewise irregular or cogwheel inspiration audible on ausculatation is highly significant, as is paradoxical breathing when the patient is asked to breathe deeply. The lung bases are often hyper-resonant due to persistent overfilling of the chest, the diaphragm is splinted downwards, and as a result a normal liver may be easily palpable.

Typicality of Personality? Lum [1] felt that the great majority of his large series of 1735 patients tended to be perfectionistic or mildly obsessional, the men showing features of type A personality. We agree and feel that many patients tend to come from the same uptight, busy, somewhat obsessional group who also suffer from migraine. IBS, aphthous ulcers, etc. But hyperventilating patients differ from the uptight group mentioned in being additionally more neurotic and phobic. A few are frank hysterics.

Typicality of Psychopathogenesis: The Importance of Loss. Recognition of this example of *typicality* is an essential ingredient in successful management. We have yet to see a patient who did not regard the symptoms as retribution for guilt, mostly unconscious, stemming from ambivalent feelings for key figures in childhood. Why, it may be asked, is the onset so often deferred for 10, 20 or even 30 years? This is because feelings of unresolved guilt are later reawakened by deaths or dangerous illnesses in friends or relatives, reminding patients of their own mortality and that they may be next on the list. "There, but for the grace of God, go I," and they fear they do not deserve the grace. It is, therefore, necessary to ask such patients whether they have lost any friends or relatives lately or if any have been ill with cancer or heart attacks. Such shocks provoke in a vulnerable patient some cardiac "awareness" so that any chest discomfort or palpitation is regarded as an indicator of impending doom. It is then necessary to find out why the patient feels it has to be him, and why he has to pay. At some point it may be useful to say, "It almost sounds as though you have to be punished?" This is where the carefully taken family history oulined in Chap. 5 is invaluable because the age of the patient at the time of a parent or sibling's death will have been recorded. Changes in voice or an averted glance may denote unresolved feelings of loss, but as patients with psychosomatic disorders tend to conceal their emotions, it usually requires a tin-opening question such as: I wonder if any of the people you have lost, such as your mother or even your daughter in Australia are ever much in your thoughts? If there is a pathological loss reaction, this will evoke a reply such as: "Never a day passes – she is always in my thoughts," usually accompanied by emotion or tears. Another tin-opener helps to cut corners in uncovering guilt over ambivalent feelings. It is: Have you ever heard the expression "God doesn't pay his debts in gold (money)"? About half the population, i.e. those brought up in rural areas, know it from grandparents or aunts, whereas those brought up in urban areas usually do not; exceptions being urban villages with much folklore. Nor is it confined to Great Britain; it is well-known in Eastern Europe and even Eastern people have equivalent sayings. Assuming the answer to the question is "Yes", the supplementary is: Do you know what it means? "Oh yes, doesn't it mean that if you do wrong you will have to pay? My aunt was always saying it, when for example some man had not treated his wife or children well." It is then a simple matter to point out that when people close to any of us die, especially if it is unexpected, we commonly blame ourselves in some way for not being more attentive or not resolving some disagreement, which we would have done had death not come so unexpectedly. In psychological jargon this is called "unfinished business", but whether it develops from normal sadness or regret into something that haunts the individual for years with ambivalent feelings will depend upon the intensity of love and hate, mostly unconscious and repressed since childhood, over loss of a key figure by death, or by abandonment as in divorce or through adoption.

Psychological Management of Loss Reactions. How doctors can help sufferers work through these reactions will be dealt with in detail in Chap. 10 in the section on RA and the AI disease. It should be read in conjunction with this section on hyperventilation, and applies equally to the management of all phobias e.g. cancer, cerebral tumour and MS phobia. Phobias and the AI diseases share a common psychopathogenesis although differing in their response to it, the one neurotic, the other psychosomatic. Whereas phobic patients punish themselves by fear amounting at times to the certainty that they will have to forfeit their lives because of their conscious and unsonscious guilt, patients with AI diseases suffer and endure their punishment by a slow, insidious and often painful attack on themselves by antibodies directed against their own tissues.

Breathing Exercises and Re-Education in Breathing. Effective management of hyperventilation involves close team work by the doctor and a competent physiotherapist or specially trained nurse. It is theoretically possible for the doctor to learn the technique and teach patients relaxed abdominal breathing and the awareness of when their chests are overfilled, and postures which reduce the ingrained response of overbreathing in the face of emotionally threatening people or situations. However, it is our experience, and that of others, that "teaching", being authoritarian, often conflicts with effective psychological management or psychotherapy.

For this reason it may be best for the doctor, having seen the patient and worried spouse or partner for 1–2 sessions and having initiated the psychological management, to refer the patient to a physiotherapist and stay in the background until the physiotherapy is over. It will have already been explained to the patient that the basis of their frightening physical symptoms lies in their unconscious overbreathing and that an important part of the treatment will include how to "unlearn" the habit. After this the doctor will see the patient again for as long a period as necessary to "work through" the basis of the phobic feelings.

However, while this is the ideal, it is not always possible with every patient. Some patients are so disturbed or suffer recurrent panic from further attacks that they need sessions with the doctor and physiotherapist at the same time. This necessitates close team work and an understanding by the physiotherapist of what the doctor is doing, the psychodynamics of the disorder, and the predilection of all psychosomatic patients to try and split their care givers (responsible agents) [7].

Patients naturally want to know how long the physiotherapy and psychological management will last. Some patients recover quickly with as few as eight physiotherapy sessions and the offer of a refresher course and 1–2 sessions with the doctor after the initial interview. More disturbed patients may need 6–8 interviews over 3–4 months. Progress is facilitated by couple therapy using the partner as a co-therapist, and helping to relieve the partner's counterproductive overconcern and/or manipulations, e.g. cases T.I. and K.S..

We find that it is only the exceptionally disturbed hyperventilating patient who needs to be seen at intervals over 2–3 years. Such patient's hyperventilation usually recurs with the advent of new phobias, set off by further deaths and disasters reawakening all their old fears of retribution (see case history K.S.).

Hypoventilation. Compared with hyperventilation, hypoventilation is rare and usually due to deformities of the chest or fixation of the rib cage, or in ankylosing spondylitis or gross obesity. The other cause is the Kline-Levin syndrome, due to hypothalamic damage from encephalitis, tumours, vascular lesions, etc. It has notable somatopsychic effects of depression, salt craving and bulimia. The only possible psychosomatic example of hypoventilation is breath-holding.

7.1.3 Case Histories

K. P., a woman aged 42 who complained of a burning sensation over the heart, tension in the neck and shoulders, headaches, palpitations, fainting feelings (as if about to pass out, especially in the street), also said she felt guilty because she was "no use to her husband". Her symptoms had started 19 years previously following her father's unexpected death from pneumonia. "I adored him; if we had not gone away for the weekend I might have saved him – the doctor said if he had been got to the hospital sooner he might have lived." She still felt responsible despite the fact that her mother and younger siblings were with him. To the question: Have you heard the expression God doesn't pay his debts in money? – she nodded. Her only son had been killed in a road traffic accident 4 years before. Later she said she had seen this as the penalty she had to pay for her own badness but she also felt guilty at not being more distressed over his death.

At first she was unable to acknowledge any double feelings for her father. An appointment was made to see her and her husband together a few days later. After repeated declarations of how much she adored her father, it was suggested that only those we love most are capable of hurting us, and it was quite possible to feel two ways. Perhaps he had been strict with her?

Her husband intervened: "Well he used to thrash you with his tongue".

P: In my 'teens he drummed the fear of VD into me so that even now I cannot sit on a public lavatory seat ... He was overprotective – my two sisters rebelled – I could not ... most of his money went on beer and there were arguments – I tried to make peace – I was angry with him for picking on my mother. He hit me when I tried to protect her and was always sorry after ... I would lock myself in my bedroom and he would weep outside, imploring to come in.

D: In a way he blackmailed you?

P: Yes.

The patient in a persistent state of hyperventilation, had exacerbations when she went out or in crowded spaces. She carried a mental map of every road or shop in the town where she had panicked and collapsed with hyperventilation and said she would arrange never to go back to the same place again. After 19 years this involved her in taking very circuitous routes, and these were becoming increasingly limited.

By releasing her angry feelings for her father and by repeatedly working through childhood feelings and events around her father's and her son's deaths –during which she wept copiously– she was able to acknowledge good memories as well as the bad and was now able to make use of the exercises to reduce her hyperventilation which she had previously had to stop because the relaxation induced frightening fantasies and made her panic. This case shows why some hyperventilating patients fail to benefit until their underlying phobia has been relieved by psychological management.

T. I., a married woman of 31, had had her first recognised attack of hyperventilation 2 years previously. Asked if she remembered any emotional stress at the time, she said she had been wound up by her big, smothering, manipulative and alcoholic mother-in-law trying to get money out of both her and her husband, telling each not to tell the other. Money had always had a particular significance because her father had died of MI when she was 3, leaving four children. Her mother had had to go out to work and from the age of 5 she remembers feeling responsible and doing everything. This experience had led her to seek security by accumulating money through hard work in business, and she accorded with Lum's impression [1] that hyperventilating patients tend to be type A personalities. "I had the need to be a secure squirrel," she said. Her initial symptoms of breathlessness, multiple ectopics and chest pain caused her to think she had heart trouble like her father. From an early age she remembered feeling faint in the lavatory, probably due to hyperventilation even then. In the 2 years before being seen she had consulted a neurologist, a physician, an acupuncturist and a hypnotist without a diagnosis other than hypochondriasis or benefit from treatment. Her husband, whose mother had always been ill, had an aversion to illness and had become angry because she could not work; he felt she was imagining her symptoms.

Management involved making the diagnosis and explaining carefully to both of them the mechanism causing her chest pains, faintness, etc. Her husband's belligerence to this wife and her doctors diminished when he was congratulated for being nearly right by urging her to see the hypnotist. The patient, initially resistant, became much less sceptical when it was suggested correctly that she also at times probably has had paraesthesia and cramp in her hands. (It is helpful to demonstrate the main d'accoucheur, and it was so in this case.)

After four joint sessions with her husband she had resolved much of her preconscious feelings of guilt dating from childhood and was able to make use of her physiotherapy whenever she felt breathless or panicky.

Six months later she was free of all symptoms but remained aware that they would recur if she again reverted to overbreathing in the face of internal or external threats.

(Therapy time 4 h plus physiotherapy)

K. S., a married woman of 52, was referred in 1981 having had psychiatric treatment for many years and consultations with various physicians and surgeons, the former mainly for chest pain, palpitations, breathlessness and faintness, and the latter for abdominal pains and symptoms of spastic colon.

The youngest of five, her mother had died when she was 9 of chronic nephritis which had worsened after her own birth (a breech). Her childhood memories were of her mother always ill and of guilt as she made demands on her. Visits to the doctor terrified her. Three weeks after her mother's death, a school friend died unexpectedly. She felt she might be the next and had her first attack of hyperventilation at night, suffering palpitations and a feeling that she was going to die. She dared not tell anyone about it in case her worst fears were confirmed. Her school work began to deteriorate, and she cut herself off from people and things she enjoyed, such as dancing. She had never been very close to her father but trusted him, and her mother's place was taken by an elder brother, only for him to die in a POW camp in Singapore when she was 12. Once again she experienced feelings of anger at being left, and guilt over her selfishness and the feeling she was bad luck to the people she loved. In her 'teens her father remarried. She resented this, disliked her stepmother and fell ill with pleurisy and other infections; she had depression at 18 and her long psychiatric career began with phobias about suffocation, heart disease, cancer, brain tumour, strokes and madness. She had had ECT and most of the psychotropic drugs. After the birth of her children, she mended some of the bridges with her father so that his death when she was 32 did not leave her with the remorse it might have done.

Shortly after referral in 1981 her hyperventilation symptoms had worsened, particularly feelings of unreality; the exacerbation was due to the deaths of four relatives in 12 months including a sister-in-law of her own age dying after a heart attack at a party. She said later on, "I fear I will die of cancer." A further reason for referral was a desire to get off psychotropic drugs which were receiving adverse publicity.

Management of this patient had taken longer than the patients already mentioned, and she is quoted for that reason. She has required psychological treatment at greater depth and for a longer period because she was so psychologically damaged, and because her hyperventilation had become ingrained because of excessive drug treatment and it's side effects over 40 years. She began to progress when her husband was encouraged to come with her, although sometimes she tried to prevent him when she sought to make him the convenient receptacle for anger which really belonged to her father and mother. She presented dreams, one of which involved a dog without a tail. Asked if she thought the body of the dog stood for her or the lost tail she said, "I am the dog and the tail represents everything I cut myself off from after my mother's death."

After 2 years' work she was able to accept re-education of her habitual overbreathing but continued to develop other phobias, e.g. for brain tumour, stroke, cancer again and irreparable damage from Ativan. Over 3 years she had had 26 sessions, latterly jointly with her husband, who thinks he would have left her without this help.

I. N., a married woman of 33, began to suffer from attacks of hyperventilation, causing chest pain and palpitations in 1984 following pain after retrograde pyelography for pseudo-cystitis. She feared she had pulmonary emboli. Previously she had had bilious attacks in childhood, migraine, pseudocystitis (detrusor incompetence) and puerperal depression. Her father, who had died suddenly in 1979 of MI was still in her thoughts daily: she was obsessively sad that he had never seen her children. Having been closest to her father and the indulged youngest child, she then added almost as an afterthought that just before his death they had disagreed over her proposed marriage. This was the basis of her unresolved guilt and mouring. Her husband said: "She always feels she is unlovable," and she added that she feared for the security of their own marriage because her husband's parents had divorced.

Psychological management involved enabling her to recognise and accept mixed feelings and consequent guilt for her father. Her husband's help was invaluable in the early identification of emotional triggers to her hyperventilation attacks, for example, when her perfectionism led to her getting irritated and tense because her sewing was not going right. Her attacks remitted after six sessions of psychological management to help her through her unfinished business with her father, coupled with re-education in breathing. (See also Chap. 6, p. 85, Mrs. M. N.)

7.2 Vasomotor Rhinitis

In their book *The Nose* [8] Holmes et al. said they were surprised to find that the nasal mucosa in reactive individuals would either swell or shrink depending on the nature of a life-threatening event. They also noted that such responses in the nose were always associated with what the individual's experiences, attitudes and emotional reactions were at the time.

The nasal function of seven men and five women were studied intensively in this way for periods of a few weeks to as much as 8 months. In a second experimental study, "a verbal threat was delivered ... in terms of the previous experience of the individual and which had acquired a special meaning for him."

For example, a 40-year-old salesman whose mother had always been unhappy and tearful and whose father had beaten him developed persistent nasal obstruction shortly after his marriage. This coincided with the failure of a business enterprise for which he blamed his wife, who had declined to work in it. His nasal symptoms improved with psychological help but flared up when his wife insisted on buying furniture with money he had saved to buy another store. He relapsed again a year later when his wife had a pelvic operation, rendering her sterile. Her failure to become pregnant had already been a source of great disappointment to him. A year or two later he left her for a few weeks but returned because he missed the comforts of home. Reddening of the nasal membranes and markedly increased secretion was noted during discussion of his conflicts and the suggestion that his wife should also come and be questioned. At this he became tremulous and tearful; asked later what he had said to her, he answered "Dr. Wolf wants you to come down," and she replied, "I am not going to see him." The patient added that she didn't want to come because she was afraid that the things he had talked about would be brought up.

Many people including the authors, have noted how commonly patients suffer from nasal congestion during interviews at points when they feel threatened or frustrated by what is being discussed. Doctors should be as aware of this as of the significance of borborygmi or belching or sighing, wheezing or coughing in asthmatics or hyperventilators. Like other forms of non-verbal communication, such responses can tell doctors that their own behaviour and/or the topic under discussion usually is the cause and be a signal to say: "I wonder what you are feeling, your nose/stomach/chest seems to be speaking for you."

J.W.P. has found that his own sneezing attacks and momentary catarrh commonly follow about a minute after thinking about something to be done such as the despatch of a letter but which cannot be done (because of the non-arrival of some additional information which has to be included). The underlying emotion at these times seems to be that of mild "frustration". That would be in keeping with what Macdonald wrote in 1888 [9], that life experiences provocative of nasal catarrh included conflicts, resentment and frustration. Holmes et al. [8] agreed with this, and further details of their studies are included in the next section on asthma.

7.2.1 Psychological Management

Vasomotor rhinitis is generally regarded as a trivial complaint but can be very distressing not only for the patient but also for close relatives. Such patients usually attend a GP and if the problem is severe, may be referred to ENT surgeons or allergists. They rarely consult internists unless they have concomitant asthma, as was the case for *James* reported in the next section. We recommend a similar form of psychological management for severe vasomotor rhinitis to that detailed in the next section on asthma. Considering the great number of patients disabled by this condition, much more attention should be given to the potential of appropriate psychological management. *The Nose* was written 36 years ago, but how many medical students have been told about it by their teachers? The number of ENT surgeons or allergists who have read it must be very few indeed. It is a deficiency which needs correction.

F. A., aged 12, lived on an isolated farm with his grandparents, whom he regarded as his parents. His birth to their daughter (then 14) was a closely guarded secret. After his birth he suffered emotional rejection and spent long periods in his pram. His grandmother was working and his real mother, whom he was led to believe was his sister, was at school. In any case she was not encouraged to be too maternal in case she betrayed the family secret.

Intractable rhinitis set in when he was 9. Despite standard treatments, antihistamines, inhalers, nose drops and desensitisation, he had not been to school for a year and had not been allowed to play with his only friend because of risk of exposure to pollens. Worse, the allergists had insisted that his dog be given away. For similar reasons he was not allowed near the farm animals which he loved, or to help on the farm.

Management involved empathising with the grandmother's feelings of guilt, and the dilemma in which she had been placed at his birth. Not to have done so, thus protecting her "secret", would only have resulted in her withdrawing the child from therapy. Commiseration was offered on the conflicting medical advice being received, but assurance was given that no attempt would be made to alter the existing drug regimen. Instead, the influence of emotional factors on variations in allergic hypersensitivity was explained [12, 13], in this case the boy's inevitable frustration at being separated from the things and people he loved, and probably feeling rejected and even outcast.

A letter of reassurance was sent to his teachers, and he was allowed back to school. Shortly afterwards he was again allowed to play with his friend and to go about the farm. Simultaneously, he came once a week to the same, quiet-voiced, motherly physiotherapist for relaxation and breathing exercises as described in Chap. 7 for asthma and hyperventilation, and for migraine in Chap. 9. His rhinitis improved dramatically, and he began to lead a normal life.

7.3 Asthma

Our standard format has been for case histories to follow psychopathology and psychological management, but in this instance we decided to start with a transcript of a first outpatient interview. Because it expresses clearly the *typicality* of coping mechanisms and provocative situations met with in asthma, it is hoped that by keeping James' responses and attitudes in mind, the reader may find subsequent recommendations on psychological management easier to unterstand.

James, aged 52, has had asthma for 3 years and vasomotor rhinitis for 30 years.
P: I can't walk; after 50 yards (45 m) I get out of breath.
D: Tell me about your family?
P: We were just ordinary people, father he wouldn't bother a lot.
D: Do you think your mother was a bit different?
P: My mother was ginger haired (laugh) that may answer a lot of questions!
D: She was firey? [Later he said he and his father disliked his mother's strident scolding]
P: Yes.
D: Are you married?
P: Yes.
D: Children?
P: Four children.
D: Are they boys or girls?
P: 3 girls 1 boy (laughs).
D: You laugh at that. (picking up a non-verbal communication)
P: Ha! Ha! I do, there must be some reason for it, I don't know it ...
D: Well, I wondered why you chuckled; what was going through your head?
P: It was the simple reason that when the children were small I used to think to myself girls are a nuisance, always a nuisance, I wanted all boys, but now I know different – girls are a lot better than boys, my word, dear oh dear! that's what went through my head.
D: When you were a boy, do you think you spent more time with anyone in particular?
P: No, no, I've been a loner all my life.
D: Have you?
P: I would prefer to be alone you know. I often wonder whether people make me allergic – allergic to people I don't know.
D: I think that is possible.
P: Honestly, present company excepted, I hate meeting fresh people.
D: Yes, what do they do to you? What do you feel when you meet somebody fresh?

P: Well, it just puts a blanket on me like that (makes a violent gesture as if pulling down a blind). I just want to get out of the way, that's all.

D: Yes?

P: That's what I feel, I've never told anybody that, but it is what I feel. If relations come in, or a person who is bold comes right up to you and shakes your hand, ooh to me, ooh (draws back in his chair.)

D: Do you think that some people or certain types of person annoy you?

P: Well, the domineering type of person does.

D: Do you know you are saying something which almost everybody who has asthma says?

P: Like I went and sat out there (points to small waiting room for clinic) that little cubicle with those people, it seemed to me … shut in, I felt shut in there, I didn't like it at all.

D: That was why I asked you to come in before your turn, I saw you were uncomfortable, but you don't have to feel uncomfortable with me. [We had met once before socially.]

P: But I do, I knew I would before I came; it's how I am.

D: When you come up to hospital and see a doctor you have not seen before, and sometimes doctors do things – they prescribe pills for you to take, they tell you to do this – they can be a bit domineering.

P: Oh yes, yes!

D: The same with nurses.

P: Yes, I know that (Ha! Ha!).

D: You know what I mean? (picking up the non-verbal communication)

P: I know exactly what you mean; there were two at St. Peter's, one on Winston Ward and one on Orwell.

D: Yes?

P: Directly she came up to me she started, "Are you all right?" I said, well … well, she was that type of person. Mind you she's all right, but …

D: Doctors and nurses are brought up to think of themselves as mums and dads, and you are OK if you are prepared to be tucked up and do what you're told.

P: Mm, mind you they're really good, there is no doubt about that.

D: Sometimes if somebody comes along and tells you to lie down and be a good boy and take your pills, some people feel, "I don't want to be treated like a child." (This was too positive and was denied)

P: That doesn't bother me that way, but when the other one comes and wants to stick a pill in your mouth with her fingers, well, phew! … I didn't like that at all, I didn't like that at all. I was so ill she got away with it that time, but she never did come and see me any more, you know.

A description of the patient's subsequent course is continued as the first case history at the end of the section.

7.3.1 Allergic and Psychogenic Causes

Medical students are still taught that there are two types of asthma, the most common caused by allergy and the other nervous or psychogenic which is felt to be less important. This ignores strong evidence that psychological and allergic factors are complementary in aetiology [10]. Wolf [12, 13] noted that eosinophilia, a pathognomonic feature of allergy, could be induced by emotional stress in the experimental subject as easily as by inhalation of ragweed pollen. He also found that during life situations involving emotional conflict, typical attacks of hay fever followed pollen inhalation, but that if pollen inhalation was not followed by hay fever, it was possible to promote it by discussion of significant emotional problems, and then by reassurance to induce the nasal congestion to subside although pollen was still being inhaled. One of Wolf's rhinitis subjects during an interview about the substantial difficulties she was currently facing developed an asthmatic attack when nasal swelling and secretion was at its peak.

Rogerson et al. [14] while studying asthma-eczema-prurigo syndrome in children acknowledged a strong hereditary disposition and found in addition that 17/23 had also experienced parental rejection and smothering arising from guilt over such events as shotgun marriages, or children coming too early in the marriage.

Dekker and Groen [15] by exposing patients to emotional situations which had a special meaning for them induced asthmatic attacks indistinguishable from those occurring after inhalation of allergens or spontaneously. Under laboratory conditions some patients were found to react to both allergic and emotional stimuli, and Groen [11] concluded that a division of asthmatic patients into *psychogenic* or *allergenic* is not justified.

Our experience also indicates that sufferers who are strongly allergic may be treated for years with only transient relief by desensitisation, aerolysers, sodium chromoglycate, oral and inhaled steroids, but remit following effective psychological management (see cases George, Alan and James). At the outset of such management many patients have a substantial eosinophilia indicative of their allergy, which eventually subsides to normal as the asthma lessens in intensity.

7.3.2 Mechanisms of the Expiratory Wheeze

Asthma is identified by the occurrence and recurrence of paroxysmal attacks of expiratory wheezing. Inspiration is not impeded except that the chest is already overfilled with air. Inspiratory rhonchi are absent unless there is much bronchial secretion or infection; expiration, however, is noisy and exhausting. Talma [16], a Dutch physician in 1898, noted that the loud expiratory wheeze in asthma was identical wherever the stethoscope was placed on the chest or neck. From this it was deduced that the wheeze arose centrally from narrowing of the main bronchi and trachea and not the small bronchioles, and was transmitted all over the chest. This has been confirmed by bronchoscopic observation of the carina during asthma or forced expiratory breathing, and by straight radiography of the trachea [15]. Gandevia [17] later demonstrated by bronchography collapse of the main bronchi during forced expiration in emphysematous subjects, some of whom undoubtedly had primary asthma. Much of this experimental work on wheezing was done by Dekker and Groen [15] who demonstrated that it was the sudden collapse of the musculo-membraneous posterior third of the trachea and main bronchi, unsupported by cartilage, which leads to the asthmatic wheeze as soon as forced expiratory effort caused intrathoracic pressure to rise above intratracheal and intrabronchial pressure. These workers even persuaded a cadaver's lung placed in a pressure jar to wheeze!

Many asthmatics and bronchitics who learn that "pursed lip" breathing eases their laborious wheezing are unaware that it does so by raising intratracheal and intrabronchial pressure, thus helping to prevent collapse of the posterior third of these large air tubes during expiration. Accessory muscles of expiration are only brought into action when the outflow, normally due to elastic recoil, is impeded. Then a high to low pressure gradient develops between the periphery of the lung and the centrally placed main bronchi and trachea, and when the pressure difference between that outside and that in the lumen is great enough, the unsupported posterior wall of these large air tubes collapses. This explains the wide range of triggers to asthmatic attacks, e.g. swelling of the bronchial mucosa and bronchiolar muscle contraction due to histamine release from allergy, or irritation by dusts, fumes fog or infections, also certain emotional stimuli unconsciously perceived by the subject as threatening, or combinations of these.

Emotional stimuli act via forced expiration by accessory muscles in someone with an already overfilled chest or by changes in responsiveness to allergens as demonstrated by Wolf's studies of the nasal mucosa.

7.3.3 Psychological Management

It follows that psychological management is just as necessary for patients with a large allergic component to their asthma as for those with a wholly psychogenic basis. As in other psychosomatic disorders discussed in this book, management will be fruitless or unnecessarily difficult if it fails to take into account the *typicality* of personality traits and attitudes as well as the *typicality* of life situations and events to which these patients are particularly susceptible.

Typical Sensitivity to Domination. Asthma sufferers are especially sensitive to people behaving in an authoritarian way (see transcript of James, Alan and George), and this applies as much to doctors and nurses as it does to spouses, employers, friends and neighbours. This sensitivity originates in childhood in relation to parental behaviour or even tones of voice, or of surrogates such as a sibling, stepmother, etc. Patients with asthma, if given the opportunity, not only admit their intense dislike of anything they see as domination or being pushed about, but visibly and audibly react by changes in posture and breathing, and by coughing in response to such threats. This is easy to confirm by audio or videotaped interviews, and will be indicated in transcripts at the end of the section. High-pitched, sharp commands are particularly resented as replays of childhood experiences of a parent or surrogate and result in audible wheezing within a minute or two.

Typical Sensitivity to Rejection. People with asthma are equally sensitive to what they regard as rejection. Doctors or nurses may therefore feel that the path they must tread is extraordinarily narrow. Sensitivity to rejection also originates in childhood, but the rejection is often provoked by the asthmatic's own behaviour, albeit unconsciously. For example, a girl of 14 when asked about things which annoyed her foster mother said: "It is because when I don't do what she wants me to, such as washing up, I just stay silent, and that really annoys her (laughs), then she gives me a dishcloth and pushes me by my neck to the sink." An unmarried man of 42, living at home with his parents, chuckled when he described how his father waited up for him every night when he came home from the pub in order to tell him that the cause of his asthma was drinking too much beer. Asthmatic children who develop attacks whenever their parents go out or on holiday or before going to school on a day when a snappy teacher is taking their class are suspected of bringing their asthma on intentionally. This may evoke parental displeasure. One of the most important things a doctor can do to help an asthmatic child is to explain to the parents that the link between what the child feels as an emotional threat and the onset of asthma is unconscious, and results from changes in breathing and/or a swelling of the respiratory muscosa, as so clearly demonstrated in vasomotor rhinitis [12]. Asthmatic children are often considered to be precocious, and this annoys some people. In adults the same behaviour is seen as cockiness. They like to challenge or contradict and in this way court the rejection which at the same time they so much dislike. For example, a doctor may suggest a new inhaler which he has found useful. The chances are that the patient will reply: "Ah, but I've tried that already, doctor, and I didn't find it any use at all." Asthmatics also irritate people and provoke rejection by non-verbal communication, i.e. hostile silence, or a posture with head and chest thrust forward, a mixture of submission and aggression, aggressive coughs, laughs, flashing eyes, i.e. a bridling form of response.

7.3.3.1 Management of the Uncomplicated Acute Attack

We have assumed throughout this book that whatever drug or physical treatment a doctor deems appropriate will be pursued simultaneously with psychological management. Asthma is no exception, with a mortality rate unchanged for 30 years [22] despite, or because of, new and powerful remedies which may have made doctors more remote.

The Atmosphere at the Bedside. This is usually tense, especially if it is a child seen at home with parents or others in the room. In the hospital, voices, looks and jerky movements of young doctors and nurses convey the same effect. Fear of asphyxia is within us all, and to the inexperienced the asthmatic wheeze also seems threatening because it is so noisy.

A doctor's first task is to allay tension by quiet words and unhurried actions, and show who is in charge. Those not directly involved should be asked politely to leave the room, and those remaining asked to sit down at some distance from the bed while the doctor takes a chair at the bedside. While noting the patient's pulse, blood pressure and colour the doctor should talk quietly and slowly with the patient, not only about the attack, drug treatment and previous episodes but about other things such as hobbies and holidays. This is as important for a child as for an adult. If the relatives interrupt, they should be reassured but asked to leave their questions until the doctor has finished the interview and examination; they should be told that their help may be needed concerning drug dosages, empty nebulizers, previous infections and attacks, etc. During unhurried examination, talking with the patient should continue; after which the course of action to be proposed by the doctor should be discussed in the patient's presence, even if he or she is a child. Hospital admission should be considered not only in view of the patient's clinical condition but also of the doctor's perception of the emotional situation in the family: anxiety, panic, hostility, oppressive overconcern, and especially when the tension within the family does not seem to lessen during the doctor's visit. Assuming admission to hospital is not indicated, the necessary drug regime will be decided, and should be explained to the patient and family. They also should be informed where the doctor can be found in the next few hours and a promise made to be visited by the doctor on the following day if improvement is not sufficient to permit attendance at the office (surgery).

Initial Management of the Severe Attack. This usually means a patient who has been in status for some hours, and as such is more likely to have been admitted to hospital. The following advice on management is additional to what has been said in the previous paragraph.

The doctor needs to find at least 15 min, preferably 30 min for the interview, sitting quietly at the bedside and encouraging the patient to talk. Young doctors are reluctant to do this because they feel the patient is already too exhausted and should not be troubled. With the patient struggling for words because of the laborious expiration, this is understandable, but in reality it is only after about 10 min of quiet conversation that the breathing begins to ease, and with it the patient's facility of speech. Talking assists rather than impedes expiration. It does not much matter what topic is introduced providing there is reasonable privacy, and that the doctor speaks slowly and quietly, always allowing the patient to reply without being interrupted. His first question might be: Do you often get attacks as bad as this? What treatment in your experience has helped in the past? or Have you ever found anything tends to bring these attacks on? Then as soon as seems reasonable the conversation may be turned to other things in the patient's life such as: Tell me where you go on holiday, or What sort of interests have you got? After about 10 min it is possible to ask: "Do you think you are a sensitive chap?" and if so, "What sort of things or people annoy you?" If the answers are negative, it is useful to ask, "How do you react to bossy people who try to push you about?" When asked whether anything like that has been happening lately, the patient often reveals the emotional cause of the present attack. Within 20 min a good idea will have been obtained of the family background, reactions to important key figures and authority, feelings about rejection, previous experience of doctors and nurses, etc. Meanwhile the intensity of wheezing has usually subsided. Having established this rapport, it is necessary to assure the patient that the doctor will return wether the same evening or the next day). The doctor must not fail to keep that appointment and if delayed should send a message. If a patient has to be transferred to an ICU for tracheostomy and aided ventilation because of dangerously high pCO_2, it is doubly important that the doctor visit and talk with the patient even if he or she can only nod. Staff in ICUs tend to pay great attention to CVPs and blood gases while ignoring the owner. Subsequent interviews can be managed in as little as 15 min, depending on the patient's progress, and then stretched out to once a week, providing this is discussed beforehand so that the patient knows what is happening. After the first interview, which may have to take place in an ICU, ward or patient's home, subsequent interviews should if possible be carried out in a side room, office or GP's surgery; such continuing management is discussed later.

Other Recommended Actions:

1. Avoid talking when patients wish to talk; ask their opinion about treatment and what they feel about the illness, rather than telling them what you, the doctor, think about it. The importance of doctors and nurses speaking quietly and slowly to asthmatic patients is supported by experimental evidence of these patients' unusual sensitivity to high frequency sound waves [18] and their own admitted aversion to noise and strident voices.
2. Standing over asthmatic patients should be avoided as fas as possible because they feel dominated. Instead, doctors should sit at a lower level than their patient, in a relaxed posture and not too close.
3. Mandatory phrases such as "you should", "you must", "don't" are to be avoided. They irritate and usually cause an asthmatic to do the opposite. Years ago a patient expressed this clearly, "We can be led but not driven," while another patient commenting on his general experience of doctors, nurses and receptionists said, "It's their methods – they tend to herd you about like sheep."
   Bridling is a term that describes this reponse.
4. Many people with asthma feel uncomfortable in small spaces such as lifts, the underground, hot crowded shops, small wards and oxygen tents, and they may even develop attacks in these situations. The sensation of being smothered or of not being able to get enough air is common to both hyperventilators and asthmatics. These situations are perceived as threatening and cause the subject to start breathing more deeply.
5. Their sensitivity to smothering applies as much to the emotional environment as to the physical. Situations in which the patient feels caged, trapped or crowded are also provocative. The asthmatic patient bridles or draws back from anyone who is effusive or oppressive, a learned response in childhood to significant persons or surrogates. Parental oppressiveness is likely to be enhanced by anxiety and overconcern for an asthmatic child, for example a mistaken belief that the child is more likely to get asthma if it gets cold, or wet or does not eat its dinner. Effective psychosomatic management of this disorder requires doctors and nurses to be aware of these things and if possible avoid them. For example, it is wise to ask an asthmatic's permission before carrying out an examination or even a procedure, such as venepuncture, whereas in other conditions it would be enough to tell the patient what is proposed.
6. Touching is better avoided, whereas for patients with other conditions when overcome by grief, a doctor's or nurse's comforting hand is appropriate. Asthmatics react to touching as an intrusion on their private emotional territory and equate it to smothering.

7.3.3.2 Continuing Psychological Management

Doctors need to be aware of the asthmatic's extreme sensitivity to rejection and to devise strategies to deal with it.

1. For example, if a doctor goes into a ward in which he has a patient with asthma, it would be wise not to pass without saying, "Good Morning", or waving

a greeting. Otherwise the doctor may soon become aware of the patient's displeasure when hearing noisy wheezing upon leaving the ward.

2. Doctors normally process clockwise on ward rounds. This may involve a wait for as much as an hour for an asthmatic patient until the cortege reaches the bed. Doctors keeping their eyes and ears open will know that the asthmatic patient is getting tense as wheezing and coughing increase. A houseman or student nurse should be despatched with an apology for the tedious suspense, and it can be worthwhile taking the next ward round anticlockwise.

3. Patients with asthma interpret a peremptory discharge by a doctor as a form of rejection and react by developing an attack of asthma before they are due to leave, or during the following night, or if the discharge has been from a GP's surgery the GP may be made to pay for this lack of understanding of the patient's sensitivity by a demand for a night call. In hospitals, apart from the pressure to clear beds, it is often some aspect of an asthmatic's *typical* behaviour that has irritated nurses or medical staff and leads them to tell the patient that as the beds are in short supply "and as you are now better, you may go". This is almost invariably interpreted by the asthmatic patient as a "rejection" and therefore counterproductive. As already stated, asthmatics should not be told but asked. For example,

D: How has your chest been?
P: Not too bad.
D: May I listen to it?
P: Certainly.
D: (The doctor then notes the type of respiration and listens to the chest. Instead of saying: "Well, that's a lot better", it is preferable to say) You're still a bit tight, but better than when you came in.
P: Oh, I thought I was a lot better (will be the reply)
D: Mm, I don't think it is quite right yet, I think you should stay a bit longer.
P: I was hoping to be able to go out ... I have a niece getting married this weekend, and I would like to go to the wedding.
D: (reluctantly) All right, provided you would be willing to come back on Sunday.
P: But if I found I was alright, could I telephone the ward?
D: (reluctantly) Yes, but if you do that I think we should check you over at the first clinic which would be on Wednesday. You will remember we sent you out too soon last time.
Patient acknowledges this with a canny smile saying he would be happy to attend the clinic on Wednesday.

The GP anxious to return an asthmatic to work will find the same strategem useful. Thus, effective psychological management of asthma involves understanding these patients' contrariness and their inclination to do the opposite of what people want them to do.

4. Pelser and his colleagues in Amsterdam discovered some 30 years ago that the best way of getting patients out of hospital was to tell them that they were going to be kept in until fit. Almost invariably the patients ask how long that will be. A suitable reply would be, "It is not possible to say, but it might be several weeks or months depending on progress." Patients then realise that they are not going to be discharged peremptorily despite being aware that their aggressive attitudes may have annoyed some members of the staff; they feel that they have nevertheless

been accepted by the doctor in charge. Feeling more secure and a little triumphant, the asthma usually subsides over the next few days, and it is at this point that they begin to feel the need for freedom from the oppressiveness of the senior doctor's wish to keep them.

Some doctors and nurses on the ward will be sceptical or critical, especially if they have not been there long enough to gain some understanding of what is being attempted. Understanding is helped by informal discussion with doctors and nurses off the ward, and by seminar teaching illustrated by video tapes. However, without the full cooperation of the head nurse as the example for the team of nurses to follow, the whole exercise may be needlessly laborious or even blocked.

5. A trained team is important in managing all psychosomatic disorders, and none more so than with asthmatics and their *typical* sensitivities. Nurses and doctors should be scrupulous about their manners, e.g. not talking across patients as if they were not there. If they do so the patients will probably show their feelings by wheezing or coughing at them. An experienced ward sister or head nurse develops a sixth sense for underlying tensions between the patient and other patients or nurses. Unless such tensions are identified early, a patient's asthma may deteriorate inexplicably, and he or she may demand to be discharged before fully fit. In such cases the patient should be seen as soon as possible and encouraged to express the cause of the upset and offered a move. Alternatively the aggressor may be moved. The team approach applies equally to GP surgeries or health centres, where receptionists' and nurses' attitudes are equally important, and none more so than when a partner or locum is deputising. Asthmatic patients are fearful of being given the brushoff (rejection) by locums, partners or doctors they have not met, or who have made an unfavourable previous impression such as by saying that the dosage of drugs prescribed by their normal doctor was too high or too low. Thus anticipation of rejection at weekends, or while their doctor is on holiday, leads a patient to hang on until they are in status and in great danger, having used their aerolysers excessively.

6. Because of this risk J.W.P. began some 30 years ago to give asthmatic patients a handwritten and signed card saying: "This card admits X to my first outpatient clinic at 4 p.m. on Monday or Wednesday without an appointment," *or* "If X cannot find his/her own GP, presentation of this card at the Emergency Department will be enough for immediate admission to one of my beds." This privilege is never abused, and patients say that mere possession of the card is of therapeutic value because it makes them feel secure. Comparable policies of self-admission have been adopted by chest centres in Edinburgh, Manchester and elsewhere with promising results.

Patients Needing Psychological Management at Greater Depth. For selected patients it is necessary to treat more intensively, as it was for two young patients who had had years of unremitting disease despite every form of orthodox treatment (George and Alan). Without remissions, not only are such cases prone to the complications of chronic chest infection, emphysema and cor pulmonale, but disruption of their social and working life will have a detrimental effect on their families' health and on schooling.

7.3.3.3 Outpatient Psychological Management

Patients who have had some psychological management in depth as inpatients will need to continue it at mutually agreed intervals as outpatients. For those presenting initially as outpatients, the management is the same as for inpatients; the transcript of George is an example of outpatient management over a period of 5 years, involving 16 hours of interview time. Doctors should always say as little as possible, and patients should be encouraged to talk as much as possible in these sessions. Couple therapy is usually contraindicated in asthma, whereas it is most helpful in disorders such as UC, Crohn's disease and MS. This is because of the asthmatic's sensitivity to be caged or trapped, even by the nearest and dearest, not in the sessions but subsequently. They suspect that their spouses may be tempted to apply what they have learned by tactlessly pointing out what the patients may be thinking or feeling whenever they cough, or wheeze, or bridle.

Physiotherapy. Treatment requires physiotherapy as well as psychological management. The importance of applying both approaches at the same time cannot be overestimated, and examples are given in the transcripts at the end of this section. The physiotherapist should, just as the other members of the therapeutic team, understand the principles of psychological management in order to know how to respond to the challenging behaviour and splitting of care givers already described. Brisk physiotherapists who resemble gym mistresses will usually be counterproductive.

Breathing exercises in the past concentrated on forced expiration squeezing the last possible unit of air out of the lungs. This reinforced all the existing errors of an asthmatic's habitual breathing. Instead, what is required is re-education to help the asthmatic patient learn not to overfill the chest, which results in air trapping, reduced tidal volume and some tracheobronchial compression at the point of forced expiration. Patients learn to shift their breathing from upper thoracic to abdomino-lower thoracic, thereby using the diaphragm instead of it being persistently pushed downwards by overfilled lungs. Attention should also be paid to the patients' posture encouraging them to relax the shoulders, neck, dorsal spine and the upper arms, which are frequently retracted in asthma. For characteristic postures in asthma see Heckscher [19].

Other Therapists. If the help of other therapists such as psychiatrists, group therapists or physiotherapists is felt to be necessary, it is most important that patients are not just sent there by their doctor because it will be seen as rejection. Such actions must always be preceded by consultation and the patients' agreement.

Group Psychotherapy. Groen and Pelser [20, 21] presented 18 severely asthmatic men and 15 woman treated by group psychotherapy for 4 and 2 years, respectively. The patients so treated did significantly better than control groups treated only symptomatically.

Typicality. The case histories and transcripts reveal a high degree of *typicality* both in the asthmatic patients' childhood, their coping mechanisms developed in response to it, and *typically* provocative life situations. For example, they illustrate that beating, or the threat of it, is a common childhood experience, whereas it is rare in patients with UC, whose most common memory is of quarrelling in the family.

The histories also depict the asthmatic's *typical* responses to anything they perceive as domination or oppressiveness on the one hand, and rejection on the other. These responses include hostile silence, "dumb insolence", the non-verbal response of "bridling", sarcastic remarks and hostile coughs. This behaviour so annoys parents and other people in authority such as school teachers that they may be provoked to physical violence. Later, the same behaviour often leads to rejection by employers, doctors, nurses and spouses. The starting point of oppressiveness/rejection is set in early childhood for reasons such as being born the wrong sex or too much similarity to a difficult parent or grandparent, being born illegitimate or at a time of dissension involving the mother, or a relationship with one parent being resented by the other. This may occur when a father returns after years of absence and is regarded as an intruder (see transcripts).

7.3.3.4 Summary

Practical points of management have been detailed in the early part of this section. By careful avoidance of behaviour perceived as oppressive or dominating, such as touching, loud voices, commands, standing over or too close to the patient, or of rejection however strong the provocation, a doctor may be the first person in an asthmatic's life to be tested who does not react aggressively.

The first essential is to be seen as a non-dominating, non-rejecting figure. The second requirement is for the doctor to act as a mirror or sounding board from which in time patients learn to discover themselves and by their own initiative are enabled to change their ingrained damaging and inappropriate coping responses. The transcripts of Alan and George illustrate how they achieved this over 2 and 5 years, respectively.

7.3.4 Transcripts

James (transcript continued). Two weeks after the first outpatient interview, he was admitted to hospital in status asthmaticus:

P: I've talked to you more than I've talked to anyone – I can sit all day and say nothing. As a child I never talked to my aunt.
D: Can you talk to your wife?
P: No, the other day when I came to the clinic she wanted to come in, if she had you wouldn't have got anything out of me. Ha! Ha!

Five days later: when asked how he really felt about his son's broken marriage
P: I don't like it, I am one to give loyalty and that is it. Mothers think they know what is best for their sons, don't they?
D: Is your wife close to the boy?
P: Yes, they've sold the house, my son was with us for 12 months, his wife was a pusher, she didn't want children and he did. (At this point he began to weep, the first time he had shown emotion except bridling and aggressive laughs. After a few minutes he went on.) He never did much

with me, and 4 months ago he told me to my face he was always afraid of me, his wife and my wife were there. They came to tell us of the break-up. He said he blamed me for it all. I have not got a son, I said to myself. (more tears) I said I would forgive him but I shall never forget, although I tell him I will to make him feel better. [The reason for his cryptic remark about preferring daughters was now evident.]

D: It sounds as though you must have misunderstood each other a good deal?

P: Yes, often, he would never come with me when he was 15, wasn't interested, only in courting, they started too young.

At the end of the interview he needed some time to regain his composure before returning to the ward. Tears had totally replaced his previous wheezing (syndrome shift). During the next few days he was weeping or on the verge of tears much of the time, especially if spoken to. Asthma had been replaced by an anxiety state. Junior doctors and nurses urged the prescription of anti-depressants; I declined this advice and explained why. At the same time I let the patient know that I understood his emotional pain but that it was better out than in, where it had been for so long. Five days later on 6th February he went for a walk and was delighted with the freedom of his breathing. On the 8th February he was tense again and said his chest was tight, he said the ward had been like Piccadilly Circus all night, patients and nurses talking. "It frustrated me," he said. He then tested me out saying that he had had some sedatives at home called Spandettes, could he have them? By all means I said. In these circumstances it is easy for doctors to make the mistake of saying no because there is something better. He then went on to say that it was the women's high pitched voices that had annoyed him. (Sensitivity to high pitched sound [18].)

By the 15th of February his anxiety state had begun to improve, and a few audible wheezes had returned. He referred again to his mother who had tried to change his father after he had retired. "I didn't like it, I hate to have a tie on or a suit and so did he."

Two days later on entering the ward it was noted that he was looking very withdrawn but was not wheezing. On enquiry a nurse said that he had been rebuffed by a patient opposite whom he had tried to talk to. He was seen alone, I told him I was sorry for the setback because he had been making such progress. He replied that he would not stay on the ward with this other patient. Offered transfer to another ward, he said he would prefer to go home. With suitable reluctance this was agreed, providing he attended as an outpatient the following week. He came saying he was a bit better; he had not had to use his aerolyser or Becotide (*typical* response to feeling rejected).

D: Is your wife pleased?

P: (pointedly) She hasn't asked.

Three months later he was in severe status and was offered immediate admission and accepted. He complained that his own doctor had been away and that he had had to see the partner who had refused to increase his prednisone, which he felt he needed. Instead he had been given a particular antibiotic which he said had never done him any good (*typical* response to feeling rejected). He came out of status more quickly on this occasion, and during his inpatient stay had two interviews, the last one on the 24th May, the day before he said he would like to go home. No pressure whatever had been put on him to go, in fact he was encouraged to stay, which as already explained is important in the management of asthmatics, who see peremptory discharge as equivalent to rejection.

He was seen at intervals over the next 3 years and steadily improved, requiring less medication from his doctor. The physiotherapist received a Christmas card in 1985 saying that he had been well for 2 years and felt he did not need any more treatment.

Alan; aged 20; had asthma for 18 years. *First interview:*

D: Can you tell me when your asthma first started?

P: I was told it started at 2 years old, but ...

D: Had you brothers and sisters?

P: No, not that I know of, no.

D: And you had a stepfather, I gather?

P: Yes.

D: When did your mother marry him? How old were you?

P: About 6 months, I never knew anybody else. I didn't know about it [illegitimacy] until I found out myself.

D: What age were you?

P: About seventeen. I didn't say anything, I just got drunk and smashed the car up.

D: You felt pretty angry?

P: Yes, they hadn't told me.

D: What sort of a chap is he? Is he easy to get on with?

P: In a way sort of restrictive.

D: You felt restricted?

P: Yes, it was *his* house.

D: Do you think that you are sensitive to feelings?

P: Yes, very. I can see things and judge things people probably wouldn't think about.

D: Do you think you were lonely as a child?

P: Yes, very lonely.

D: Did you have many friends?

P: I had my mother's brother, he was about the same age as me. We more or less grew up as brothers. We went to the same school, and then I began to see differences, like I didn't seem to grow, and I felt slightly inferior and he shot up to about 6 ft 2 in (1.90 m).

D: Do you get angry about things? I mean obviously you were angry when your parents hadn't told you about this?

P: I get angry, but it's a very passive anger, you know I don't – like as I say, my uncle has grown up bigger, and he goes out drinking. He's a man's man you know. We all go down in his van, and I sit in the back and two sit in the front and they are always laughing and joking and saying, oh, about girls and things you know, and because I don't go out that sort of gets to me a bit you know.

D: Yes, sure. Do you find dealing with girls a bit difficult?

P: Yes, because I am slightly sort of inhibited, I suppose it would be all right, but I don't know.

D: I expect you would be fine. Do you think you were strictly brought up?

P: Fairly strictly.

D: Who was the stricter one of your parents?

P: Oh, father, obviously. Mother was just the opposite.

D: Mother was kind and protective of you?

P: She is a very fussy and worrying sort of person.

D: Did you get beaten at all?

P: No, just a clip. Now it is more sarcasm in front of people.

D: Do you think your mother had a sharp tone of voice, or was she rather gentle?

P: No, she wasn't sharp except when concerned with my health.

D: So she would get protective then, and she might get anxious?

P: Yes, anxiety would make her sharp.

D: You have been treated for this asthma by many doctors?

P: Yes.

D: Of course, one has to say this about asthma, there is no cure for it.

P: No? Well, there is a cure for the psychological asthma, isn't there? In yourself. I mean, change of situation probably brings about change of attitude, and probably you could change yourself.

D: You are right. What I was trying to point out, though, is that one is always oneself, and certain things which are very distressing might always cause an attack of asthma, but they would become much rarer and you would probably know why they had happened, and be able to get out of it. What do you feel about being pumped full of tablets? What is your response?

P: In a sense it doesn't change much. The tablets don't work after a while, because tension just takes over.

D: So you are saying that if you are very tense, no tablets really work?

P: No.

D: Well you started the conversation by saying you found situations upset your asthma?

P: The attitudes with which I am treated and the background which I can see, like the background of my mother and that of my father, the way they treat me, I just come home and watch the TV.

D: It upsets you I suppose?

P: Yes.

D: Well now, the ward is a funny place, you will find funny people, you will find people who will annoy you. You have been in hospital, I expect?

P: Yes.

D: Where, at Bealings or St. George's?

P: St. George's

D: Then you will know what it is like, there are people who are all right, and there will be people who will be a bit awkward. Well you can talk to me, Mr. X you will find an easy chap to talk to I suspect, because he understands this trouble, and you may want to let off a bit of steam every now and then, but I shall be here from now until September 7th, and we shall be meeting each other; then I am going to go on holiday. I thought I would tell you that now, because I hope by then we may have got you on the right road.

Writing to his GP after he left hospital J.W.P. said: During his 10 weeks' stay he received re-education in breathing and relaxation exercises from the physiotherapist, and ten therapeutic sessions with me. His asthma recurred twice on the ward, once when a nurse rather tactlessly asked him to show her a photo of his girlfriend, and the second time when a senior nurse made a sarcastic remark in front of him about her doubts and his need to be in hospital at all. Gradually we managed to get him going home for weekends. Some of these weekends were very traumatic, and he developed asthma in response to them. The last occasion was when he announced to his mother that he was going to have a test at a racing driving school at Snetterton. Your partner was called to see the mother on that occasion when she had clearly had an attack of hysterics. The hospital stay may have seemed rather long, but when one thinks how long this patient has had asthma, and how much medical and nursing time he must have taken up over the years, then 10 weeks were not very long. I was anxious not to discharge him before he felt ready to go, because these patients always interpret peremptory discharge as equivalent to rejection. In my case it would, of course, have been equivalent to the parental rejection to which he is so sensitive.

For some time Alan had felt it might help if his mother could express her point of view. Several appointments were offered which she failed to keep, making a variety of excuses. Ultimately, however, she accepted one on the 23rd October.

Interview with Mother and Patient:

M: They taught me how to breathe myself so that I could show Alan how to breathe and I used to spend hours trying to teach Alan how to breathe, how to hang him over a chair.

D: You probably hammered the base of the lungs?

M: I did everything they told me, you know. I was just a confused mother. They had me so confused that I didn't know what was best, because I saw one doctor and he said, "Oh you must pamper him, you mustn't correct him." I see another doctor who says, "Give him a damned good smack on the arse, it will do him good," but I am only a mother and I do get worked up. You get worried if you can't see your son progressing. He wasn't having any life, he wasn't going out anywhere enjoying himself, all he could do was to sit and watch television. My father and I did have a feud over Alan. I mean he turned me out of the house. He never referred to Alan as Alan or your son, but as "that" and he used to say, "What are you doing here with *that*? ... you can get *that* out of my house." Alan does get annoyed, if in the pouring rain I say, "Put your coat on."

D: Do you think it is a good thing to say that to somebody of his age?

M: Well, I say to my husband, "Put your coat on."

P: If it is raining I have got the level of intelligence to put a coat on when it is raining (annoyed).

M: But they haven't always, you know, and he has been given a free choice.

D: Yes (doubtfully).

M: He has been able to come and go as he pleases, you know [patient laughs] and he just doesn't decide to go.

P: You can't do as you please when you have got your mother sitting up to about 2 o'clock in the morning, Ha! Ha! "Where have you been?"

M: But to say, suddenly "I want to drive a racing car," well why the hell a racing car, I just felt that because we had said we didn't like the idea he was hell bent on proving that he would do it anyway.

P: Not at all.

D: I am glad you came, thank you very much, because it has helped me a great deal.

M: I don't really know. I came tonight, and I said if he starts on the track that all the other doctors have that I am a possessive mother, I have caused your asthma, then I am going to get up and I am going to walk out and I am going to say, "Do what you like with my son."

D: Have I said that?

M: No.

11th interview, 14th December, just after starting carpenter's training course 40 miles (64 km) away:

P: The first Monday I telephoned, and it seemed when I heard her voice I could just picture where she was and the house and everything, you know, which made me feel closer. Therefore, I telephoned every night, but well she telephones me most now.

D: You are going to have ups and downs, you will undoubtedly get another attack of asthma from time to time.

P: The main thing I want is to get conditioned to people. More than anything I would like to be able to sort of stand up and tell a joke in a crowd.

D: Have you had any more dreams? You know you had one or two rather frightening ones when you first went home?

P: Not frightening.

D: But nothing quite so frightening as the one you had when you couldn't find the walls? [In this dream he had described terror when unable to find the walls of his room. It was suggested that this represented his increasing freedom, and that the disappearing wall of his cage was frightening.]

P: Oh no, nothing like that.

At the fourteenth interview in January 1975 he said that he had had slight wheezing while at home at Christmas but added, "If I had been at home longer I would have had an attack because there was no scope, you just cannot get through to my stepfather, there is a coldness there." A month later he arrived in a beard. "Mother doesn't like it," he said, "but I am learning to be more aggressive."

Five weeks later at the fifteenth interview he came with severe asthma, saying that he had been wheezing for a month and had been back to the Chest Department which he had previously derided, and this despite open access to me and my department at any time if he relapsed. He spoke in parables which clearly indicated his negative transference to me which I had been expecting. I said I fully understood his resentment at having to be dependent on anyone, which applied to me just as much as to his mother, but that his dependence on me would be transient, while my door would always remain open to him. At the end of the interview his chest was quieter.

I saw him 4 days later. His chest was normal, and his anger at my oppressiveness had subsided. At the eighteenth interview in May, just before the end of the course, he came in with a substantial Viking beard and moustache, not a wheeze audible, and ran downstairs at immense speed, something he could not have done a year before. In June he relapsed after experiencing denigration while applying for jobs. He discovered that 5-years apprentices referred to Government trainees as "6-month wonders". It was therefore not surprising that Alan at home, out of work and exposed to this level of aggression from his mother should relapse severely. He said the atmosphere was claustrophobic. I offered him a bed, apologising that there was not more suitable accommodation, but he could treat the ward as a hotel and come and go as he liked. After initially rejecting the offer he came in on the 5th August, 1975. When seen the next day he was better. "I did say to her I would like to live away from home, and she burst into tears ... She feels if I say I want her to be less concerned, she thinks I am taking my love away." The patient stayed for 5 weeks. No attempt was made to discharge him, and the nursing staff needed a good deal of briefing because many of them could not understand why he was there apart from having breathing exercises. Their displeasure reached a peak when he came in one night at about 11 p.m. a little drunk. He became more and more independent and took his discharge 1 week after I had gone on holiday.

30th and final interview, 19th June, 1976: [As the patient had missed or cancelled two previous appointments he was sent a letter suggesting a further appointment to decide how to leave things (termination).]

D: The attacks have not been quite so prolonged like you had last summer?

P: Oh, nothing like it, I think mainly because I have been concentrating on my work and things. I don't know if I had my beard last time, did I?

D: Yes, you have got a different shaped one now.

P: I haven't got one at all (laugh) I have just got the moustache. I shaved my beard off – my girlfriend didn't like it.

D: Tell me about her. When did you meet her?

P: Oh, last December. [Discussion of girl friend and attitudes of mother and stepfather to her followed.]

D: Yes, perhaps you feel freer and able to do things in your own right whereas before you felt a bit restricted?

P: Yes, I wasn't sure of anything before, but now I am, sure that I could do anything really.

D: I don't know what you felt when I wrote to you suggesting this appointment? (embarrassed, non-verbal movements and coughs at this) You still probably have mixed feelings about coming to see me. We discussed this once before, do you remember, when I suggested that in any sense being dependent on me is just as difficult for you and irritating for you as was your dependence on your mother?

P: It is not irritating in the same way.

D: No?

P: Sometimes it is a bit like coming back, walking up the steps today the heart started to pound a bit, and then you see the facts and it is just (pause) ...

D: It takes you back into a situation your were in long ago?

P: Yes. Yes, I think my girlfriend, Julie, is a great passport really because before when I used to go on my own and that wasn't the same, mother noticed I was going out, but now it is different.

D: Yes. She wants you to make progress, but she will also have the double feelings of losing you which we have talked about before. I think we ought to discuss whether you need to come and see me, or whether you want to come and see me again, and if so, when, or whether you would like to leave it open, and what it would mean to you if we didn't make a fixed appointment, I mean, so these are psychological things.

P: Well, on the first point I would have to regard my attitude towards coming here.

D: Yes, that's right.

P: When I was ill I knew that I had to come. I think the worst part was when I started to get better and had to come back again then, but now that I am on the road to recovery I can see that it doesn't matter at all, you know, I would rather ...

D: You can come or not come on your own. You don't feel that I am pushing you or that you have to?

P: Oh no. I think we could set a date and in the meanwhile a longer date, and if anything does come up then I could ring or write, and now it has got to the stage where the only time I really need to see you is if I have a crisis, or when I feel I need to see you, so I think from that point of view now I could sort of leave it open.

D: Good, I think that's fine.

P: Another thing with a fixed appointment is you feel that you may enjoy yourself in between but you always feel drawn back.

D: As you rightly said, if you have a fixed appointment then you have to take some positive action to cancel it, and if you were to cancel it, am I going to feel hurt?

P: Yes, (laughs)

D: As your mother feels hurt when you want to go?

P: In a way, sort of rejecting you?

D: Well, that might worry you?

P: Yes, that would be my worry, and the next time I did come, or if I did come you would feel ...

D: Yes, so the very fact that you had to cancel would be difficult for you perhaps?

P: Yes, I think the best way is to leave it open and then I know that I can always come back.

D: The French say, "Au revoir," that means not goodbye finally, but goodbye until we meet again.

P: Yes.

D: Which may be a long time.

P: In some ways I hope it is, because it will mean that I have done well.

D: Yes, that's right. It is a step, well, it is a step in your independence. [Long silence, 35 s. It was very important not to interrupt it.]

P: (Sigh!) It feels strange in a way.

D: Does it?

P: Yes. (pause)

D: How does it feel? (pause)

P: Well like you said, you know. I hadn't got another appointment and ... (pause)

D: Does it feel like the dream you had where there are not walls to the room?

P: It is like a feeling where the father say to his – well, this is metaphorical – but where the father says to his son: "There, son, there's the world," you know it's that sort of thing, and by now I have to take it, so that's all there is to it.

D: It is a bit like your mother said, you know, "Why don't you go out?" and, of course, every time she said that you had a feeling you didn't want to go.

P: Yes, (laughs) it was strange.

D: Perhaps you feel that a little bit about this, but I think you know very well that ... that it is a step; rather than actually having to come you could write. or you could telephone. All right?

P: Yes.

D: Good. Goodbye, Alan

P: Thanks a lot anyway.

D: Not a bit. (shake hands)

P: O.K.

D: Goodbye.

(Therapy time 32 h over 2 years)

The following letter was received from the patient's GP nearly 2 years after termination of therapy:

> Marvellous news about this boy. He seems to be totally normal, bright and cheerful, is to be married in a fortnight's time, and his fianceé is already pregnant. He plans to buy a new car next year and is to spend a fortnight's honeymoon at Blackwater near Aldershot in the bungalow of his fiancée's uncle, who is temporarily posted away. Everything in the garden looks marvellous, and I am grateful to you for all you did for him. His mother's influence upon him is minimal, but it was a hard battle to achieve this state of affairs.

George, aged 32, an only child and a diesel fitter who had had asthma since infancy. His asthma was persistent with severe exacerbations and had been treated by his GP with all standard inhalers and Ledercort for some years. He was unable to run any distance and had an overfilled chest with elevated shoulders and arms retracted. Before treatment, which included physiotherapy, his breathing was almost entirely restricted to the upper chest. His mother had RA which had come on a few months after his marriage a few years previously, of which she disapproved and destroyed within months. The patient then returned home.

D: Do you think you are more like mother or father in temperament?

P: Similar to my father, my father is very good tempered but my mother is quick tempered.

D: What sort of things upset her?

P: I do sometimes if I don't clear away you know, sometimes I will leave things in the bedroom and she gets at me but I still do it. (said with a triumphant grin)

D: I think you are old enough now to be able to leave things? Do you tell her that sometimes?

P: If I do, she gets upset. My mother worries, she likes to know where I go sometimes and of course I won't tell her. Probably that's my way if people keep asking me questions about things, I dry up. My mother gets upset, she gets angry because I don't clean my car a lot, you know.

D: Do you think that attitudes ever fire your asthma off?

P: No, I don't really think so (denial is totally opposite to what he says later) ...

D: Some people ask: "How can feelings affect asthma?"

P: Well, if I forget my inhaler that seems to cause an attack you know.

D: O.K. that should tell us something, shouldn't it. What is your reaction when you feel you haven't got your inhaler?

P: I start to panic in a way ...

D: Do you think your mother worried a lot about you as a child?

P: Yes, if I wanted to go out with my mates like you do as a boy and I had been wheezy, mother wouldn't let me go out.

D: What did you feel about that?

P: I used to play up, of course, my mother would see my father and he would say you're not going out and that was that.

D: How did they discipline you?

P: I would get a hiding, you know, if I did anything wrong my father would do it, my mother as well,

D: Really?

P: Yes, my mother she used to hit me a lot when I was 8 or 9, she hit me with a broom.
(Challenging behaviour is illustrated by the following:)

P: You see when I mentioned to my mother I was going camping in Scotland she was against it. She said the cold would get in on me, but for once my father stuck up for me and told her.

D: So consciously you may have been pleased to be able to go to camp and do the things that other people do and get away with it?

P: I was, you know, I was amazed because my mates are both hard workers and when we got wet they expected me to crack up and were surprised when I didn't and they did.

D: What did your mother say?

P: The tent blew away one night and I telephoned and told them – I shouldn't have really (smile) – all the clothes got wet and I told my Dad when he answered the telephone and he said from that time until I got back home she was worried sick over me, and yet I was as right as rain. It was really good (triumphant grin!) ... if anyone gets on to me to do something I don't want to do it, as a child I used to get hidings for that.

A few months later he said that there had not been so many arguments at home, and when asked why replied, I've said something, and added, "Mother's arthritis is no better." A few months later, Mother moans a lot, they are decorating and expect me to do it, I hate the job and won't. It's little things like that she always gets on to me about, if someone tells me not to do something I tend to go and do it.

A year after the first attendance:

P: I feel on top of the world and am on a very low dose of steroid, I've just got back from holiday and got wet again. There's been less aggravation, she has stopped nagging me, I think my father had a word with her about it.

At 18 months:

P: Definitely the best summer I have had for years.

Some time later he spoke of a car accident and having to pay the fine:

P: Mother wanted to know all about it and things like that, I just walked away you see, it *sets me up,* I mean it's the constant questioning; father doesn't even bother to ask.

D: How do you mean, sets you up?

P: Well, it gets me

D: What do you feel?

P: Tense really, if they didn't ask I would tell them.

D: Does your mother have a positive voice?

P: Yes, positive and talks quickly, she gets very irritable, like you tell me people with arthritis tend to feel sorry for themselves. Sometimes she will want something, and if I don't get it at once she says, "Oh, I'll get it myself." She tries to make you feel guilty. I don't think she means to but that's just the way she's got.

A little later he came and said he was very well and thought the main reason was because he had met a steady girlfriend, and this was taking him out of the house more.

The following is an example of the way patients try to split their care givers:

P: I've not had any time off work, but the only thing is Dr. M. will always give me prednisone while Dr. E. won't let me have it and always thinks that I should get down to 0.5 mg a day. (It seemed that the time was right to ask him how he felt about continuing to come and how often, i.e. anticipating termination.)

D: Perhaps we should discuss how you feel about coming up, we've been seeing each other now for about $2^{1}/_{2}$ years.

P: What do you mean?

D: I wonder how you feel about it, I mean it's getting to a point when you may be saying, "Is there much point in all this?"

P: I think since I have seen you my asthma has been better because I used to take between 2 and 3 Ledercort before, I've definitely been better, and feel better being able to come and tell you things, I look forward to coming actually.

Discussion then turned to his girlfriend and what she might feel about his asthma and whether she would want to come to interview. The patient's expression showed that this was dangerous ground, probably because he didn't want his future wife to replay his mother's oppressiveness; J.W.P. retreated rapidly.

D: Why not then leave it until after you are married?

P: I think she would have liked to have come in this morning.

D: Well, ask her in if you want to, but I thought perhaps it was a bit early?

P: Yes, I think I'll leave her out there! (cagey grin)

D: You don't like people pressing you?

P: No.

D: "Crowding" is the word you use?

P: Yes, I don't like being told.

D: It makes you tight?

P: Yes, tensed up.

D: Unconsciously, you probably fill your chest a bit fuller when that happens; people, like animals, do that when they feel threatened.

(After marriage and just before the first baby was born he was seen again).

P: I would like to get rid of it (asthma).

D: You're never cured of asthma but you don't have to have it so much, and I think I've said that to you before. [It is important that physicians "allow" their patients to keep some of their asthma as it has been for many of them the only avenue of emotional expression in certain circumstances. Question of termination is once again approached.] Well perhaps we should talk about whether you feel you still need to come up here.

P: I think I would still like to, maybe once a year, I don't feel as if I can talk to my family doctor because he is so busy.

D: They are always busy, family doctors.

P: You seem to take a bit more time.

D: Well, we've talked a good deal over the last few years although the actual total time we have spent is probably not more than about 16 h, which is not much over 4 years.

P: Five years, isn't it?

D: Oh, it's 5, is it? Well, if you would like to strip your shirt off to see how your chest is, because it looks pretty good from the breathing point of view.

P: (while dressing) I can run now, I was never able to run. The other day, I chased a young boy at work and caught him; I thought to myself if that had been a couple of years ago I would never have been able to do it. Four years ago if I had run really hard and quickly I would get so tight I would think I was going to die, I wouldn't be able to breathe.

D: As I said before you will still be prone to attacks of asthma under certain circumstances, certain emotional tensions will probably get through to you.

P: I think that is it more than anything. I'm definitely better than before the treatment when I was tensed up; I was contracting myself all in but I don't do that now, you see I can stand normally now.

(Therapy time 16 h over 5 years)

Late Onset Asthma. Late onset asthma has always puzzled clinicians, especially those who think that all asthma is due to hypersensitivity to inhaled pollens, mites or other allergens and if the patients' environment has not apparently altered for 30–40 years. It is then that a new deodorant, a farmer's insecticide or the cat next door gets the blame when in most cases it is due to stressful recent changes in the domestic environment. Examples are the husband's retirement leading to increased tension because he is always in the way, or the death of a mother who had previously held the balance of power between rivalrous sisters – the power vacuum is then filled by the dominant sister and the dominated/rejected sister is the one who may develop asthma.

Maria, aged 50, late onset asthma. She had first experienced asthma 2 years prior to admission to hospital in severe status in 1973 when her eosinophil count was 20% of 8400 white blood cells. She was treated with corticosteroids, reeducation in breathing and psychotherapy. Her extreme hostility to her mother was first revealed when the physiotherapist asked why the parcel she had received that morning (from her mother) remained unopened in her bedside locker. Later she told J.W.P. she had been born at a time when her father was dallying with a Spanish nursemaid, and it seemed that from then on she had been the receptacle of her mother's anger, whereas her sister, born later when the marriage was more tranquil, had never been able to do wrong in her mother's eyes. The patient recalled been given a penny on Saturday mornings to go out and buy a cane for her mother to beat her with. Despite all this, she did quite well at school and made a successful marriage, and had a son and lived happily for years 100 miles away from her mother, until the latter moved to live a few miles from the patient. Mother now telephoned her daily with all kinds of complaints and requests, whereas previously she had only telephoned once a month because the cost of a long-distance call was too great. After psychological management and breathing exercises Maria's asthma improved.

She was referred 8 years later for an opinion because of lower chest pain. The following transcript is from that interview and illustrates clearly the patient's psychopathology and resulting typical passive – aggressive coping mechanism in dealing with her oppressive mother and the experience of being beaten in childhood that is so common in asthma.

D: The trouble you had 8 years ago was related to having your mother coming to live much closer?

P: Yes, and when we moved to H. she moved too, so we have got her right at the bottom of our long garden. She lives in a beautiful bungalow, Dr. P. but she absolutely hates it. Twelve months she has been there, nothing I do is right, nothing I say is right. My husband has just stopped going over there –.

D: I remember he is very tolerant ...

P: He is a very tolerant man, but you see 5 min before I came out, her sister came and said she had accepted a transfer back to F., but mother doesn't want to go now. What *do* you do? So when I get back home I've got to go and see her – so I'll send my husband (wheeze).

D: She has always been difficult with you as I remember?

P: Yes.

D: Whereas your sister coped with her?

P: Yes, my sister can get round her – I'm afraid – I just can't any more. Nothing I say is right, my son won't go near her.

D: When your mother moved from L.K. it was the time you got your asthma?

P: That's right – every place she's been, Dr. P., we have decorated, we've done the garden, but got nothing but grumble, grumble, grumble.

D: You have had worries with your mother all your life (wheeze) but you didn't get your asthma until you were 48, and I remember you saying that when she was at L.K. she couldn't keep telephoning because it cost too much.

P: Yes, that's right.

D: But when you got to F. she was on the telephone every day.

P: Yes, that's right. Yes, and its the same again now you see (wheeze). She won't leave me alone – I know it's wicked but I heartily dislike her at the moment (wheeze).

D: Do you remember when you were in the ward with the very bad asthma you had a parcel?

P: Yes, from my mother (wheeze) and I didn't want to know – she never buys a thing – so what do you do with the old b. ... – lady. Now she's going back to F. I know I will be backwards and forwards there (wheeze).

D: I really wanted to know what has changed because –

P: She's wicked now (cough).

D: The difficulties you had with her of course started in your childhood?

P: Yes.

D: When you couldn't do right, your sister could, I think?

P: My sister still can't do anything wrong, although she lives so far away, not that I begrudge it because I love my sister.

D: I remember a time when the garden wasn't right.

P: The garden isn't right here but she won't have my husband do it.

D: When did it all go wrong? I seem to remember you got off on the wrong foot when you were a little girl. Your father left didn't he?

P: Yes, I was about 4 or 5.

D: Do you remember your father being kind to you?

P: (wheeze) He couldn't have been all that bad.

D: Was your mother strict with you when you were little?

P: With me? Yes

D: Not your sister?

P: No.

D: What sort of things did she get strict about?

P: Well, we had a great big coalburner and I had to scrub it every Saturday morning, and once I had done it she said "do it again." I got a hiding if it was dirty, I wasn't allowed to go with a friend, I never went out, Dr. P

D: Your sister could?

P: My sister could.

D: You must have felt that as a child?

P: Of course I did, I bottled it up and I suppose it's coming out now, because I shall tell her one day, I hate her.

D: You never have yet?

P: Not as yet – I told her I dislike her when she gets in these horrible moods every morning (wheeze).

D: Yes?

P: But I shall tell her one day, but I mustn't because she's 86.

D: I know its very difficult for you. Did she beat you as a child?

P: Yes, I had the cane but I had to go and buy it myself every Saturday morning at the corner shop, where penny canes hung on the wall.

D: And she made you go and get it?

P: Yes, I had to go and get it.

D: How old were you then?

P: Before I went to school and after I went to school – used to get a good hiding every week.

D: Do you remember what you felt when you were being beaten?

P: Yes, I hated her. My sister will tell you Dr. P that they used to have to drag my mother off me before she murdered me, and I was little. Can you wonder its all coming out now?

D: No I don't, I'm surprised really you are as well as you are.

P: I wish she would leave us alone, if she's going to be nice that is alright. We took her out last week to B. for the day, she grumbled when we brought her home.

D: Your sister thinks it unfair?

P: Oh yes, she does because we do get on well together (wheeze).

Her recent chest pain and possible causes and tests which would be needed were then discussed.

D: Have you any other things you would like to mention?

P: No I don't think so, just wish she wasn't here. She tortures you.

D: Do you think she has any idea she does that?

P: Oh I think so, but we've often said, my sister and I, just the two of us, that when mother goes there's a skeleton in the cupboard somewhere. Until she goes we shan't find out what it is.

D: Um. Do you remember Mrs. H. the physiotherapist?

P: Yes, I still do her exercises.

D: You think the exercises helped you?

P: Yes, because I only have had one bad attack since and had to ring the doctor (wheeze), that was last Sunday.

D: Well that's not bad.

P: No, I can cope with the little ones.
D: Have you had any more presents from her lately like the parcel you had in hospital?
P: I have had to give them all back ... the engagement ring she had given me as a keepsake.
D: And you had to give it back to her?
P: Yes, and the powder bowl and ebony mirror.
D: Do you think she will go back to F.?
P: If my husband says "go", she will, but of course he won't because he's too nice.
D: But you won't be able to tell her?
P: No, because I am her daughter.
D: I think that is why he has to be strong for you.

References

1. Lum LC (1981) Hyperventilation and anxiety state. J R Soc Med 74:1–4
2. White PD, Hahn RC (1929) The symptoms of sighing in cardiovascular diagnosis. Am J Med Sci 177:179–188
3. Weiss E, English OS (1949) Psychosomatic medicine. Saunders, Philadelphia
4. Meller WF (1972) History of Second World War: casualties and statistics. HMSO London, p 59
5. Lum LC (1975) Hyperventilation: the tip of the iceberg. J Psychosom Res 19:375–383
6. Lum LC (1982) Total allergy syndrome. Lancet 1:516
7. Winicott DW (1966) Psychosomatic illness in its positive and negative aspects. Int J Psychoanal 47:510–516
8. Holmes TH, Goodell G, Wolf S, Wolff HG (1950) The nose. Thomas, Springfield
9. Macdonald G (1888) The mechanism of the nose as regards respiration, taste and smell. Br Med J 11:1810
10. French T, Alexander F (1941) Psychogenic factors in bronchial asthma. Psychosom Med [Suppl]
11. Groen JJ (1970) The mechanism of the disturbance of respiration in the asthmatic attack. In: Proceedings of the 6th world congress of psychotherapy. Nederlands Genootschap voor Psychotherapie, Amsterdam, pp 371–375
12. Wolf S (1952) Causes and mechanisms in rhinitis. Laryngoscope 62:601–614
13. Wolf S (1956) Life stress and allergy. Am Med 20:919–928
14. Rogerson CH, Hardcastle DH, Duguid K (1935) A psychological approach to the problem of asthma and the asthma-prurigo syndrome. Guy's Hosp Rep 85:286–308
15. Dekker E, Groen JJ (1957) Asthmatic wheezing. Compression of the trachea and major bronchi as a cause. Lancet 1:1064–1068
16. Talma S (1898) About nervous asthma. Ned Tijdschr Geneesk 34:390–403
17. Gandevia B, Atkins EF (1963) The spirogram of gross expiratory tracheo-bronchial collapse in emphysema. Q J Med 32:23–31
18. Mason RK (1967) Asthma and high frequency sound perception. Nature 214:99–100
19. Heckscher H (1942) Emphysema of the lungs and its significance to relapsing bronchitis, cardiac and respiratory neurosis and bronchial asthma. Munksgaard, Copenhagen
20. Groen JJ, Pelser HE (1959) Verdere ervaringen en resultaten van groep psychotherapie bij lijders aan asthma bronchiale. Ned Tijdschr Geneesk 103:65–75
21. Groen JJ, Pelser HE (1960) Experiences with, and results of, group psychotherapy in patients with bronchial asthma. J Psychosom Res 4:191–205
22. Burney PGJ (1986) Asthma mortality in England and Wales: evidence for a further increase 1974 – 84. Lancet 2:323–326

8 Cardiovascular Disorders

8.1 Essential Hypertension

It is easier to understand psychological management of this disorder if one is acquainted with the main strands of research on hypertension in general. For a comprehensive review the reader is referred to Brod [1]. In animals and man variable vascular reactivity to stressors such as pain and cold has long been felt to be in part genetically determined, and the same is felt about individual variability of response to emotional threats. Racehorse owners and breeders of dogs and cattle would be amazed that anyone should think otherwise. However, it has been fashionable for some doctors, sociologists and psychologists to attribute human behaviour only to environmental factors. After Dahl et al. [2, 3] had shown that one strain of rat was sensitive (S) and another resistent (R) to experimentally induced hypertension, Groen et al. [4] decided to find out whether the two strains differed in behaviour; they found that R rats were exploratory and aggressive and S rats the reverse. It had been Groen's clinical experience of *typical* behaviour in hypertensive people which led him to pose the question in the first place.

Extrapolation from behaviour in rats to humans is clearly unjustifiable, but this work suggested that future research should look at inherited differences in behaviour *as well* as pressor reactivity, which itself might be influenced by abnormal docile behaviour frustrating the expression of natural aggression.

8.1.1 Psychological Management

First are the reports of Saul [5], Alexander [6], Binger [7] and Dunbar [8]. Dunbar's clinical, longitudinal and psychoanalytically based studies led her to describe a premorbid personality profile for hypertension. This was followed by experimentally designed clinical investigations [9, 12]. (The titles of the first two of these papers are illustrative, i.e. "Clinical and experimental observations on the lability and range of blood pressure in essential hypertension," and "Hypertension as a reaction pattern to stress: summary of experimental data on variations in blood pressure and renal blood flow".) The consistency of these workers' findings and others since [13] continue not to receive proper acknowledgement. This may be because too many workers since have lacked the necessary interviewing skills or have asked the wrong questions. Rarely have they given their subjects enough time to lower emotional defences, which in practice takes weeks rather than days.

The 1960s was a decade dominated by questionnaires and personality inventories. For reasons explained elsewhere (Chap 18), this proved to be a blind alley.

Physiologically based research has employed physical stressors such as cold or pain or allegedly psychological stress such as mental arithmetic, frustrating puzzles or discordant sound [14]. When results lack uniformity psychophysiologists usually fail to ask themselves whether the subjects' perception of what was being done to them or asked of them could be responsible, e.g. whether the doctor is seen as a dedicated scientist, a "persecutor" or a vivid reminder of a key figure. Indeed, for some subjects mental arithmetic is a pleasure and not a challenge. A clear review of the methodological difficulties implicit in this field of research has been given by Weiner [15]. In the behavioural field the seminal contribution was that by Miller [16]; since then there have been several reports of biofeedback-aided autogenic learning in the treatment of hypertension. Mild hypertension may be lowered by such means [17], but recent studies describe high drop-out rates and failure to maintain improvement. Moderate or severe hypertension rarely responds to such methods and usually requires hypotensive drugs. It is when these fail, or when hypertension enters the accelerated phase, or in young men with their bad prognosis, that psychological management is called for in addition to drugs. Case histories at the end of this section illustrate a form of psychological management which we have found to be effective. Follow-ups show that patients so treated may remain in remission for a period of years.

8.1.1.1 The Profile

The first requirement is for doctors or therapists to be aware of those aspects of the hypertensive patient's profile, which concatenate in case after case and constitute typicality. Likewise, they need to be aware of the *typicality* of provocative life events and situations. The main features are summarised as follows and appear repeatedly in case histories.

1. Ambivalence for Key Figures and Surrogates. Although emphasised in all the reports quoted, readers will note that ambivalence is common to all disorders described. This may sound ridiculous, but for each disorder, or group of disorders, the individual's response to these double feelings differs, e.g. in intensity and how much is conscious. What distinguishes hypertension from other disorders is that the anger is often so great as to be of murderous intensity. It is also conscious or close to consciousness. Van der Valk (personal communication), compared the anger of one of his patients to that of a "caged tiger". Another distinction is that loving behaviour from a parent has been minimal, which often leads to the parental figure being idealised and therefore made unattainable. This results in surrogates such as spouses being bound to fail. Another disorder in which anger is conscious or close to consciousness and is voluntarily controlled is pharyngeal spasm (Chap. 6), but here the anger is less intense and countervailing love greater.

2. Origins of Anger and Hostility. Findings which recur in the reports already mentioned are: (a) childhood experiences of death leading to hypertensive patient's *typically* overvalued fear of dying themselves, or of others close to them dying; (b) early experience of accidents or illness: parental alcoholism and violence, resulting in rage at actual or anticipated deprivation of infantile needs during adult life; (c) authoritarian, repressive parents or surrogates making heavy demands for compliance and low tolerance for expression of anger; (d) conflict with a sibling favoured by parents.

3. The Childhood Response to Ambivalent Feelings. Reports in the papers quoted, and our experience, show that many hypertensive patients' early response has been to act out their aggression with temper tantrums, violence to siblings, getting into fights at school and trouble with authority. Such behaviour leads to the frequent use by hypertensive patients of the term *black sheep of the family* to describe how they were regarded, or saw themselves in childhood.

4. Control. The above behaviour leads to further repression and rejection by authoritarian key figure(s). Penalties, actual or anticipated, or threats to the child's or adolescent's level of security, however tenuous, lead ultimately to a conscious decision to control their anger. This may occur after brushes with the police, actual or threatened retaliation, the need to hold a job down or fear of a spouse's withdrawal or desertion.

5. External Friendliness. Most observers have reported external friendliness from adult hypertensive patients, resulting from conscious control of their aggression, especially when they fear they may be, or have been, unfairly treated by an admired or loved person.

8.1.1.2 Typically Provocative Life Events

Reisser et al. [11] commented that onset or relapses of hypertension occurred "When individuals encounter life situations which evoke unresolved conflictual feelings which could not be adequately handled through normal channels of expression or behaviour." We and others have drawn attention to the following:

1. Deaths of key figures (transcripts F. D., S. Q.)
2. Dying key figures for whom the hypertensive subject has strong ambivalent feelings and where expressed anger is not possible without fear of killing (transcript R. K.)
3. Rejection/denigration by surrogate key figures replaying childhood experience, siblings, spouses, and people in authority, employers, police, doctors, nurses (transcripts K. A., W. A.)

8.1.1.3 Comments on Main Points of Profile

Dunbar said of hypertensive subjects:

> They have a problem in working off their rage on the one hand, and on the other of doing things well enough to be liked and admired ... they have a history of unresolved conflict with authority and try to *cope* by making themselves

important, but pent up resentment breaks through at awkward moments ... preoccupation with death and destruction is prominent in nightmares antedating the traumatic deaths of relatives and friends (case R. K.).

Binger et al. [7] found death or separation of a parent in 12 of 24 patients, and in 23 of 24 the finding of hypertension was first made after the death or illness of a relative or separation of parents.

Weiss and English [18] and Reiser et al. [11] support Saul [5] on the recurrent finding of control of emotions and fear of loss of control. Weiss and English use the term *throttled aggression* to describe the state of chronic rage. Reiser et al. [11] found "ambivalence to parental figures the predominant central conflict ... and we encountered in 11 of the 12 patients (that) ... conflictual attitudes towards siblings were important in 8."

In a paper given to the British Society for Psychosomatic Research in 1966 D. Paulley quoted remarks of three severely hypertensive patients she had studied in depth for 2 years:

"I try not to feel at all."
"I trained myself to cope."
"I had to be strong."
"I kept (anger) to myself."
"I did not answer back, I am afraid of loving but I am explosive inside."
"I am bottled up – I suffer inside anger – it's too terrible, it's like I am going to burst."
"I had to take the burden."
"I will blow my top and go off pop."

On Murderous Intensity of Anger. For example, a professional man with severe hypertension walked into the consulting room grinning and making jokes like a theatrical compère. When asked what he did on holidays he said he had not been able to take one for 25 years because his wife suffered from ozaena (atrophic rhinitis), the smell of which was so bad that staying in hotels or any social contact was impossible. She had refused to see a doctor because of a traumatic memory of tonsillectomy on the kitchen table as a child. Asked whether he had told her of his feelings regarding her intransigence he answered, still grinning broadly, "I am afraid that if I started I would not be able to stop." [murderous feelings]

Another example is Hambling's [12] patient who, faced with the possibility of damaging allegations by his sister-in-law at an inquest on his mother-in-law, said: "If I could do away with her without getting found out, I would do it tomorrow."

On "Black Sheep" and Rage at Preferred Sibling and Denigration

Mr. K. A., aged 52 presented with accelerated hypertension and encephalopathy. When cerebral function had sufficiently recovered he said he was the "black sheep" of his family and had never been able to please his strict and rejecting mother, whereas his devious younger brother, whom he had hated and attacked physically whenever the chance arose, had been indulged. Both brothers served in the Second World War; the patient came back although he had served in a parachute regiment whereas his brother, conscripted into the pay branch of the Army, had unfortunately been torpedoed and drowned. His mother told him that she wished he had been killed and not his brother. His long-standing rage at women found an outlet at this point when he discovered that his first wife had been unfaithful, and he divorced her. Accelerated hypertension had developed when his second wife, a nurse who stood for a "good mother" to him, invited her invalid mother to live with them. His rage at being displaced yet again became intense but had to be controlled because of fear of losing his wife.

8.1.2 Case Histories and Transcript

S. Q., a married woman of 42 was first diagnosed as hypertensive in 1973 (BP 220/120). Her father had died shortly before onset. In 1979 after hypotensive treatment from her doctor (oxprenolol and a diuretic), she was admitted with accelerated hypertension, left hemiparesis, papilloedema and BP 210/140. Nurses remarked that she was withdrawn. J.W.P. first saw her on a ward round and, being aware of the need to find out about any recent losses, he asked attendant staff except for the house physician and nurse to leave for a few minutes. After drawing the curtains and sitting on the bed he asked quietly: "Tell me about your family, sometimes this sort of thing comes on after the shock of losing people close to one." The patient lowered her head and began to weep. Comforted with an arm around her shoulders, she was encouraged with quiet words: "Take your time," and after weeping for a minute or two: "Perhaps you can now tell me what you are feeling."

P: I lost my eldest sister a month ago – we were very close – she was like a mother to me ... it was a terrible shock because she had kept the fact that she had heart trouble from me until a week before she died.

Later, out of the ward she told of her feelings of guilt that she had not done more, and because death had come suddenly she had not been able to "finish her business with her".

After this release of emotion the nurses reported that she was no longer withdrawn and would talk to them. She said that previously she had been too bitter and remorseful to do so. At subsequent joint interviews with her husband, she expressed fears that he worked too hard and might die too. [NB overvalued fear of death and anticipation of death]

Over the next few months she gradually accepted some of her feelings of guilt over her anger for her primary key figures and surrogates, such as her sister and husband. By the third interview after leaving hospital, eye contact between herself and her husband was seen for the first time. Her BP remained at 140/100 until a neurologist changed her drug regimen to a powerful β-blocker which made her feel as if she were "going to die", and BP rose temporarily to 200/120; it rose also briefly on the occasion of the anniversary of her sister's death. As with other patients with prolonged mourning reactions she was given annual appointments a week or two before the anniversary date. Her blood pressure was still 140/100 when last seen in 1983 (medication; methyldopa and a diuretic).

R. K., a man aged 49 who was found to be hypertensive in 1980 (220/150) when he complained of headaches for 6 months after visiting his mother in a distant hospital. She had become senile following a leg thrombosis, and he had found visits distressing; he had become especially depressed after his last visit. He said he was a man who always put 100% into everything he did, and his wife confirmed this [NB driving temperament and work addicted]. Memories of childhood included that his mother was strict, a dislike of his older brother who was favoured by the grandparents while he felt denigrated, and anger with his mother for not standing up for him. "She did as my grandparents told her ... My brother never wanted to know me, I used to fight him and although he was bigger than me, I could master him, and I only stopped bashing people when I met my wife [NB *black sheep,* overt childhood aggression and subsequent control and sibling envy] ... I wouldn't cry because I wouldn't let them see I was beaten."

His father had died in an accident when the patient was 14, "He was a great fellow – a soldier – rather strict, but he thought I was the neglected one. I was separated from him by the war." [NB death and loss].

At his marriage 33 years previously his mother had not wanted him to leave her and said she felt she would never see him again. Ever since he had felt guilty about leaving her. "Whenever I visit her she fingers her wedding ring which she has promised I should have at her death or if she gets old." He had never been able to accept it because it would have meant accepting her death. This illustrates anticipated mourning – ambivalent and dependent feelings for mother and grandmother, which were transferred to his wife as revealed by dreams he had a few weeks before he was seen, and which he had found very disturbing.

The first dream was of an incident years previously when he was courting his wife. They had gone to separate parties, but on his way home he met her with another boy. There was a row, but they made it up. However, he had found the dream terrifying, whereas the original event had not been. The second dream was a nightmare in which he and his wife had had intercourse, and she had then said: "The chap is in the garden." The latter nightmare had recurred regularly until he was seen, and terrified him because he felt he might kill the man in the garden or his wife, or both.

The first interview released a lot of emotion and tearful expression of fear of his anger. He was helped to see that his wife was standing for his mother for whom his anger had always been repressed. In this way he was able to admit his guilt about finding every possible reason for not visiting his mother, guilt that was increasing as her death approached. Seen a week later without any major change in his hypotensive drug regimen, his blood pressure was 120/85. The highest subsequent reading in the clinic or in his GP's surgery was 160/110. His mother died a month after he was first seen. At an interview 6 months after the first, he added that his trouble began when his mother took ill and "every time I was due to go and see her I couldn't, making excuses like the car wasn't working or had no petrol".

He said he now felt pretty good and had only had two of his bad dreams. "Talking has helped." Six months later, before returning him to his GP's care BP was 130/85, and he had had no more nightmares. At telephone follow-up 3 years later his GP said his BP was 120/90 and the only medication was Moducren, 1 tablet per day.

W. A., another man of 60, was referred with hypertension and right hemiparesis in 1974. For 10 years he had served on his local council with much dedication but a month previously had been voted off it. He felt this to be an injustice, and the night before admission had been to an emotional evening given by his friends and old colleagues in appreciation of his efforts.

His anger at this treatment by the electors was a replay of what he had experienced in childhood. An only child of restrictive, quarrelling parents who split up when he was 7, he spent the years between 7–13 with grandparents who were also authoritarian. Mother then remarried, but he found his stepfather cold and obsessional.

Externally friendly and jolly, he said that since his teens he had been a striver and a coper and had learned to control his anger at injustice which had got him into trouble as a boy. However, it was only just under the surface because he said that when Harold Wilson (Prime Minister) came on the TV screen he dared not stay in the room for fear of breaking the TV set.

F. D., a married woman whose blood pressure had been normal a year before her father's death, was found to be hypertensive 6 months after it. Her GP had given her methyldopa, propranolol and a diuretic, but despite this, accelerated hypertension developed shortly after the first anniversary of her father's death (BP 240/160). A registrar's comment in the notes in 1979 has a familiar ring, "Spoke to husband – no obvious friction, family upset, financial or otherwise. She has two sisters. One brother died 18 years ago." *Her father's death a year previously, the cause of her brother's death, which was suicide, and the patient's feelings about her father's death were not mentioned.* Had an adequate family history been taken or had the question been put: "Are any of the people you have lost much in your thoughts?", the registrar's findings would have been quite the opposite. This became evident on the ward round as the patient was unable to control her tears when asked about her feelings for her father and brother, both of whom she said were constantly in her thoughts. For reasons apparent in the following interview a day later, her father's death had reawakened powerfully destructive ambivalent feelings and guilt over her brother and her mother.

One day after ward round:

D: What sort of temperament do you think you've got? What sort of person are you?

P: Well, I am not a person who loses my temper – I have quite a lot of patience.

D: When you were younger, do you think you had less patience?

P: Yes, I was a bit of a tomboy because I was always with my brother. We were not allowed to mix with other children and had to come straight home from school.

D: Who was the stricter of your parents?

P: Oh, my mother, father went along with what she said. Well, my mother idolised my brother and my father and I got on very well when I was younger.

D: It sounds as though you didn't get on very well later on?

P: No, after he was left alone, he altered a bit. Whatever I did for him began to be compared unfavourably with my sister.

D: That was rather hurtful? (She lowers her head, remains silent.) What are you thinking? You were thinking something then?

P: (begins to weep) Well, he changed so much.

D: Tell me when you can; it's all right, take your time.

P: We were so close.

D: You and your brother?

P: In the war – I helped Dad – when my brother did come home he married and had two lovely girls, and he always wanted a son of his own and made a lot of my son – then there was jealousy over another woman (sobbing).

D: This is the hurt is it? You feel you should have done something when he stopped coming?

P: Yes ... in my bedroom one day I heard people talking outside – talking about him and this other woman – I hadn't seen him for a long time and one day I saw him in town, he passed me and wouldn't look at me and I ran after him ...

D: Didn't look at you?

P: ... went right by, but he promised he would come again. Then 10 days after it happened – they couldn't find him – he had drowned himself.

D: (Comforting patient with an arm round her shoulders) I felt it must have been something nasty (said gently, followed by pause during which patient weeps).

P: It was terrible because I think if I could only have talked to him perhaps I might – then after Dad died a year ago, I was turning out the house and found several diaries – he didn't leave a will ... he had had all Dad's money – there was nothing there at all.

D: When was it your Dad died?

P: Thirteen months ago

D: So then he went after your father for money?

P: A fortnight before he drowned himself – Dad had said he hadn't got any more then ...

D: I suppose he felt desperate because he felt perhaps he was going to be exposed by this woman's husband?

P: Yes.

D: How many years ago did you lose your brother?

P: Just over 14.

D: Possibly losing your father brought it back?

P: ... everything in connection with the farm he had sold, everything – all the papers were destroyed – everything, and he had been so deceitful.

D: You must have had very strong feelings perhaps when you discovered this deceit?

P: I felt terrible. There was so much we could have done for him – there was no need to deceive us ...

D: That was very hurtful, I think?

P: Yes.

D: You were angry?

P: I felt – I felt horrible really towards my father ...

D: You must have felt very angry.

P: I did, I resented everything.

D: And still do?

P: I do, after all the 58 years that I thought he was a marvellous man ...

D: He let you down?

P: It's an awful thing to swallow really.

D: And you also loved your brother but he really let you down too, to be truthful?

P: Yes, really.

D: And you felt guilty that you might have been able to help him if you could have gone to him sooner?

P: Well, I feel that if only he had talked with us.

D: You said earlier on, you are not a person to lose your temper.

P: I did.

D: But you must have had to contain a lot of this bitterness and anger?

P: Well, you know when he died we didn't know – he hadn't told us – anything at all until we went through my father's papers. My sister is more happy-go-lucky.

D: You said she shrugged this off more easily and she'll weep?

P: I don't.

D: I felt perhaps it was difficult for you to cry?

P: ... it is difficult really – I don't –.

D: When you were little, could you cry as a child, do you think?

P: Not really – I think because my brother told me off (laughs).

D: You had to be a tomboy and tough like him?

P: Yes.

Subsequent Course. The patient was seen 13 times over the next 6 years. During the last 3 years it was mutually agreed that the appointment should be annual but booked for the anniversary months of July and August, always her difficult time. Her BP has remained at 150/100 until the time of writing and medication is methyldopa and a diuretic.

At her last visit she said she no longer woke every day with feelings of dread, e.g. of her husband dying which had led her to seek an emergency interview in 1981, or of developing cancer herself. She still had a horror of death and avoided funerals but, "I face things better, am starting to drive again and have opened a joint bank account." She meant by this she had overcome some of her earlier fears of her husband dying and coping with widowhood.

Summary. Accelerated hypertension precipitated by loss. Management and acceptance by physician standing for key figure(s) of patient's rage and guilt.

8.2 Cardiac Arrhythmias

Increased electrophysiological excitability of heart muscle is felt to be the basis of most forms of cardiac arrhythmia. Accepted causes in the absence of underlying heart disease include toxins, such as nicotine, caffeine, alcohol and drugs, electrolytic imbalance, thyrotoxicosis and infections. To these such an eminent authority as White [19] added "forced respiration and breath holding" as a cause of ectopic beats, and "vomiting, exertion and emotion, excitement and fear" for auricular fibrillation.

The advent of cardiac monitoring, 24-h ECGs and resuscitation for malignant cardiac arrhythmias has greatly stimulated research into arrhythmias and sudden death occurring in both the damaged and the normal heart.

For research on emotional factors promoting arrhythmias the reader is offered the following references [20, 26] and for the behavioural approach [21, 27]. Most of these emphasise the critical importance of an individual's perception of an event or events. This is a refreshing change from previous studies which had concentrated on the external stresses of modern life.

Full understanding of the role of neural as opposed to hormonal or chemical links between brain and heart in the arrhythmias depends on further research, as does the possible effect of the long Q-T syndrome [28], and whether or not there is a genetically determined element.

The initial promise of β-adrenergic blockade in preventing malignant ectopic rhythms has been disappointing, as have been the benzodiazepenes and anti-depressant drugs. Orth Gomer [26] concludes: "A preferable approach is to use the patient's own resources, avoiding the inevitable side effects of most pharmacological therapy." This underliness the importance of the part to be played by various forms of psychological management, not only in the benign arrhythmias, but also in the malignant forms, e.g. ventricular fibrillation. The latter are particularly important in the acute phase of MI and its aftercare. This will be dealt with in detail in the section on IHD

8.2.1 Premature Contractions (Ectopic Beats)

When someone first becomes aware that his or her normal cardiac rhythm is disturbed, it usually occasions anxiety. Later, when accustomed to the irregularity, alarm may diminish.

Paul D. White [19] pointed out that half the people with premature contractions (ectopic beats) are unaware of them, a finding amply confirmed since by 24-h ECG recordings. Massie [29], Cook and Cashman [23] and Calvert et al. [30] found ventricular ectopic beats in 62% of 283 healthy, middle-aged men compared with 85% of patients with coronary heart disease.

Injudicious Medication. James Mackenzie [31] drew attention 70 years ago to the mismanagement of such patients "made miserable for life by vague prognostications of danger and who have been subjected to *prolonged or quite unnecessary treatment*" (p. 199). Unfortunately, his teaching was not sufficiently heeded, and many patients, especially the elderly, have suffered malaise and nausea as a result of their low tolerance for digitalis, while the injudicious use of β-blockers – "the modern scourge" – has caused unnecessary feelings of debility not only in the old but also in the not so old. β-Blockers favoured by some in the treatment of hypertension are also prescribed for post-MI patients with the intention of reducing cardiac load and irritability especially in patients with multiple ectopics. Post-MI debility is emotionally damaging enough without increasing it by unnecessary use of β-blocking adrenergic drugs. Where these have been prescribed, reducing or stopping them often results in improvement and a grateful patient.

8.2.1.1 Psychological Management

In all the disorders discussed in this book we have stressed the need for clinicians to think, listen and investigate at two levels simultaneously, the physical (soma) and emotional (psyche). This applies especially to a patient with numerous ectopic beats either in the presence of heart disease, e.g. after MI, or in an otherwise normal heart.

It is our experience that many patients with ectopic beats are also hyperventilators and that if they can reduce their hyperventilation (see transcript T.I), their ectopic beats remit or become less numerous. This accords with White, already quoted, on "forced respiration and breath holding", and also with the view of Lum [32] that "alarming dysrhythmias may occur" and with that of Gottlieb [33].

Patients who suffer angor animi after MI frequently hyperventilate, which in turn results in symptoms of chest pain, breathlessness, weakness, as well as in frequent ectopics, leading them to think they are about to have another MI. How to recognise this and its clinical management will be dealt with in the next section on coronary heart disease.

Psychological management of troublesome ectopics of which the patient is conscious and in the absence of organic heart disease or accepted toxic causes is as for hyperventilation syndrome (Chap. 7): re-education in breathing combined with a relaxation technique, and psychological help for guilt and fears of retribution.

Where hyperventilation is superimposed on top of organic heart disease, the same measures apply in addition to standard medical treatment, avoiding β-blockers if possible because the side effects of fatigue and postural hypotension cause some patients to panic and hyperventilate. It is also worth mentioning, as Heckscher did in 1942 [34], that oedematous lung bases in left ventricular failure also are a cause of hyperventilation and a factor to be considered in the mechanism of cardiac asthma.

8.2.2 Paroxysmal Auricular Tachycardia

This is the second, most common cause of patients presenting with disturbed cardiac rhythm. White [19] lists the same causes as those responsible for ectopic beats and considers it an allied condition. Although usually it is also associated with a normal heart, the incidence of associated heart disease was more common than when ectopic beats were the sole presentation.

Case histories of paroxysmal cardiac and effort syndrome quoted by Dunbar [8] are informative because they are detailed and include full biographical anamneses.

Not only were most of Dunbar's cases phobic about their symptoms, but reading between the lines it seems certain that most were hyperventilators. There is a striking similarity between her cases and those described in Chap. 7.

Most patients with paroxysmal auricular tachycardia respond to standard medication or tricks they find will stop it. Those patients in whom attacks are so frequent as to be a nuisance often do well with psychological management as described for hyperventilation.

8.2.3 Auricular Fibrillation and Flutter

These arrhythmias are usually due to disease of the heart such as mitral stenosis or ischaemia or to thyrotoxicosis. Classical physical signs of thyrotoxicosis are frequently absent in the elderly, and diagnosis may depend on sophisticated tests involving TRH-TSH. Psychological management is therefore likely to be less relevant than in the arrhythmias discussed previously.

Emotional stress combined with a command to overbreathe provoked auricular fibrillation in two middle-aged men, one a senior police officer, the other a managing director of a business firm, both authoritative characters, used to giving orders and being obeyed. Both were undergoing a pulmonary function test, which was carried out by a young, attractive, blond, female laboratory assistant. Both developed atrial fibrillation during the assessment of the maximum vital capacity, when this until now sweet, soft-voiced woman suddenly began to shout: "In – out – in – out," like a military drill master. They later confessed that this sudden and totally unexpected change in attitude from her came as an emotional shock, to which they could not react with angry protest or by telling her off because they realised that she was just doing her job.

8.3 Ischaemic Heart Disease

8.3.1 Psychological Management

To be effective *psychological management* depends on physicians understanding these patients' *typical* personality and vulnerability originating in their childhood upbringing, and on an understanding of certain social and cultural factors in contemporary Western societies, which enhance this vulnerability, e.g. lower male dominance over women and children. Physicians must recognise the patient's *typical* coping mechanisms, e.g. of work addiction. Type A behaviour is one aspect of this. They must also note *typically* provocative threats to the expected rewards for this ingrained rigid coping behaviour, leading the individual to feel cut down or "chopped", hopeless and exhausted, e.g. enforced retirement, redundancy or failed promotion. It is these coups or "chops" which antedate MIs by days or weeks in addition to the possession of type A behaviour.

Personality and Vulnerability. The mythological figure of Sisyphus typifies the feelings and attitudes of the 70% of people with coronary artery disease who have type A behaviour, and are the "willing horses" who characteristically are appointed foremen and are also disposed to DU. Sisyphus' task was forever to push a large stone uphill only to have it fall down again as he was about to get it to the top. Of the 30% of people with IHD who do not display these type A work-addicted characteristics, many will be predisposed to arterial disease because of diabetes or hyperlipidaemia, or have an AI disorder such as polyarteritis, giant cell arteritis [35] or scleroderma. Hypertension is another predisposing factor, but here there is an overlap with IHD in childhood emotional deprivation and subsequent compensatory striving to achieve. This has been described in the section on hypertension with illustrative case histories. It must also be remembered that MI and cardiac deaths from sudden ventricular arrhythmias may occur without evidence of coronary artery disease at autopsy. Currently, wider recognition that ventricular arrhythmias may be promoted by severe emotional stress has led to increased interest in their psychological management (see [21, 26, 36, 37]).

Research. For the past 25 years psychosomatically orientated research has been dominated by social studies and the measurement of and prevalence of type A behaviour, which was first reported by Friedman and Rosenman in 1959 [38]. The high incidence of IHD in Western societies has, during that period, been mostly attributed to social evils such as the rat race, the demands of the conveyer belt and the habit of excessive smoking. However, an article by Davies and Wilson in 1937 [73] describing behaviour and attitudes in DU sufferes shows that type A is not really as new as claimed. The main features of both reports are here placed side by side for convenience of comparison:

Type A (1959)

1. An intense and sustained drive to achieve
2. Profound inclination and eagerness to compete
3. Persistent desire for recognitions and advancement
4. Continuous involvement in multiple ... functions ... subject to deadlines
5. A propensity to accelerate the execution of many physical and mental functions
6. Extraordinary mental and physical alertness

DU (1937)

Peptic ulcer is common in the cities ... in the young and vigorous and those dynamic in outlook. The typical patient is a restless, active man of spare build ... is a man of aggressive alertness and readiness to tackle any job or any problem ... [and citing Robinson]. They display enthusiasm for any project in hand and execute their task with zeal and sometimes with a degree of excitability.

With the overlap of behaviour and emotional attitudes which have been regarded as significant in both IHD and DU, it was not surprising that follow-ups of a large series of DU patients showed that more than the expected number developed IHD [39, 40]. One of us (J. W. P.) reported personal experience of this crossed incidence in 1979 [41] as follows:

It is commonplace to find, on a single round of 20 male patients with assorted disorders, that out of the 5 or 6 with myocardial infarction, 3 or 4 have had previous DU, and on one occasion 3 patients in adjoining beds had their gastrectomy scars bearing testimony.

So many words have been written about type A that it is not possible to summarise them; however, some references to the alleged influence of social class on type A behaviour and therapy to reduce it have been included [48–50, 5]. Of many sociological and cultural studies on the incidence of IHD the following limited selection reveals how complex is the problem.

In an investigation [42] of IHD in 250000 employees of the Bell Telephone Company it was found that it was not the tycoons at the top who were most at risk but people in the middle echelons. The highest incidence in this group was among those who had had a college education but had not progressed beyond middle management. Possibly the greatest surprise was that personnel who had not had a college education but by sheer ability had reached top management, showed the same relative immunity from IHD as their college-educated, high-flying colleagues.

Then there was the low incidence of IHD among the Rosetans reported by Bruhn, Wolf, et al. [43]. This isolated group living in Pennsylvania came originally from southern Italy and had succeeded in keeping the customs of their homeland by isolating themselves and discouraging intermarriage. The males were accorded the same esteem as in southern Italy. While the women did most of the work, the men spent much of their time sitting, talking, eating, drinking and smoking, all considered by health educators as high risk factors in IHD! This finding lent support to Groen et al. [44] who had suggested that erosion of the traditional status of the male in Western societies had led some of them to a "work addiction" to try and compensate for loss of esteem, which they equate with loss of love.

Third came the finding that Japanese immigrants [45] to the United States of America continued to share the low incidence of IHD of their own homeland provided they maintained their native customs and way of life. However, Japanese who adopted American attitudes of life style experienced the same rate of IHD as their American neighbours; intermediate was a group who maintained some, but not all, of their old traditions, and had an incidence of IHD that was also intermediate. Assessment of dietetic fat, calories, smoking and alcohol in the three groups showed no material differences.

Next, studies of social class in the United Kingdom have shown a higher incidence of IHD in unskilled and manual workers [46]. The anti-smoking, healthy diet and inequality lobbies [47] have made much of this but have ignored childhood emotional deprivation. We have previously suggested [48] that the latter is more likely to be relevant to disease-prone behaviour of IHD and DU patients and do so again here.

Paradoxically, type A behaviour has been thought until recently to be less common in social classes 4 and 5 (manual workers), but reports [49, 50] now suggest that self-rating questionnaires are unsatisfactory in this group, and we think that questions about being on time for work and keenness at work, in a group whose work is often repetitive and dull, may be inappropriate and that the answers may be misleading. For example, many IDH patients from classes 4 and 5 regard their work only as a means of earning money or a place at which they can indulge in trade union or political activity. Only when questioned: "What do you do with your spare time?" would come the type A answer: "You must be joking, I don't have any spare time." One such man looked after thirteen gardens, another mended all his neighbours' cars, others made violins, bred caged birds or were heavily involved in the "black economy".

What Can Be Learned from This? There appears to be a clear clinical relationship as well from the surveys between type A behaviour and the incidence of IHD (for example, see transcripts G. N., T. I., R. K., L. Q.). Yet by no means everyone with type A behaviour develops IHD. Other factors such as genetic disposition or protective cultural factors are probably influential. After all, Japanese people work harder than most but have a low incidence of IHD. It seems likely that over the past 25 years external social factors, relevant though some may be, have received too much attention, and that too little has been given to the childhood background which programmes all subsequent behaviour, including excessive application to work, amongst those men and women who ultimaltely develop IHD when the compensation of work and achievement is frustrated.

Why This Lack of Inquisitiveness? Considering the millions of words written about type A behaviour and the money spent on researching it, the lack of interest in the possible motivating factors in childhood is astonishing because it is generally accepted that it is then that the good and bad habits of a lifetime are laid down. The reason for this seems to lie in the wind of antipathy to psychodynamic concepts and mechanisms which began to blow about 1960 and is still blowing [51]. Wittkower and later Kubie [52] felt that the baby had been thrown out with the bath water. Without some understanding of the psychopathology and psychodynamics of patients with IHD, as with other psychosomatic disorders, a doctor trying to treat them effectively is rather like a navigator without a compass or radar.

Typical Childhood Background. The most comprehensive description of the *typical* early cnvironmcnt is probably still that of Mittelmann and Wolff [53] for the related disorder DU (Chap. 6). Groen [54, 55] observed that the background of behaviour and conflicts in IHD was similar to that of DU and that both disorders shared the same double level conflict. "Most patients described their youth as having been filled with hard work ... and little time for play and cosiness ... The patients had often had severe conflicts with their fathers." Groen's co-author, Treurniet [44], observed that patients tended to compensate for feelings of dependency by hard work, needing to dominate those around them, some by being compulsively sexually hyperactive. He considered that such promiscuous behaviour had a pseudomasculine quality. (See the case history T. I. and also what Cassem and Hackett [56] said about the psychological management of inappropriate behaviour by some patients towards nurses after MI.)

An earlier article by Arlow [57] also portrayed the coronary patients' psychopathology very clearly. "The incomplete, spurious identification of the patients with their fathers, leading to overcompensatory mechanisms of defence, such as compulsive competitiveness and subsequent traumatic effects of failure ..." The case histories he quoted showed how close in time failure preceded coronary occlusion. Another valuable contribution on the topic was made by Dreyfuss [58].

Other Influences: The Protestant Work Ethic, Unemployment. Apart from denigratory parents (see transcript L. Q.) cultural influences are likely to play a part in child rearing through pressure towards achievement and work, for example, Mr. G. N. His father spent 2 years in Canada because of unemployment in the 1930s. Another patient's father, who was a stickler for work himself and never praised his son, had previously been an out-of-work miner. We referred in 1979 [41] to the combination of a powerful Protestant work ethic with long-standing high unemployment as a feature of west central Scotland, an area with the highest incidence of DU in the United Kingdom and now the highest incidence of IHD in the world.

Parental Death or Divorce. Should either parental death or divorce occur before a child reaches adolescence, it usually means being brought up by a step-parent or an elder sibling. While material care may be good, emotional warmth is often lacking [48]. It is not only clinicians treating IHD who should be aware of provocative factors in childhood, but also research workers studying type A behaviour and sociologists assessing cultural stresses, because these may only be provocative when they reawaken sensitivities and attitudes acquired in childhood.

8.3.1.1 Prophylaxis

Because patterns of behaviour predisposing to IHD are established long before the clinical presentation, in theory at least prevention might be possible. For example, anything that might reduce emotional deprivation of the most exposed members of a sibship would be expected to pay dividends, not only in the prevention of IHD, but of other psychosomatic disorders, neuroses and delinquency. It would involve education of potential parents about the destructive effects of broken marriages and one-parent families, and/or the rejection of a child for any reason, some of which we have already listed. Unbalanced indoctrination towards high performance in a world where there is no longer enough work to go round may soon be seen as undesirable. Potential parents should be helped to understand that while ambition for their children to do well is both right and biologically necessary, pressure, albeit unconscious, on their children to make up for what they feel were their own failures at school, is still common and undesirable. Children need to feel that they are loved for themselves and not only for what they do. This requires that in their upbringing rewards have a higher place than punishment or undue criticism.

Prophylaxis Shortly Before Infarction. Symptoms of tiredness, exhaustion and depression a few days or weeks before a patient develops an MI have been noted by a number of clinicians. An example of this is the case of G. N. (see transcript). Perhaps the most common view is that the exhaustion is secondary to the IHD, possibly enhanced by hyperventilation [44, 59, 21], but we and others [55, 44, 41] suspect that it is due to psychological entrapment without possible exit, the result of the individual's realisation that he or she lacks coping mechanisms other than work and type A hyperactivity when these compensations are finally blocked or rejected. Greene et al. [60], interviewing close relatives of 54 victims, mostly dying of IHD, reported that 76% of them were considered to have been depressed for weeks or months before the sudden death, apparently precipitated by the definitive type of life events we and others have described (next section).

It has been suggested [61, 26] that if diagnosis of impending MI could be made during the prodromal phase of exhaustion, then the attack itself might be staved off by first identifying the threatening life event and then offering social support and psychological insight. Alternatively, as Freeman and Nixon have suggested [62] rehabilitation and re-education in breathing for those who are hyperventilators might be preferable to the current overdependence on drugs and β-blockers, (see, Chap. 7 for hyperventilation and this chapter on arrhythmias).

However, even if proved effective in reducing the risk of re-infarction, such measures would seem less applicable to the first attack because people with the typical attitudes described are very unlikely to heed the warning symptoms and seek help or listen to their spouse.

8.3.2 Psychological Management After Infarction

Pioneering work was carried out by members of the Psychosomatic Unit at Ulm [63]. They were trained both as internists and psychotherapists and were trusted by their cardiological colleagues to carry out psychologically orientated interviews in the Coronary Care Unit. Initial fears that this might precipitate relapse of dangerous arrhythmias were found to be groundless, a finding confirmed by Cassem and Hackett [56], Pelser [64] and others.

We recall MI patients whose recurrent arrhythmias and cardiac arrests continued to frustrate all efforts by medical staff to control them with drugs until they were encouraged and enabled to talk. One such patient, and electronic engineer, initially all smiles and denial, started to weep within a few minutes, as he told of his denigrating father whom he could never please despite substantial achievement, and his recent dismissal without a word of thanks after 20 years of devoted service by an employer whom he had always regarded as the "good father" he had never had. After this emotional interview in the ICU the patient had no more ectopics and no further cardiac arrests, and made an uninterrupted recovery.

Another reason why patients need to be encouraged early to talk about feelings and any emotional tensions in the days or weeks prior to the MI is that in as little as 48 h their *typical* defence of denial and need to appear strong takes over from the openness shown in the first 24 h when they are still anxious and defenceless. By the 3rd day it is usual for them to say: "I am a fraud, doctor; when may I go home?" They are then likely to say that anything said previously, really meant nothing or was untrue.

Such manifestations of denial conceal deep anxiety for the future, the most important being: "Am I going to be able to work? Am I going to be able to keep my job? Am I going to be half a man? Is it going to affect my sex life?" See earlier comments about how important their masculinity is to these male patients.

Nursing and medical staff should be helped to understand how damaging the casual remark such as: "You will have to think about changing your job" can be to a stevedore shortly after a MI. This may be true, but the patient will need time to be able to accept it, with the support of family and peers, perhaps in a rehabilitation group.

Nurses also need to be warned about what Cassem and Hackett [56] termed inappropriate behaviour. This leads to male patients who fear loss of masculinity trying to reassure themselves by sexual innuendoes which female nurses, understandably, find tiresome. Rather than the cutting reply, it is reasonable to suggest to these nurses an alternative and less damaging response such as: "Oh, you naughty boy!"

Patients after MIs are usually terrified of another attack and sometimes lie like graven images waiting for the sword of Damocles to strike again. They particularly fear an attack during sleep, and for this reason fight to remain awake, however heavily sedated. This can be damaging and exhausting, and psychological management calls for clinicians to recognise it and inform their MI patients that they need not worry about a relapse during sleep because this does not happen. Fortunately, this assurance is also true.

Clinicians should recognise hyperventilation in this phase. It frequently results in ectopic beats, especially during visiting hours and ward rounds, which alarm both the patients, their relatives, nurses and junior doctors, and which calls for reassurance, explanation and re-education in relaxed abdominal breathing, using the diaphragm rather than the thorax, by a competent physiotherapist.

After the First Few Days. As patients begin to move about, they are frequently surprised and frightened when they feel so physically weak. It is useful to warn them about this beforehand, and that it will not last long. In some centres they may have the chance of joining a rehabilitation group under skilled supervision, in which they will learn through graduated exercise that their tolerance often returns to what it was before their MI. Where a rehabilitation group is not available, patients may initially carry out a few simple exercises while their GP watches, takes their pulse, etc., and then practise them for longer periods on their own.

This is also the time to encourage patients to talk more about their work or domestic problems and about previously unexpressed childhood difficulties with parents or other key figures, pointing to likely parallels in their feelings for frustration experienced in the days or weeks prior to the MI. The transcript of G. N. tells of his hopelessness and frustration; although exhausted, he would force himself to go out in the evenings to avoid telephoned accusations from his aunts that he was neglecting his mother, who had always refused to do what he suggested in any case. This domestic stress coincided with lack of support at work from his seniors, resulting in this very conscientious man having to let down an old customer and friend. The last straw was his car, and his chest pain came on as his long pent-up anger and frustration reached a climax with this inanimate object.

How Much Advice?. Doctors should resist the temptation to tell MI patients *not* to overdo things because they are unable to change their lifelong coping mechanisms quickly. Instead, psychological management, individually or in groups, should be designed to help them change gradually and then to make their own decisions as far as possible free from hitherto unconscious emotional drives.

One useful analogy is that of the *diversion* of tide and waves by building groynes at *angles* leading the sea to build up its own shingle banks rather than *straight* walls, however powerfully constructed, which the sea usually undermines and destroys.

Management of Spouse's Anxiety and Guilt. Spouses and children of work-addicted people have often felt, and sometimes expressed, their annoyance at always seeming to come second to work, politics, trade unionism, philandering or even golf. Following the MI with its imminence of death, such ambivalent feelings result in guilt and exaggerated overconcern. This is often evident when a patient's every movement evokes a spouse's anxious question to the nurse or physician, for example: "Do you think his (or her) colour is all right?" The patient usually gives a sickly grin but dares not ask for the visits to be shorter. Doctors can help here by suggesting that shorter visits are better as they place less of a load on both the patient and visitor, the exception being relatives coming from a distance. Doctors need to control the annoyance they may feel about a spouse's tiresome behaviour and resist being punitive by restricting visits. Instead spouses should be allowed to express their feelings in privacy, and by accepting their overconcern and guilt and empathising with their resentment at the patient's previous behaviour, damaging tensions around the bed can be greatly reduced.

Three examples from a great many are offered. A patient (T. I.) when asked how he had been sleeping prior to his attack said: "Rather poorly for 2 years." Pressed for reasons, he said that work had been heavy, and he had rarely been able to leave his office before 11 p.m. His wife appeared extremely anxious and was seen alone in the manner already suggested. Regarding her husband's overwork she said that he had resented her bringing her mother to live with them 2 years before. He had always demanded and had had all her attention prior to that. She felt that his MI might have been provoked by questions she had put to him a week before it had occurred. The questions related to stubs she had found in his pockets of cheques paid to jewellers, and then she understood why he had been spending long hours at his office with his secretary instead of coming home. In other words, she had administered the coup, and the outlet offered by his secretary for this vulnerable man's masculinity and need for recognition had been blocked.

Another man (L. Q.), the only one of six brothers to succeed academically and leave his father's farm, had never been forgiven for doing so by his father. For years, in one of the armed services, he had worked far beyond the call of duty in voluntary activity, by which he obtained some of the esteem (love) to compensate a little for that which he had not received in his childhood. However, the price he had to pay for his industry was a DU which ultimately led to him being invalided out. He then took a degree in management and was doing well as a member of a team at an institution whose job was to organise residential seminars and courses. His hard work was appreciated by all, and he was told that he was in line for promotion, which led him to redouble his efforts. His wife empathised with him but nevertheless became rather lonely in the evenings and took up some social work. To avoid feeling distanced from her, husband joined her in this, leaving him no rest at all. A week before his MI he heard that a less able colleague, who had been currying favour with the boss, had been told he was to be given the promotion the patient had been working for. That, in his case, was the coup, leaving him feeling hopeless and unable to win, in the same way as he had always felt with his father.

A third example (R. K.) is a man whose intense pride in his own efficiency was cast in doubt when an aircraft, for the maintenance of which he was responsible, crashed. Rumours circulated that the crash was due to negligent maintenance, and his MI occurred 3 days later. During recovery he said he did not want his condition discussed with his wife because he did not want her worried (characteristic show of independence [44]). He also said that if he was not going to be fit enough to play golf, he would rather die. It was suggested that his golf must mean a lot to him, and he said he was a scratch golfer and represented his service. His recovery was greatly assisted when his Commanding Officer came to tell him that the inquiry revealed that the crash had been due to pilot error.

Convalescence. It has been fashionable for some time in various quarters to attribute slowness in recovery from illness or operations to *illness behaviour,* a term coined by Mechanic (Chap. 2). Yet advocates of this concept seem more interested in the concept itself than in the quite simple causes apparent to most clinicians, for example, factors such as a trade union official or friend encouraging a patient to put in for compensation, or the overanxious spouse discouraging any physical activity, including sex, laced with old wives' tales. The most important factor is the sensitisation of a patient in childhood to exaggerated parental responses to trivial illnesses, doctors, or even visits. On the other hand, a child's fear of illness can be only too real when a parent is suddenly taken away to hospital or when memories of childhood are coloured by visits of doctors and nurses and a parent always ill. Another factor in Western societies are the actions and warnings of some health educationists and others who have a vested interest in creating fear in their listeners, particularly the media who also create unnecessary anxiety and introspection. These are some of the factors which retard recovery from MI and other disorders. Doctors who understand some of these adverse influences can do much to defeat them [64].

Rehabilitation Groups. The quality of life of survivors from MI has been improved through rehabilitation groups, but to date membership has not apparently reduced the rate of re-infarction. Our own experience is that such patients gain more from the support and example of their peers in the group than from the graduated exercises alone. The most careful assessment of rehabilitation groups, with and without biofeedback reinforcement to try and reduce type A behaviour has been reported by Price and Friedman et al. [65].

Rehabilitation Groups for Spouses. There is growing evidence that rehabilitation for spouses are helpful, and our experience supports this, particularly when they are led by a competent group leader with some understanding of psychodynamics. However, as such activities must compete for funds increasingly stretched by other demands, it is likely to be some time before they reach their maximum potential. A comprehensive account has been written of such work by Adsett and Bruhn [66].

8.3.3 Transcript

Mr. G. N. aged 56, had migraine in 1940, DU in 1945, vagotomy in 1976 and MI in 1980

First interview for migraine (1975):
P: ... right side of face went all blurred – I sort of covered one eye ...
D: You made a career in the RAF and you married, at what age?
P: At 24.
D: How did that go initially?

P: Very well for about 10 years, then, unbeknown to me, she began having various affairs.

D: That was the time you first got your ulcer. Are you the sort of chap who can let your work go?

P: No, no I can't; it's impossible, I try very hard. I always feel guilty if something is not done.

D: Do you know where that started in your life?

P: Not really, unless it was when I first became an NCO in the Air Force.

D: As a child were you expected to be tidy or on time for things, or do things properly?

P: Yes, I was expected to be on time.

D: Your father was rather a particular chap, a draughtsman, wasn't he?

P: Yes.

D: Do you think he was fussy about his job or not?

P: Yes, very fussy about his job. It *had* to be right; everything *had* to be right.

D: The attitude to work then was rather different to what it is today, perhaps because of the slump and the unemployment of the 1930s.

P: That's true. In fact he did go to Canada when I was about 2–3 years old to try and find work.

D: How long was he away?

P: About 2 years – a very short time really.

D: What about the clock?

P: Five minutes early rather than 5 min late, and of course I had been late this past week at work on two or three mornings simply because of hold-ups of traffic.

D: Yes?

P: … I don't take it out on the traffic itself or the car; I just sort of get upset when I do get to work – geared up.

D: Of course, this punctuality was a feature of your mother – it was important to her?

P: Yes, it was indeed, and in the services as well; it was always. You'd never be late for a parade.

D: No. So, what sort of job are you doing now?

P: Service manager with an engineering company.

D: Is it a demanding job?

P: It is indeed, there are so many aspects to the job.

D: Do you take a lot of the work home with you?

P: I do, yes.

Attended clinic in October 1967 alone, saying the tensions between himself and his wife were worse, which was why she had not come.

Following the case up in 1980 it was discovered that he had recently suffered a MI, thereby fulfilling psychosomatic expectations (DU to MI). He was offered a further follow-up appointment, which he gladly accepted, and was accompanied by his wife.

D: I heard you had had a vagotomy.

P: That was in 1976.

D: With regard to the heart attack, did you have any indication that you might get one, I mean had you had any chest pain or –?

P: Nothing at all, it just came completely out of the blue. I was a little late coming from work, something wrong with the car (speaking rapidly) – I ran to the car, I had a little plate to put on the car – to get about – in a bit of a hurry – the screw had fallen out so I had to run back to the warehouse, got the wrong one, had to run back again and they had locked the back door so I had to run round the front – it was just, you know, a lot of circumstances. (voice angry – frustrated)

D: Yes.

P: By the time I got back to the car, the pain caught me.

D: Yes?

P: I just sat there with the window open, and then I went and picked up my wife, and the pain became worse. It had sort of come down the arms by then; the lack of oxygen made me feel terrible.

D: Surely, and you went to the hospital. I remember you were always a pretty acitve chap, and your description of running around and getting things out of the car fits in with your temperament.

P: Yes, well now I've slowed down.

D: Have you?

P: Oh yes, if I'm late, I just walk.

D: You don't hurry like you did?

P: No.

D: Do you find that difficult?

P: Yes, very. I start up and have to stop again.

D: Yes?

P: Fortunately, we are now under new management. You could never telephone the old management to get backing for a decision; make it yourself, he said. I had been going on all day, then at 4:40 when I went to look for someone to help this lady and gentleman, old customers of ours, I didn't get any help from the management at all.

D: Very irritating.

P: Yes, especially if you are trying to help a customer, and of course I finished up in hospital.

D: Things didn't go the way they should have gone; at any rate, you've got a better set up now, more appreciative, too.

P: Yes.

D: Your mother was alive, in the north of Scotland when I last saw you.

P: She's still alive but she's in a home now.

D: She used to worry you a bit – she had good neighbours but would not accept help.

P: Yes, that's right. Well, things got worse in the past 2 years. It became very worrying because my aunt used to ring me up and say she's doing this or that, and ask when are you going to do something about it.

D: So you had this additional worry going on, when did that cease?

D: After my heart attack. They kept ringing me up. When they rang me up after my heart attack, my wife got on the phone to them.

P: That was good. She must understand some of the pressures you have been under?

D: Yes.

D: Good. Is there anything else you would like to say? I have a feeling it might be worthwhile asking your wife what she thinks of your progress, if she would like to come in.

P: Yes, sure. [Patient brings wife in.]

D: Your husband was getting badgered a bit by telephone calls?

W: Yes, he was. I said: "Do you really want me to answer this one", but I knew if I did, it would be: "You know I have to …" There was also a lot of pressure from work – I think that triggered that heart attack as well.

D: What do you feel about that work pressure he has told me a little bit about?

W: I mean he would come home and talk to me and I would let him because I … every day … and he would be sitting there, and I could see he was mentally fatigued, and *that* is worse than physical, I think.

D: Yes?

W: He felt frustration at work when he couldn't get an answer.

D: Yes, he had nobody to help him, you know, which he should have had.

W: He's got a different manager now.

D: Well, prior to the heart attack you had had the pressures at work and pressure over your mother. I wonder which you feel was the major pressure at that time?

P: Work I would think. I was able to, I think, put my mother out of my mind at work – the only time I used to find I could. I wouldn't even think about it. But at home the telephone would ring, and it would by my aunt – whenever I came off that telephone after I had talked with her I would be upset. She used to ring every Saturday because – they were getting old –they were 20–30 odd miles away from my mother and I was 500 miles away.

D: The indications were you could do more, I presume?

P: Yes.

D: But you couldn't?

P: How can you?

W: Before Christmas he wasn't feeling very well and I kept worrying then and I said: "Go to the doctor and tell him *how tired* you feel." I said it was not natural because I knew the symptoms actually were not like him, and the doctor sent him for a blood test ... I think if he had had treatment or got time off, I don't know if it would have made any difference, but that is when I answered his auntie, and I got so uptight with her because I said I knew George was not well. Then he got a letter saying there could be redundancies, and then I had a nasty letter from his aunt which at first I hid from him.

D: How often did his aunt phone him up?

P: About once a week, I think.

W: But not any more. That is when she wrote this nasty letter.

D: When you have worries in the family do you often unconsciously go and work a bit harder to keep the worries at bay?

W: Yes.

D: But then, unconsciously, you find yourself doing more without realising it?

P: I didn't want to stay in, did I? I didn't want to stay in in the evenings. No – I take the easy way out – probably I feared the telephone ringing and it being my auntie again.

D: Yes – I understand it – you couldn't resolve that problem. How long have you been feeling that you didn't want to be sitting at home – you wanted to be out?

P: ... about 6 weeks before my heart attack.

D: Six weeks – so you had been pushing yourself?

P: Yes – I used to have a sleep when I came in, didn't I? That was quite new, and I used to sit after tea in a chair and go to sleep, didn't I?

W: Oh yes.

P: And wake up and then want to go out.

W: You were especially tired then – worn out.

P: I used to sleep at lunch time as well.

D: So you then went out to the bowling and to see friends?

P: Yes, some times go up and watch the bowling – things like that.

D: Yes – just to find something to do to avoid your auntie's telephone calls.

Summary. This patient illustrates (a) syndrome shifts from migraine to DU to MI; (b) type A personality common to DU and IHD as we have described, and perfectionism in migraine; (c) exhaustion prior to MI as his work addicted coping behaviour failed to attain rewards at work and his inability to cope with the demands and accusations of his aunt over his mother; (d) the final coup or "chop" came in the two nasty letters, one from the aunt and the other from the employers warning of redundancy, culminating with being put down by his employer the evening before his attack.

8.4 Raynaud's Phenomenon

This is a genuinely psychosomatic disorder whether present on its own or when associated with migraine (Chap. 9). AI disease, such as SLE, scleroderma, RA and MCT may also present with Raynaud's phenomenon. The form of psychological management which benefits these disorders in general has been described in Chap. 10, but we have no clear evidence that it relieves patients' symptoms of Raynaud's phenomenon once established.

Raynaud's Phenomenon Not Associated with an Autoimmune Disorder. Research done on the psychopathogenesis of this form of the disorder has often been impressive [67–69]. A questionnaire revealed that approximately 50% with migrainous headaches had suffered from Raynaud's phenomenon [70]. Drugs such as ergotamine and β-adrenoreceptor antagonists being taken for migraine did not appear to be responsible for the incidence of Raynaud's although they tended to increase its severity. It has also been suggested that hemicrania (migraine) and Raynaud's phenomenon may be manifestations of the same disease [71].

We have not treated enough of these patients to be able to recommend any particular form of psychological management, but suggest it would be reasonable to try the same form of group therapy and relaxation found to be effective for 80% of patients with migraine, particularly as autogenic and/or biofeedback training has been reported by Freedman et al. [72] to be of some benefit.

References

1. Brod J (1971) The influence of higher nervous processes induced by psychological environment on the development of essential hypertension. In: Levi L (ed) Society, stress and disease, vol 1. Oxford University Press, London, pp 312–323
2. Dahl KL, Heine M, Tassinari L (1962) Effects of chronic excess salt ingestion. Evidence of genetic factors part in susceptibility to experimental hypertension. J Exp Med 115:1173–1190
3. Dahl LK, Heine M, Tassinari L (1964) Effects of chronic excess of salt ingestion on vascular reactivity in two strains of rats with opposite genetic susceptibility to experimental hypertension. Circulation [Suppl] 11:11–12
4. Groen JJ, Welner A, Ben-Ishay D (1970) Exploratory and aggressive behaviour in rats with and without experimental hypertension. Psychother Psychosom 18:326–331
5. Saul L (1939) Hostility in cases of essential hypertension. Psychosom Med 1:153–161
6. Alexander F (1939) Emotional factors in essential hypertension. Psychosom Med 1:175–179
7. Binger AL, Ackerman NW, Cohn AE, Schroeder HA, Steel JH (1945) Personality in arterial hypertension. American Society for Research on Psychosomatic Problems, New York (Psychosomatic medicine monographs)
8. Dunbar F (1943) Psychosomatic diagnosis. Hoeber, New York
9. Reiser MF, Ferris EB (1947) Clinical and experimental observations on the lability and range of blood pressure in essential hypertension (abstract). J Clin Invest 26:1194–1204
10. Wolf S, Pfeiffer JB, Ripley HS, Winter OS, Wolff HG (1948) Hypertension as a reaction pattern to stress; summary of experimental data on variations in blood pressure and renal blood flow. Ann Intern Med 29:1056–1076
11. Reiser MF, Rosenbaum M, Ferris EB (1951) Psychological mechanisms in malignant hypertension. Psychosom Med 13:147–159
12. Hambling J (1959) Essential Hypertension. In: The nature of stress disorder. Hutchinson, London, pp 17–40
13. Groen JJ, Van der Valk JM, Welner A, Ben-Ishay D (1971) Psychological factors in the pathogenesis of essential hypertension. Psychother Psychosom 19:1–26

14. Steptoe A, Melville D, Ross A (1984) Behavioural response, cardiovascular reactivity and essential hypertension. Psychosom Med 46:33–38
15. Weiner H (1977) The psychobiology of human disease. Elsevier, New York.
16. Miller NE (1969) Learning of visceral and glandular responses. Science 153:434–454
17. Patel C, Marmot MG, Terry DJ (1981) Controlled trial of biofeedback – aided behavioural methods in reducing mild hypertension. Br Med 282:2005–2008
18. Weiss E, English OS (1949) Psychosomatic Medicine. Saunders, Philadelphia
19. White PD (1937) Heart disease, 2nd edi. Macmillan, New York, pp 857–:887
20. Lown B, Desilva RA, Reich P, Murawski BJ (1980) Psycho-physiological factors in sudden cardiac death. Am J Psychiat 137:11:1325–1335
21. Lown B (1982) Mental stress, arrhythmias and sudden death (editorial). Am J Med 72:177–180
22. Theorrell T (1980) Live events and manifestations of ischaemic heart disease. Psychother Psychosom 34:135–148
23. Cook TC, Cashman PMM (1982) Stress and ectopic beats in ships' pilots. J Psychosom Res 26:559–569
24. Reich P (1985) Psychological predisposition of life threatening arrhythmias. Annu Res Med 36:397–405
25. Kornfield DS (1980) The intensive care until in adults: coronary care and general medical/surgical. Adv Psychosom Med 10:1–29
26. Orth Gomer K (1982) Evidence of psychological influence on the formation of ventricular arrhythmias: implications for preventive therapy. Acta Nerv Super (Praha) 2 [Suppl 3]:498–503
27. Millar NE, Dworkin BR (1977) Effects of learning on visceral functions – biofeedback. N Eng J Med 296:1274–1278
28. Schwartz PJ (1980) The long Q-T syndrome. In: Kulbertus HE, Welleus HJJ (eds) Sudden Death. Martinus Nijhoff, The Hague
29. Massie E (1970) Palpitation and tachycardia in signs and symptoms, 5th ed. Lippincott, Philadelphia
30. Calvert A, Lown B, Gorlin R (1977) Ventricular premature beats and anatomically deferred coronary disease. Am J Cardiol 39:627–633
31. Mackenzie J (1913) The extra systole. In: Disease of the heart, 3rd edn. Frowde London, p 199
32. Lum LC (1975) Hyperventilation: the tip of the iceberg. J Psychosom Res 19:375–383
33. Gottlieb B (1969) Non-organic disease in medical outpatients. Med Update 1:917–922
34. Heckscher H (1942) Emphysema of the lungs and its significance to relapsing bronchitis, cardiac and respiratory neuroses and bronchial asthma. Munksgaard, Copenhagen
35. Paulley JW (1980) Coronary ischaemia and occlusion in giant cell (temporal) arteritis. Acta Med Scand 208:257–263
36. Haughey BP, Brasure J, Moloney MC, Saxon G (1984) The relationship between stressful life events and electrocardiogram abnormalities. Heart Lung 13:405–410
37. Engel GL (1976) Psychological factors in instantaneous cardiac death. N Eng J Med 294:664–665
38. Friedman M, Rosenman RH (1959) Association of specific overt behaviour pattern with blood and cardio-vascular findings. JAMA 169:96–106
39. Watkinson G (1956) Relation of chronic peptic ulcer to coronary sclerosis. Gastroenterologia 85:201–204
40. Watkinson G (1958) Relation of chronic peptic ulcer to coronary sclerosis. Gastroenterologia 89:292–301
41. Paulley JW (1979) Ulcers, heart disease, and type A behaviour. Lancet 2:1238
42. Hinkle LE, Whitney LH, Lehman EW et al. (1968) Occupation, education and coronary disease. Science 161:238–246

43. Bruhn JG, Chandler R, Miller MC, Wolf S, Lynn TN (1966) Social aspects of coronary heart disease in two adjacent ethnically different communities. Am J Public Health 56:1493–1506

44. Groen J, Van der Valk JM, Treuniet N, von Heijningen HK, Pelser HE, Wilde GJS (1965) Acute myocardial infarct, a psychosomatic study (Summary in English). Bohn, Haarlem

45. Marmot MG (1983) Stress, social and cultural variables in heart disease. J Psychosom Res 27:377–384

46. Marmot MG, Mcdowell ME (1986) Mortality decline and unlearning social inequalities. Lancet 2:274–276

47. Working Group on Inequalities in Health (1980) Black report. DHSS, London

48. Paulley JW (1975) Cultural influences on the incidence and pattern of disease. Psychother Psychosom 26:2–11

49. Matthews KA (1982) Psychological perspectives on the Type A behaviour pattern. Psychol Bull 91:293–323

50. Byrne DG, Rosenman RH, Schiller E, Chesney MA (1985) Consistency and variation among instruments purporting to measure Type A behaviour pattern. Psychosom Med 47:242–261

51 Wittkower ED (1960) Twenty years of North American psychosomatic medicine. Psychosom Med 22:308–316

52. Kubie LS (1971) The retreat from patients. Arch Gen Psychiatry 24:98–106

53. Mittelmann B, Wolff HG (1942) The emotions and duodenal functions. Experimental studies on patients with gastritis, duodenitis and peptic ulcer. Psychosom Med 4.5–243

54. Groen JJ (1951) Emotional factors in the etiology of internal disease. J M Sinai Hosp NY 18:71–89

55. Van der Valk JM, Groen JJ (1967) Personality structure and conflict situation in patients with myocardial infarction. J Psychosom Res 11:41–46

56. Cassem NH, Hackett TP (1971) Psychiatric consultation in a coronary care unit. Ann Intern Med 75:9:14

57. Arlow JA (1945) Identification mechanisms in coronary occlusion. Psychosom Med 7:195–209

58. Dreyfuss F (1959) Role of emotional stress preceding coronary occlusion. Am J Cardiol 3 [5]:590–596

59. Engel GL (1971) Sudden and rapid death during psychological stress. Ann Intern Med 74:771–782

60. Greene WA, Moss AJ, Goldstein S (1974) Delay, denial and death in coronary heart disease. In: Elliott RL (ed) Stress and the heart. Futura, New York, pp 143–162

61. Nixon PGF (1976) The human function curve: with special reference to cardiovascular disorder. Practitioner 217:765–770, 935–944

62. Freeman LJ, Nixon PGF (1985) Chest pain and the hyperventilation syndrome. Postgrad Med J 61:957–961

63. Karstens R, Kohle K, Ohlmier D, Weidlich S (1970) A multidisciplinary approach for the assessment of psychodynamic factors in young adults with acute myocardial infarctions. Psychother Psychosom 18:281–285

64. Pelser HE (1967) Psychological aspects of the treatment of patients with coronary infarct. J Psychosom Res 2:47–49

65. Price VA, Friedman M (1986) Modifying Type A behaviour and reducing coronary recurrence rates. In: Lacey JH, Sturgeon D (eds) Proceedings of the 15th European conference on psychosomatic research. Libby, London, pp 178–183

66. Adsett CA, Bruhn JG (1968) Short term psychotherapy for post myocardial patients and their wives. Can Med Assoc J 99:577–585

67. Mittelmann B, Wolff H (1939) Affective states and skin temperature experiments study of subjects with cold hands and Raynaud's syndrome. Psychosom Med 1:271–92

68. Graham DT (1955) Cutaneous vascular reactions in Raynaud's disease and in states of hostility, anxiety and depression. Psychosom Med 17:200–207
69. Freedman RR, Ianni P (1983) Role of cold and emotional stress in Raynaud's disease and scleroderma. Br Med J 287:1499–1502
70. Zahavi I, Chagnac A, Hering R et al. (1984) Prevalence of Raynaud's phenomenon in patients with migraine. Arch Intern Med 144:742–744
71. Atkinson RA, Appenzeller O (1976) Hemicrania and Raynaud's phenomenon: manifestations of the same disease. Headache 16:1–2
72. Freedman RR, Ianni P, Werig P (1983) Behavioural treatment of Raynaud's disease. J Consult Clin Psychol 51:539–549
73. Davies DT, Wilson ATM (1937) Observations on the Life history of chronic peptic ulcer. Lancet 2:1353–1360

9 Central Nervous System

9.1 Migraine, Vascular Headache and Premenstrual Tension

Approximately 10% of people in Western societies suffer from migraine or a variant at some point in their lives, but Crisp et al. [1] in a community of 5000 at Shipston-on-Stour reported the high figure of 25% in women. The incidence is higher than average in occupations demanding precise and sustained application of hand or brain, e.g. school teachers (about one in three), nurses, accountants and cashiers on the one hand, and tailors, embroiderers, watchmakers and lathe workers on the other. This appears to be due to autoselection [3]. People lacking the ability or willingness to maintain high standards, especially under pressure, gravitate to work that suits them better. Many patients with migraine also suffer from vascular (tension) headaches between attacks. These may be unilateral or bilateral and without nausea or visual phenomena. Because they may persist for days or weeks, sufferers find them very tiring and usually say they would prefer to have classical migraine which while of greater severity is of shorter duration.

In his book [2], Wolff recorded the most comprehensive account of the psychosomatic aspects of migraine to date. In it he said it was justifiable to include those "kindred headaches ... or migraine variants ... having in common vascular mechanisms". He added that restricting the definition of migraine to classical migraine "results in profitless subdivisions of an overlapping headache syndrome". We agree; these other syndromes include cluster headache, trigeminal migraine and hemi-anaesthetic and hemiplegic migraine. Had Wolff included the word migraine in the title of his book it would have greatly assisted retrieval by research workers and doctors who have followed him, and he would have received proper recognition for his outstanding contribution. Readers wishing to extend their knowledge of this disorder and its management are advised to read the 1948 and 1963 editions of Wolff's book because editions since his death have omitted much of value from the original account. The relevant chapters are 11 entitled, "The relation of life situations, personality features and reactions to the migraine syndrome", and 12 on "Migraine therapy". In these chapters he describes *typicality* of personality and attitudes and also *typically* provocative life situations,and illuminates the path a doctor or therapist needs to follow in order to achieve success. He stresses that a more direct approach than is acceptable in orthodox psychotherapy is more likely to succeed. Apparently Wolff himself had migraine, which may account for his unusual understanding. The following advice before starting any patient on treatment is as relevant today as when he wrote it in 1948: "The patient ... must appreciate that anything out of a bottle can offer no more than transient help."

Paulley and Haskell [3] reported their experience of over 800 patients, and since then a further 800 have been treated by the same methods. The following recommendations are based on that experience.

9.1.1 Diagnosis and Examination

We have repeatedly emphasised the importance of full history taking and examination. This is never more important than when faced with a patient with migraine or migrainous headache. At the end of a comprehensive history, providing it includes some of the detailed enquiries and facilitations to be described, a doctor should be 95% sure that the diagnosis of migraine/vascular headache is correct. This must be followed by a full examination including the CNS, and it is nearly always advisable to X-ray the skull and to explain to the patient that although no abnormality has been found, it is almost certain that friends or relations will ask what tests the doctor did and if the answer is none, then the common reply is: "Well, that's what happened to Uncle Bill, and he had a brain tumour." Only once has a patient questioned whether this X-ray would show the brain, and he was sent for a CAT scan! This investigation is rarely necessary, but unfortunately in some parts of the world the nadir has already been reached of patients being referred to physicians or neurologists as "headache – CAT scan negative"!

Some Essentials in History Taking for Patients with Headache. Although "organic" non-migrainous causes account for no more than about 5% of patients presenting in general practice or hospital with headache, the doctor's first responsibility is to exclude these by detailed questioning and examination. This enquiry must cover the characteristic features of the headache in such conditions as raised intracranial pressure, sinusitis, giant cell arteritis, retrobulbar neuritis and glaucoma. At the same time one will be listening for clues pointing to a diagnosis of migraine, migrainous equivalents or vascular headache. Some of these clues can only be elicited by taking a psychosomatically orientated history in which the presence or absence of the *typical* personality traits and attitudes found in migraine will be of paramount importance. If these are absent, clinicians should suspect some cause other than migraine. However, many patients with migrainous/vascular headache are told without supporting evidence that they have sinusitis or sinus headache and as a result may suffer for years with the wrong diagnosis and without appropriate treatment. Such patients attend saying: "I've got my sinus again" ([4] p. 665). The reason why many patients with a history of attacks of classical migraine also suffer between attacks for days or weeks from persistent vascular (tension) headache is unknown. However, it seems to be related to the fact that classical migraine occurs *after* periods of tension and overactivity in the "let down" period at weekends, the first day of a holiday or even heavy sleep, whereas vascular (tension) headache seems to be associated with periods of unremitting tension without intervening phases of relaxation.

Typicality of Profile and Multicausality. It has been questioned whether there is a *typical* profile in migraine on the grounds that other people may have it, or may appear to have it, without having migraine. While this may be true, it does not mean that the profile is irrelevant to migraine, only that an additional determinant may be involved, such as inherited disposition or that the individual has yet to come up against a *typically* provocative life situation. Patients with migraine share certain traits with obsessional neurotics, and it is often asked why the obsessional neurotic does not also suffer from migraine. One reason appears to be that tension in the obsessional patient is temporarily relieved with completion of a particular ritual, e.g. handwashing or shutting doors, whereas patients with migraine are seldom satisfied with their performance and are always striving to do better. Another difference is that obsessional neurotics score highly on personality inventories whereas migrainous patients may not [1]. This is because although both groups are obsessional about such things as cleanliness, tidiness and punctuality, patients with migraine expend a great deal trying to attain perfection in one or two areas of their lives and yet be unconcerned about others. As a result migraine sufferers score as many minus as plus points on an inventory or questionnaire designed to measure obsessionality [1].

Inherited Disposition. Patients with migraine have about three times more first-degree relatives with the disorder than would be expected by chance. The incidence of blood group O is as high in migraine as it is in DU [3], that is, about 6%–7% above expectation against controls. Other genetic markers such as HLA may be influential but have yet to be identified.

9.1.1.1 The Typical Profile

Uptightness. Patients with migraine are ready to admit that they are often uptight whereas they may deny being tense – a term they sometimes feel is pejorative.

Striving. They strive whatever the cost to approximate to whichever standard they have set for themselves, domestically, at work or at play.

Guilt. They feel guilty over anything seen as laziness or failure to attain such standards. At the same time they may tolerate low standards about things considered unimportant, e.g. poor cooking and an untidy house set in a weedless garden defended with rigour against cats and children. Guilt also ensues if the subjects allow themselves to feel pleased at their performance, i.e. guilt over self-satisfaction at high marks in a competition or examination.

Perfectionism. The above attributes may be summed up as perfectionistic, a term which many patients with migraine resent, seeing it as derogatory and irritating because they are tired of family or workmates telling them so.

The Clock and Deadlines. Most, but not all, migraine sufferers' lives are dominated by the clock. It they fall behind the clock at work or while travelling from A to B they become tense, and if held up in traffic they experience guilt that they may keep someone waiting. In these circumstances their grip on the steering wheel tightens and when they reach their destination they are often exhausted.

If migraine sufferers are not set deadlines by their employers, they are likely to set them for themselves. One housewife kept a stop watch to time herself doing her routine housework. Unless she could improve on her previous best time she felt dissatisfied.

Tensions Arising from Change of Routine or Previous Arrangements. Because of their need to maintain high standards and also to meet deadlines, interruptions and changes of plan intensify existing "uptightness". For example, a secretary given additional work because someone is ill or on holiday may also have many more telephone interruptions. Their inflexibility over changes of social arrangements, even if unavoidable, only increases their uptightness. For example, a husband says: "Sorry dear, but Bert and Daisy say they can't make tomorrow and wonder if they can come on Thursday, is that all right?" Or an agreed holiday has to be altered because of a spouse's failure to book soon enough.

Travelling and Inflexibility. Sufferers from migraine often say that journeys by train or bus, even if relatively short, are followed by migraine the next day. They sometimes describe tension building up the evening before but cannot at once explain why. Underlying it is a fear of being late and missing the train, a connection or an appointment and then anticipating the resulting muddle. They feel more secure on their own territory. Strange places mean strange people, and these "unknown" factors are seen as potential threats to their secure routine which they prefer to run like clockwork.

Holidays. First there is the packing and not forgetting to put in the children's favourite toys, then the house must be left clean to appease their own standards, but also in case mother drops in while they are away. This is followed by anxiety about getting away in time, the uncertainty of the journey and whether their hotel or boarding house will be suitable. Not surprisingly, migraine attacks are notoriously common on the first day of a holiday in the let-down period after the tension of getting away.

Origins of Perfectionism and Compulsive Activity. A disposition to obsessional behaviour is probably partly inherited, but as patients with migraine repeatedly testify, nurtural experiences in childhood are a major cause. It is usually then that the standards described in the profile are acquired from one or other parent or surrogate, either by example or by firm indoctrination with penalties for failure to perform. Surrogates may be an older sister, grandmother or the woman next door who deputises for a working mother, or later an employer or one of the armed services. It is the conforming (albeit reluctant) members of a sibship in each family who may develop migraine; non-conformers escape.

Unfavourable comparison with a sibling doing better at school is often quoted as a reason for a less bright child having to strive hard to gain approval and then to do so for the rest of his life.

Patients with migraine thus *internalise* the standards of the key figure and from then on recurrently or persistently "fight" to meet them. They say they are never happy unless occupied, or are bored or uncomfortable if not doing something useful.

However, migraine sufferers often say they would *like* to be able to sit down for a while, but if they do, they immediately feel guilty. So they drive themselves to find things to do at home or outside even when they are tired. In interview, migraine sufferers more than any other psychosomatic sufferer are always saying: "I feel I *should*", "I feel I *must*", "I *ought*", "I've *got* to", with emphasis on the italicised words.

9.1.1.2 Refinements in Interviewing and Observation: Suggestions

Features such as the quality, site, duration and frequency of the headache, whether there is a family history and whether the patient has suffered from travel sickness in childhood (75% of migraine sufferers have been travel sick) may have already pointed to the diagnosis. However, if the doctor at this point is still unaware whether the patient has any of the important attitudes described in the profile, paying attention to certain non-verbal messages may help in considering the probability. The following are examples of these non-verbal messages:

Talking fast – many such patients translate their dislike of wasting time into the way they talk.
Vibrant voices.
Emphatic speech – e. g. I work *very* hard, I feel I *should, ought, must*, etc.
Sitting on edge of chairs – before learning to relax, most migraine sufferers do this.
Tense muscles round jaw (masseters) and shoulders and neck (sternocleidomastoids easily visible).
Looking at watches during interview even if it is running to schedule, i.e. clock domination.
Quick undressers who often add: "I am ready now, doctor" – while other patients will wait until the doctor has finished writing.
Tidy piles of clothes – clothes are usually very clean and neatly folded on the chair and shoes at attention under it.

9.1.1.3 Suggested Questions to Explore the Profile

D: I wonder if you are someone who can sit for long?
P: You mean, doing nothing?
D: Yes
P: No, I become restless and *must* find something to do.
D: Do you find it easy to relax?
P: No, I can never relax *or* Yes, but only if I have got something to do like knitting or needlework.
D: Would you stand on an escalator or walk up it? (Most migraine sufferers walk up escalators).
D: Can you leave things at the office or at home, for example dirty dishes in the sink overnight?
P: (The answer is usually) No, I can't *bring* myself to do that – it would worry me and I would feel guilty.
D: How do you feel if you are stuck in a traffic jam and through no fault of your own are going to be late for an appointment?
P: I feel terrible.
D: Do you find yourself getting more tense and gripping the steering wheel?

P: Yes – I often find I do that even when I am not late but have a tight schedule.

D: How do you feel if other people keep you waiting?

P: (Some patients say they do not mind, but most do.) I wouldn't do that to them, why should they do that to me?

D: How about people at work who waste time and talk a lot?

P: They drive me mad; I don't say anything, but they make me very tense.

D: Can your husband sit down and twiddle his thumbs?

P: Yes, and that annoys me (others may add although I know I shouldn't as he has had a hard day).

D: (Enquiries about recreations, such as needlework, knitting, gardening, collecting stamps, entering competitions for jam making, etc.) If you make a small mistake when you are knitting can you leave it?

P: Oh no, I have to have it all out and start again. (perfectionism)

D: If you are making clothes for the children and it's getting late, can you leave it?

P: No, I *have got* to finish it.

D: Can you leave the cotton threads on the floor until the morning?

P: No, I have *got* to clear them up there and then, or I wouldn't sleep.

D: How do you feel if you go to sleep in your chair after supper?

P: I feel terrible, I feel guilty that I am not doing something useful.

D: Even if you are tired?

P: Yes.

D: If you do win a competition at the flower show or institute, do you feel pleased about it?

P: Well yes, but I always feel I should have done better, and even if I were to get 100 marks I should feel I did not deserve them. (see transcript at end of section)

Questions may also be directed to any recent additional pressures, such as having to visit relatives and friends in hospital or at a distance during the weekend. These things may provoke exacerbations of migraine and can be equated to "the last straw on the camel's back".

9.1.2 Treatment

Many people who have had migraine or migrainous headache do not go to doctors because of it. Instead, they take acetylsalicylic acid or some other analgesic, or put up with it. This may apply more to males than females, who for various reasons such as premenstrual exacerbation may suffer more severely. If migraine does not occur more often than every 3 months, and vascular headaches do not occur between attacks, it is better to advise the patient to take analgesics and if necessary go to bed for half-a-day than to pursue the programme of psychological management to be outlined. The reason is that patients need to be so disabled by their migraine that they are prepared to do anything to obtain alleviation. "Anything" in this case means a moderate change in their ingrained perfectionism and other attitudes described in the profile. Motivation has to be great enough for them to do things wholly alien and to accept things hitherto unacceptable.

GPs will see many more early or mild cases than in a hospital clinic series such as that described by Paulley and Haskell in 1975 [3]. The average duration of migraine at consultation in that series was 13.5 years. They were mostly patients who had failed to respond to all their GP's tablets or diets, the exceptions being young people with short histories of severe headache in whom cerebral tumour was feared by the patient, their relatives or their GP. Such patients may be phobic and have a psychopathogenesis such as that described in the interview in Chap. 5.

A GP, having reassured the patient and themselves that hypertension, raised intracranial pressure, etc. are absent, will probably prescribe a drug of his choice. For the milder case this may be enough. Even the severe case is likely to experience the transient help described by Wolff [2], only to return 2–3 months later saying, "The pill does not work anymore," thus demonstrating that it was the placebo of the consultation and the GP's reassurance and personality which had been therapeutic and not the drug. The placebo effect (discussed in Chap. 2 with references) may be expected to peter out within a few months after a single intervention.

We suggest, therefore, that the psychological management of the type we are describing should be reserved for the frequently relapsing or severe case.

9.1.2.1 Preparing the Patient

When patients with migraine are just sent to learn to relax, whether by standard methods, hypnotherapy, autogenic training, biofeedback, yoga or transcendental meditation, the drop-out rate is wastefully high. This is because the first step of psychological management is rarely carried out, as the need for it is not understood. After eliciting some or all of the traits or attitudes described in the profile, patients should be asked whether they have migraine following such pressures, and then to point out that the subset of the population (10%) of which they are members is far too large to be dismissed as neurotic, and that probably there are no more neurotics with migraine than in the rest of the population. This is important because they will already have been given the idea by relatives, workmates or doctors that they are imagining their headache or it is "their nerves". Nor should the doctor in any way appear critical of their behaviour; better a congratulatory remark such as "It's good job that there are still some people left in the world like you, or everything would stop." Without their feathers being ruffled they are able to look at the possibility of changing a little instead of becoming annoyed and not coming back. Initially, it is better to avoid the term perfectionism unless the patient offers it, because many migraine patients resent it even if it is true. Instead, they will happily accept that they have high standards.

What Type of Relaxation? When a relaxation technique is recommended, it is necessary to observe the patient's non-verbal response to the word relaxation. The doctor has to understand that for individuals with migraine it is near to sin, even though as with other sins, they may be envious of those who can! At this point the doctor can draw a parallel with an Olympic sprinter, diver or acrobat who loses if too tense before competing and has to learn a relaxation technique. Migraine patients, just like long distance runners, need to pace themselves if they are to win. Winning is very important to them, and a justifiable selling point for patients who are hesitating is that they can be just like athletes who after learning to pace themselves are able to achieve more, and do more, without in this case being impeded by frequent headaches. By such means they begin to see the possibility of being more efficient and not less. He may then be told that the treatment should enable him to choose whether he does something instead of having the feeling dating from childhood that he must, whether he wants to or not, and that such a choice applies equally to the treatment recommended – it is not something done to him and which he cannot avoid.

When it comes to what form of relaxation technique is acceptable to people with migraine we have found that these very matter-of-fact *superstable* people, who like their t's crossed and i's dotted, dislike transcendental meditation. Yoga is accepted if it is not too orientally flavoured, and biofeedback machines are too coercive. These patients are already competitive enough without adding to it, and some describe how the machine to which they are connected, by buzzing or blinking engenders a sense of failure which may lead them to strive to placate it. In the series of 800 patients reported by Paulley and Haskell [3], since extended by a similar number, relaxation exercises were taught by the physiotherapist once a week for 6–8 weeks. A transcript of such a session is appended. Patients were then asked to practise what they had learned every day for 20–30 min, recalling the physiotherapist's word picture to help them. Some request and are given audiotapes to reinforce this. When treatment is finished, patients are always offered refresher courses if necessary, and it is stressed that support from the physician and physiotherapist is never withheld.

9.1.2.2 Outcome

A follow-up [3] on a sample of patients treated individually was carried out 3–8 years after the therapeutic intervention. Two-thirds reported major improvement over the frequency or severity or both of their migraine compared with their experience before such treatment. (Wolff [2] found the same.) It was considered that the gap of 3 years after the intervention was sufficient to exclude placebo effect. Since 1971 approximately 25% of these patients were offered treatment in a group. Such selection was left to the physiotherapist, although the physician can indicate that a patient might do well in a group at the time of referral. In our experience from 1952 to 1985 many patients who found individual therapy difficult to accept, however carefully prepared by the physician and physiotherapist, were subsequently able to accept it in a group setting.

In other words, when "permission" to reduce their high standards was given by their peers, they were able to accept it more readily than when given by a doctor or physiotherapist, still clothed with the aura of (parental) authority. Being able to incorporate a less severe superego than their original is essential to a successful outcome. The doctor and physiotherapist can bring this about, and circumstances may leave no alternative, but a group of the patient's peers does it better. On follow-up of patients treated in groups, major improvement rises from two-thirds when treated individually to four-fifths despite the fact that the most severe and intractable cases found their way into groups.

9.1.3 Summary

We recommend that after helping patients to identify the areas of their life in which they cost themselves too much, and when and from whom their inflexible attitudes were acquired, they should then be led by means of a form of preparation such as that described to accept the relaxation technique to which they are best suited. In a district hospital there is usually at least one physiotherapist or nurse who has had some training in these methods. However, at present few have the training needed to run a migraine group effectively. Some physiotherapists or nurses think they can teach people to relax but those resembling tough physical education instructors are unsuitable. Preferably, they should be over 30 and have quiet voices and a relaxed manner. Apart from the qualities described, the group leader, whether physiotherapist, nurse or doctor, needs a prior knowledge of the *typicality* of the migraine patients' attitudes and *typicality* of provocative life events and situations as described in the profile. Indeed, they should have read and digested the two chapters by Wolff [2]. It is suggested that someone wishing to be a leader of a migraine group would be wise first to see such a group in action. Otherwise, apart from the basic rules for leaders of groups, i.e. turning back questions to the group to answer, avoiding premature intervention and asking the group to say what they think about it, they will learn as they go on. It is usual for a group to anticipate a feeling of loss in the week prior to their last meeting, and the tension engendered may provoke a return of the headaches which until then had been lessening. This, of course, calls for interpretation, and the group is never slow to do so. We have found that some groups arrange a reunion for themselves, but the sharpness of the cutoff can be alleviated by enabling the group to talk about it from session 5 onwards and if they are given an assurance that after about a year they may apply for a refresher course and, when indicated, join another group. This and the restriction of each group to eight sessions has alleviated the problem of overdependency.

Lastly, patients so treated often say that the greatest change has been in their awareness of when they were becoming uptight, usually felt in the muscles round their jaw, shoulders and neck. "Before treatment I thought I could relax, but now I realise I never did."

9.1.4 Premenstrual Tension

The most effective form of psychological management for this condition (PMT) is the same as that for migraine and vascular headaches. Diuretic treatment and dangerously large doses of progesterone fail to provide long term relief. Most women who suffer from PMT also have, or have had, migraine or migrainous headache, and most migrainous women suffer at some time from degrees of PMT. Water retention is common to both disorders. Anti-diuresis preceding migraine and diuresis marking the end of an attack are frequently mentioned by patients with migraine.

In a New Zealand trial of biofeedback-induced relaxation on its own versus standard relaxation training, the latter did best. However, the drop out rate was unnecessarily high and that will always be the case unless accompanied by the type of psychological preparation and management described for migraine.

9.1.5 Transcripts

An accountant; male aged 45.

D: Can you forget the clock?

P: Well, I'm a bit of a stickler for time keeping. Even going out to my friends and relatives, if I say I'm going to be there at eleven I don't like to be there at ten past.

D: No? So you are really punctual, what about other people keeping you waiting; does it annoy you?

P: It would annoy me yes, I don't like being kept waiting at all.

D: How about relaxation – I mean sitting down and twiddling your thumbs? Do you find that easy to do?

P: No, I can't sit down and do nothing, I do crosswords, I read.

D: What happens if you do sit down, say in a deck chair, and say look at the sea, I mean what happens to you?

P: Well, in no time I'd be walking along the beach, I'd go 2 miles one way and turn round and come back, or I'd go in for a swim.

Relaxation and sitting about are intolerable because they are equated with laziness; this is due to internalised example and precepts from key figures in childhood.

P: My father was only a labourer.

D: Did he sit down and twiddle his thumbs?

P: No, I've never known my father to sit around because – I do take after him in that way – he was always very fond of gardening, he used to enter for all the flower shows and so on.

D: You don't like a garden unless it is neat and tidy?

P: No, I can't bear the *sight* of a weed.

D: Not at all?

P: No (laughs), if I see one I have to bend down and pull it up.

D: You don't look out of your window and see one sometimes?

P: Oh, I see plenty in my neighbour's garden ...

D: But you can't do much about it?

P: I can't do anything about that – no.

D: Obviously things happen at work – like getting an extra load of stuff in, getting interrupted – and you can't finish what you want to finish that day, what do you do about it?

P: Well, I would take it home nine times out of ten.

D: You wouldn't find it easy to leave it over until the next day?

P: No – it would worry me if I – if I was getting out a monthly trial balance and it was a few pounds out – I would have to find them – I couldn't rest until I found it.

Female patient, aged 16, with recent severe migraine.

D: How long have you been prone to headaches?

P: Since I started work.

D: So four attacks which shut out the visual field, is it one side or the other? So you can't see sideways?

P: Mm.

D: What's your job?

P: I work in a poodle parlour.

D: Does anybody else get headaches or migraine in your family?

P: Only my mum.

D: Are you a person who finds it fairly easy to relax, do you think?

P: Not really.

D: Can you tell me what you mean by that?

P: Well, I've always got to do something.
D: Why?
P: I don't know – I don't like sitting around doing nothing.
D: Can you say why you don't?
P: Not really ...
D: Think.
P: Just bored.
D: Can your mother sit and put her feet up?
P: No.
D: Can your sisters?
P: Yes.
D: Which one?
P: All of them.
D: So, you're the odd one out?
P: Yes.
D: What do you think when they are sitting around?
P: I just think they are lazy.
D: You say you feel bored if you're doing nothing?
P: Um, um.
D: Do you feel it is a waste of time?
P: Well, it is really, you could be doing something useful in that time you're wasting. Well, I do rush about a lot at work.
D: Do you?
P: It's just that we have to pick up heavy dogs and carry them around everywhere because they are so lazy.
D: Dogs are lazy too?
P: (laughs) Some of them are – they don't like going to a certain place to get their fur clipped.

Four months later after relaxation exercises, she sits in a very relaxed posture:
D: And of course you were losing your vision, you were losing half the field weren't you?
P: Yes.
D: Have you had any more of those kind?
P: No – well, I am very relieved that they are not so bad as they used to be.
D: They may come back when you start to do too much against the clock.
P: Yes, I've found that already. (laughs)
D: Have you?
P: Yes, I got up late yesterday morning I had – it caused a headache then.
D: You rushed?
P: Yes. (laughs)

B. A., female, aged 45
P: I work fast, I want to get everything done, I'm never satisfied until I've finished – if a thing is worth doing, it's worth doing well, isn't it?
D: Well, perhaps that is something your aunt taught you?
P: That's right. Well, I think it's a waste of time to sit down and do nothing, like if I go out I take my knitting with me.
D: What about punctuality – do you mind being late for things; does it bother you?
P: No, I like to be on time, I don't want to keep anybody waiting, I don't like people keeping me waiting, therefore I don't like keeping anybody else waiting.
D: When you were brought up, by your mother or by the aunt?
P: Very punctual, yes, my aunt who brought me up, she is very particular and very punctual.

D: You cannot quite measure up to her standards?

P: No, I'm afraid I can't because she never had any children you see.

D: But it sounds as though you might have incorporated some of them?

P: Well, yes, I think I took a lot off her really.

D: Does she show her feelings much?

P: She's very abrupt, she doesn't show her feelings.

D: No?

P: And when I get these headaches I have to give up in the end and go to bed with them because I can't stop being sick, that's the trouble you see.

D: How do you react to people who annoy you?

P: Oh, I speak my mind, if I'm cross with anybody I say what I've got to say and then forget about it afterwards. I am happy-go-lucky, I never brood over anything, never sulk.

B. C., female, aged 35, another dissatisfied perfectionist.

P: I do a lot of secretarial work in the village you know, I'm secretary of quite a few organisations – I do quite a lot of social work and that sort of thing, and as I said before I like to get things done before I can relax, I always wish that I could have perfection in everything that I do – I wanted to be able to do *perfect* embroidery and *perfect* cooking and I've kept that up *all* the time. I want to learn to do these things, and I want to do all these things, and I want to achieve perfection, and I find I can't. I enter in every class in the Women's Institute because I am interested in everything that goes on, you see, and I never get top marks for anything, and it makes me irritable and worried. I'm not satisfied with anything I do – and I work very hard too – I'm very fond of hosting parties and I go to a lot of trouble to do something different.

(Asked about mother)

P: She wouldn't relax until everything was done that should be done, and mother worked well, you know. I never heard her say that she worried about obtaining perfection, but in everything she did, like country people are proud of, she made bread and her linen was very white you know, and she would have been worried if it hadn't been.

D: Can you sit down in a chair and do nothing?

P: No – I feel guilty if I'm not doing something, I can think of all the things that need doing.

D: Does your husband say that you ought to be sitting?

P: Well, sometimes I feel very irritable because I feel my husband should be worrying about something – and he isn't you see. He doesn't worry about getting ready, while I feel I must look as well as I possibly can and ...

D: Would you have a reputation for being rather abrupt or outspoken, do you think?

P: Well, could be, because I want to get things done and not harbour them.

D: That sounds as though you like getting things tidy in your mind.

P: I *do*, I *do*, I like my *mind* tidy and my *house* tidy ...

D: Yes, I understand that, I think that is very well put.

C. H., female, aged 50, has migraine and had early responsibilities because of her mother's illness.

D: What age were you then, do you remember?

P: Twelve and a bit.

D: And if you did things in the house, did she like them done properly?

P: Oh yes, just so, if they weren't done she would probably go over them again.

D: Did she?

P: And if I'd got any needlework to do or dressmaking I'd come in and get right on with it, you know, I can never let it lay, just carried on with it.

D: You don't feel comfortable sitting down?

P: I can't sit and do nothing.

D: What do you feel like?

P: I *must* have a piece of knitting or something to do. I should feel dreadful with nothing to do and just watching TV.

D: How do you mean dreadful?

P: Feel I'm wasting my time, just doing nothing.

In addition to her housework she is employed 6 h a day as a machinist.

D: When you are at work do you work piecework?

P: Yes.

D: Are you a quick worker?

P: Yes.

D: How many girls are you working with?

P: Oh, there are different sections, I think about 15 in my section, some of them don't care about the work, I like mine to look proper.

D. H., female, aged 30.

P: I couldn't really sort of … sit for hours like some people – I couldn't do that.

D: No? What do you do then?

P: Well, as I say, I couldn't sit for long – I'm usually walking around or either talking to somebody, or I used to go round the shops, you know, just to sort of take it off; my husband says for goodness sake go and sit down.

D: That's what he says?

P: Yes – he says you've got plenty of clothes, you just keep wash, wash, wash, washing, but I can't sit still for long – I must keep on the go – I *must* do this job – little job, I must do this – tonight.

D: Why do you feel you must do it?

P: I don't know. Sort of eases me for the next day, you know.

(An important factor here was that her mother was a polio victim and shared her house.)

9.1.5.1 Transcript of Haskell's Word Pictures

These word pictures [3] are spoken in time with the patient's *abdominal* breathing. The physiotherapist rests a hand on the epigastrium, which rises and falls to the rhythm of her voice. A heat lamp is placed to keep the patient warm on the couch.

"Now I'm going to describe some places to you with gaps in between. So if you want to listen to the whole lot, you can without a break; if you just want to listen to one scene you can do so, and you can pick the scene out to practise relaxation when you are on your own:

"It is a beautiful day now / and you've gone right up into the mountains / and you come to this stream / and you can hear the water wander past you very quietly / right down to the valley below. / You see the lake lying still and quiet in the sunshine. / There is a farm on the other side of the lake, / with the farmer on his tractor going backwards and forwards across the field / making deep furrows in the earth. / You see the farmer's wife out in the yard collecting eggs / you can almost feel the warm brown eggs in her hands. / These two work tremendously hard, / They've always had to make the farm pay. / But they don't worry about things they can't change, / things that don't matter, / and if they've a problem to deal with / they try to deal with it as well as they can / and put it behind them and forget about it. / When they relax, / they relax completely / and don't feel guilty / and think they ought to be doing something else," etc.

"It's a beautiful day now / and you are lying on the beach / moving the sand under your fingers cool and soft / you see the sea stretching in front of you for miles/ a lovely calm blue sea / you hear the sound of the waves breaking on the shore / very rhythmically and quietly. / You see a lot of boats at anchor in the bay / and the seagull perched on the mast of a yacht / moving backwards and forwards with the tide. / You see the village on the cliff. / There's a boatbuilder making his boats in the corner / you can hear the sound of his hammer as he hammers the nails in. / You watch his son painting broad splashes of red paint / across the bows of the boats. / These two have learnt to relax as they work / the man doesn't hit the nails so hard that their heads fly off / the son doesn't paint everything in sight with red paint / but they still manage to get more done than their neighbours / who work flat out the whole time / and are exhausted by the evening / and the more you watch them the more relaxed you are. / Now you see the big, black Persian cat / waking up and stretching, and arching his back / and only because it looks a nice thing to do / and when you want to do it / you take a slightly bigger breath / and stretch your legs and arms right out like a cat / and then go completely limp and relaxed."

9.2 Multiple Sclerosis

Psychological management for MS is rarely listed as a form of treatment. In the first place doctors are unaware of the extensive literature relating psychological factors to the onset and relapses of MS, and consequently the fewer reports evidencing the benefit from psychotherapeutic intervention have also escaped their attention.

Langworthy [5] was the first to describe the essentials of psychological management for MS 40 years ago. He wrote:

> The hope of therapy is to influence recently acquired abnormalities and prevent the development of further symptoms. These patients show a great need for a physician to interest himself in their problem. They tend to relate themselves to him in the same *passive* and *childish* [our italics] emotional pattern which they have shown to other significant people in their lives. The physician's problem is to challenge this attitude ... and endeavour to help the patient towards a more mature and satisfactory relationship.

We agree ,and J.W.P. reported his own experience with more than 300 cases of MS seen over a period of 25 years in 1976–1977 [6], and a further 58 cases in 1985 [7]. Case histories and transcripts were used to illustrate the need for doctors to appreciate these individuals' pathological vulnerability to threats of separation and engulfment (entrapment), the life situations in which such threats most commonly occur, and the sensitive methods of history taking required in the majority of cases to uncover them. Physician, GPs or neurologists will be less likely to miss the hidden treasure in the history if they are already aware of the *typicality* of the MS patients' emotional make-up, attitudes and coping mechanisms to the emotional threats already mentioned.

Those interested are asked to read this section in conjunction with the two previous reports [6, 7], especially the case histories in the first article. What follows contains new case histories and other facets of management. We have felt it better to do this than describe again previous studies on psychopathogenesis, extensive and important though they are.

9.2.1 Typicality

Evidence that the *typical* emotional make-up and coping mechanisms are premorbid may be obtained from siblings, parents, friends as well as the patients themselves, and if it is suggested to these witnesses that a patient's degree of euphoria and "belle indifférence" seems inappropriate to the dire physical disability with which he or she has been stricken, the usual reply is that the patient has behaved in the same way since early childhood.

People who suddenly find they cannot walk, urinate, or see normally show some anxiety or concern, but during history taking and examination of patients with MS doctors often find them smiling or joking (the smiling mask) as they speak of their alarming symptoms, or show no emotion at all (the flat mask). MS sufferers often recall such inappropriate emotional responses as embarrassing. For example, a patient remembered, when still at school, laughing instead of crying when her friend fell over and broke her leg, and a nurse, her uncontrollable laughter when horrified by the injuries of a man after a traffic accident.

When asked if they can give reasons for hiding feelings even to the extent of smiling when they felt like weeping, they often say that they had found it was better to do so because if they wept or showed temper, the parental shouting, weeping or fussing that followed was so disturbing, they *learned* that to show emotion was dangerous. Another reason patients give for this particular coping mechanism is that they *learned* early not to rock their frail boat of security, i.e. even as toddlers not doing anything that might incur maternal or paternal alarm or displeasure.

Separation. Whereas most children at the toddling stage of development are in effect saying to their mothers: "I am no longer part of you, I am *me*," and achieve this degree of separation by displays of independence, such as not putting their boots on, not finishing a meal, or not going to bed when told, patients with MS rarely, if ever, successfully negotiate this stage of normal development because their revolt is defeated, either by the severity of the response or by displays of maternal distress, both of which they prefer to avoid.

In this way the "giving-up" response is learned early as a means of reducing tension and a return to a womb-like homeostasis. "I could never cross my mother," they will say (Mrs. D. D.). Mother's inability to let go sufficiently for her child to take these important early steps towards independence lies in her own insecurity, usually the product of her own upbringing. Skynner and Cleese's book, *Families and How to Survive Them* [8] is recommended as a clear and most readable account of this stage of development, which Erikson had described earlier [9].

Engulfment/Entrapment: Why One Child and Not Another. As children, MS patients accept the excessively restrictive bond with their mother and surrogates as a requirement for emotional homeostasis and security. (case Mr. S. M.) [6]. Some remember both surprise and disapproval at the greater independence permitted to their siblings, by reason of their sex or position in the family, or because mother was less fraught during pregnancy and the neonatal period than in their own case, or just because the other siblings seized it and ignored the consequences [6].

My sister always had the licence, my younger sisters were more modern. I was always too frightened to disappoint my parents – I remember them taking the "mickey" out of me because I was different ... I would never have been wicked enough to pinch an apple off a tree like the others did ... I was always the child, although the eldest – I could not tell her off, and had to swallow my pride; mother is like a big protective eagle, even to stand up for myself would hurt her. Something within me just can't say "No", yet I could not bear to live on my mother's doorstep.

The patient's birth had occurred at her grandparents' house at a time of great maternal anxiety just after the war, and the double-bonded relationship resulted. The patient when aged 40 said: "It seems as if my mother and I are the same person – when she feels something, I feel it."

Puberty: The Next Stage of Separation. At puberty an individual says in effect: "I am no longer a child, I am an adult." Just as at the toddler stage MS patients describe great difficulties in surmounting this hurdle, and we have yet to meet one who has achieved it, although some may claim to have done so by confusing geographical distance with emotional distance.

For the patient already described, and for others with MS, the giving-up coping mechanisms learned in infancy are found at adolescence to be less effective. This is because chronological age, courtship, marriage and parenthood demand degrees of independence and emotional separation from key figures which they had been unable to achieve earlier. Some awareness that they lack an alternative coping mechanism to the giving-up response begins to reach consciousness. Also as adulthood approaches, separation, previously threatened, becomes a reality with ageing, sick, or alienated parents or surrogates. This inhibits patients making moves towards independence, particularly when parents exploit their age and infirmity as a means of bringing the straying lamb back to the fold, i.e. engulfment (entrapment) resulting once again from the threat of withdrawal and separation. Thus they find the symbolic "womb" is no longer as safe or comfortable as it was, and to have to go back to it becomes as horrifying to them as separation.

[Readers may note that in UC and Crohn's disease (Chap. 6), with comparable psychopathology to MS, it is also at adolescence and early adulthood when conflicts over dependence, e.g. marriage, leaving home, etc., reach consciousness and lead to disease.]

A cocooned child fails to negotiate adolescent independence because it fears displays of parental emotion vividly remembered from infancy, whereas the child who has been cowed by physical means or penalties, fails because it expects them to be repeated. Mrs. D. D. illustrates this:

P: I had to share my parents' bedroom up to the age of 10, so whether that caused a rift in their marriage I don't know.
D: Had you ever crossed your father as a child?
P: I never hated him.
D: No, I know, but could you ever stamp your foot or say I won't?
P: Oh yes.
D: You could do that?
P: Oh yes.
D: Could you do it to your mother?
P: No.
D: You could not?
P: No.
D: Why not?
P: Because she would belt me one, she would put me to bed as a punishment; as a result I did nothing in bed, so she thought to herself, well, that's not a punishment. So she used to tie me in a chair.
D: Do you think you could cross your mother now?
P: No, if I get a bit irritable down there, she would say to me: "You might be 33 years old, but you are still not too big to have a clout."
D: Good heavens. Do you think you were closer to your parents than some of your friends were to theirs or not?
P: I wasn't but I am now very close to my mother
D: So when did you come so close to her?
P: After my brother died – it seemed to draw us together. I was a very selfish girl when I was a teenager you know – when I sort of walked out – I just packed my bag, met my mother from work and said: "Cheerio," which I think was a cruel way of doing it. Well, when me and my Mum are together now, we're more like sisters.
D: Yes?
P: Now, you know – I love her.
D: Can she hurt you these days?
P: No – I am hurt being away from her more than anything.

Dynamics: Engulfment → Rebellion → Separation → Engulfment

Finding acknowledgement of adult independence barred, MS patients may then make what for them are outrageous rebellions, e.g. such as suddenly leaving home, or throwing up a career chosen for them by a parent, marrying against parental wishes, becoming pregnant, etc. Unfortunately, these rebellions do not succeed because it is the dilemma of these vulnerable people to want to be "in" when they are "out" and when they are back "in" then to be "out" again. In other words recurring separation and engulfment (entrapment).

How Threats of Engulfment Are Perceived and Conveyed. Engulfment is the reverse of separation, e.g. from the mother or surrogates. Theoretically, if separation is never achieved, the child may be said to be engulfed permanently or not born. One patient aged 42 came near to this when she said speaking like an infant: "Doctor, I just know

I never wanted to be born<u>ed</u>." Being born obviously involves some separation, but when the subsequent stages are never negotiated adequately, the individual finds threats of separation or engulfment terrifying. Further attempts to be free are either not pressed or take the form of rebellion as already mentioned, only to be put down by parental distress or by anger and threat of withdrawal (separation). Both evoke hopelessness and giving up, "back to the womb", as one patient put it.

For patients with MS, one of the most common forms of threatened or actual engulfment is being put down, or verbally admonished, and thus made to feel the child again. This may be done directly to the patient by the primary key figure, or just as often indirectly by someone seen by the patient as standing for the parental figure because of similarity in their behaviour, sex or appearance. Alternatively, the person admonished may not be the patient himself, but a spouse, a friend, a parent or a child with whom the patient identifies so strongly that it is as if it is happening to them-selves (see Chap. 4 on "Identifying with"). Lastly the threat may come from feeling someone is taking them over. Neighbours or friends as well as relatives may do this.

9.2.2 Case Histories

The following were examples of attacks following within a few hours or even minutes of patients being put down, admonished, made to feel the child again, engulfed.

Mr. K. C. A sensitive young man starting at university complained to his moral tutor that the student with whom he had to share a room was usually drunk, did not wash and brought women back to share his bed. His tutor advised him not to worry and that he would soon be doing the same. He felt put down, and his legs gave way as he descended the stairs – his first attack.

His second attack occurred after a lecturer abused two of his friends with whom he was talking. Although he was not being reproached himself, he identified with his friends. Asked what he felt at the time he said: "Frozen".

Mrs. E. Q. The childhood memories of a woman who was the youngest by some years were of her mother suffering the tyrannical behaviour of her asthmatic father. This continued until her wedding day when he threw a tantrum in an effort to prevent the patient leaving the house. She was seen after her second episode of MS which had occurred shortly after the shock of her husband's dismissal by his managing director. Asked why it had been a shock as there would be no difficulty in her husband finding another job she said: "It was the way it was done, you see his managing director was a little man and my father was a little man; in my experience little men behave like that." Thus, the overriding psychodynamic is identifying with her husband who had been put down (= engulfment), and identifying his employer with her father because of his appearance and behaviour.

Her first attack had occurred 6 years previously when her legs went numb on walking with her husband to a hospital where her only son was about to have an emergency operation. This dynamic involves the separation threat by possible death of the son.

Mr. S. M. An only child, he spent his first 9 years engulfed by his unhappy mother, herself forced to live in her parents' house where she and the boy were tyrannised by a Victorian grandfather. Eventually, although academically and financially successful, he failed to attain emotional independence because his mother refused to let go and blackmailed him whenever he tried displays of emotion. His first attack occurred within days of a domineering and boorish man telling him after years of success "that if he had been consulted he would never have employed him". The dynamic is being put down (= engulfment) by an authoritarian figure whom he identified with mother and grandfather. Another attack occurred when his mother announced her intention of coming to live near him so she could look after him (the dynamic: engulfment).

Mrs. N. M. A sensitive, recently married woman of 22, she had been the spoilt, cocooned child of a very close family. She had her first attack a day or two after her husband had turned her out of the car. On returning home he went out, taking with him the dog which had shared his bed until the marriage and did not come back for many hours. Subsequent attacks over the next few months related to the patient's fantasies of his infidelity every time she was alone. "I could not bear him out of my sight."

A year later an unwanted pregnancy was terminated on the grounds of bilaterally impaired vision from attacks of optic neuritis. The day after the termination she had a further episode of MS. A month later she said she knew the reason, which was that the gynaecologist, initially kind and empathetic, had told her just before the procedure that he didn't feel it was warranted. She said "It was his attitude – I wasn't ready for it – everyone had been so kind and sympathetic at the hospital. When he started saying things, I was at a loss – I was completely unprepared – I couldn't say anything." Like a naughty child she felt put down. It was not surprising that this patient had a hang-up over babies. She had been the centre of attention all her life and said she had always been eaten up with jealousy at parties if any other prettier or better dressed woman attracted attention.

Four years later a relapse followed disharmony in the marriage over her husband's unwillingness to have the children which she now wanted. He ultimately agreed, and she had her first child a year later. This necessitated her husband's dog being put down while she was in hospital because it had always resented her since she had insisted on it sleeping in a basket after the marriage. It had bitten her on the breast, and she feared it would harm the baby. She knew how distressed her husband was about the dog, and she felt he was silently displeased with her because he would not talk about it, and she was in mild relapse.

Mrs. M. L., an only child, had rebelled against a possessive mother and domineering father by leaving home at age 16. However, emotional independence escaped her, and her parents continued their hold on her via her husband whom they first reviled and then recruited. After her parents' divorce she attended the wedding of her father to a stepmother. During the speeches the stepmother got up and said that it was no longer a man's world and she was going to speak. The patient empathised with her father whom she felt had been put down (humiliated) just as she had felt put down by him in childhood. MS attack followed a week later, and further attacks over the next year related to similar overbearing behaviour by stepmother.

Mrs. N. C. An only child of 39, terrified of her bad-tempered father for as long as she could remember she said: "I have always felt as if I was never really loved – they never showed affection." Her first MS attack occurred 3 months after agreeing to her husband having custody of her two children aged 15 and 11 following the breakdown of their marriage as a result of violence. ("I felt it was the best thing, I couldn't fight him any longer.") The dynamic is a giving-up response but it also entails the separation threat of her daughter being turned against her, and not visiting.

With psychological management she overcame minor relapses over the next 7 years mostly related to what she felt were threats to her hard-won independence by another man, whom she eventually married.

The circumstances of a severe relapse in 1980 were typical and occurred the day after the following stress. She had never told her parents that she had MS because she feared the likely response to be blamed for having it. However, as the news that she had helped to raise a lot of money for an MS project was about to be published, she felt she had better tell them. "Mother was tearful when I told her, then father came in and said, 'Now look what you have done to your mother,' and he began to shout and go on at me."

As always she could not win, she felt hopeless and put down.

9.2.3 Childlike Appearances and Behaviour

In view of what has been said, it is not surprising that even to unskilled observers MS patients often appear childlike. Charcot [10] described this in 1877 as "puérilisme mentale". Langworthy [5] noted "emotional immaturity" and "an entangling neurotic relationship with the mother". Grinker [11] wrote, "The premorbid state of the multiple sclerotic is that of great immaturity since early infancy," and Mei Tal et al. [12] "Interpersonal relationships are characterised by strong dependent needs", Harrower [13] reported a "high incidence of passive dependency", Philippopoulos et al. [14] "emotional and psychosexual immaturity" and Paulley [6] "a pathological dependence on a parental key figure transferred wholly or partly to other key figures" (surrogates).

The Smiling or Unsmiling Mask. Patients conceal their sensitive cores behind one of the above masks. The smiling mask has long been recognised by neurologists as euphoria or the "belle indifférence" usually associated with hysteria. The unsmiling mask has sometimes been mistaken for depression, and Charcot [10] described it very well: "The look is *vague and uncertain*, the lips are hanging half open, the features have a *stolid* expression" [our italics]. J.W.P. [7] observed after longer acquaintance with such patients that they are neither truly euphoric nor depressed, rather they find it better to hide their feelings from infancy onwards. It is rare for them to weep, and then not for more than a few seconds, with a single tear at once replaced by a smile to repair the crack in their emotional defence. Indeed, some weep and smile at the same time!

It is now generally agreed [7, 12] that the childlike behaviour, moods such as "belle indifférence" and the masks in MS are premorbid and date from childhood long before the onset of demyelination. In the few severe cases in which cortical atrophy and dementia develop, the patient's previous mood becomes exaggerated as in GPI or pseudobulbar palsy, i.e. either depression or gross euphoria. These patients may become abusive and violent, to the distress of their close relatives who are unaware that underneath the patients' usual docility is concealed a great deal of pent-up anger against frustrating key figures dating from childhood. Doctors can help those who have to bear the brunt of this release phenomenon by explaining that although they are the unfortunate recipients, this rage did not belong to them.

9.2.4 Life Event Research

Studies [15, 12] have reported significant life events in about 30% of people with MS prior to onset or relapse of the disease. Although advances have been made in this method of research by trying to score the meaning of an event for the individual [16], a more sensitive interviewing technique is needed to elicit the provocative emotional threat in 70% of cases of MS. Until interviewers recognise the importance of "identifying with" and the use of facilitating methods in taking histories, life event researchers will continue to underscore.

Identifying the Provocative Event and Its Intrapsychic Meaning. The first step in the psychological management of MS is to pinpoint with the patient, as soon as possible after the first attack or relapse, the provocative emotional threat. As this is unconscious or preconscious in 70% of cases, physicians and neurologists may think that uncovering it will be too difficult, but it is not, given patience and above all the knowledge where to look. What gardener digs for potatoes in the rose garden?

At the first consultation, if a diagnosis of MS is probable although unconfirmed, it is useful to ask: "Would you be surprised if this trouble you have with your eye and your leg 6 months ago had been brought on by emotional stress?" About 50% of cases reply that they would not be surprised, and when asked why, they frequently describe the actual provocation. For those replying negatively, questions such as: "What sort of temperament have you got?" or "Do you think you are a sensitive person?", will in MS, just as in IBD, be answered affirmatively. Then the answer to the question: "Can you give any examples?", frequently provides an important clue. Even if it does not, it should have been possible by the end of the interview to establish whether the patient is sensitive to separation. An open-ended question we have found valuable is: "How do you feel about goodbyes?" MS patients say that they find goodbyes particularly upsetting. The type of family history may also provide leads, e.g. position in the family, family strife, alienated siblings not on speaking terms, remarriages, relationship with parents and in-laws and which parents they are most like, as can their reasons for a particular answer. Other questions: "Is your family a close one?", "Are your parents easy to help?, "Are they a cause of concern because of ill health or age?", are also frequently productive.

Pets as Surrogate Figures. When seeking possible separation threats it is important not to forget pets, particularly dogs and cats which may have replaced the child they have not had, or the parent they have lost or from whom they feel alienated.

For example, a woman who went on holiday had to leave her dogs in kennels for the first time. She could not stop thinking of them and suffered an episode of MS. Another patient [7] who had just moved house fantasised that her cat returned to the old house and was killed as it crossed the main road. Both she and her husband thought this was the reason for her relapse.

Pregnancy, Childbirth and Babies. Long recognised by doctors and neurologists to bear a close temporal relationship to onset or relapse in as many as 25% of MS patients, a baby poses a separation threat to the patient's position as the dependent child of the spouse [6].

One such woman who had felt cheated of her childhood because she had spent it looking after her younger brothers and sisters, made it clear when she married that she did not want children: "I had had enough of them." She was 39 when her husband said he wanted a son. Unfortunately, she had a daughter, who, as she put it, became a competitor even before birth, because from the time of conception her husband refused to sleep in the same bed with her and never did again. As soon as the nappy stage was over, he began to take the child everywhere. "He cared next to nothing for me. I felt left out and have felt left out ever since." Her first episode of MS occurred when the child was 18 months old.

It is less well known that fathers may be affected by the same threat of being displaced by their own child. W. N. P. Barbellion (pseudonym B. F. Cummings) in his autobiography [34] described it clearly:

> [p. 277] July 1916. The cradle came a few days ago, I had not seen it until this morning when I unlocked the cupboard door, looked in and shuddered. ... [p. 290] September 26, 1916, the numbness in my right hand is getting very trying. The baby puts the lid on it. ... October 5th. Our love is for always. The baby is a monster. ... [p 313] December 20th, 1916, the advent of the baby was my coup de grâce – more than once a senseless rage has clutched me ... the thought of a baby in exchange for my ambition, a nursery for a study.

It was the same for a vulnerable and sensitive only son whose childlike attempts at independence were crushed by a mother who kept a cane. He had clearly looked for some compensation for the bleakness of his own childhood when he married. Unfortunately, he was unsuccessful, and he developed MS shortly after the birth of his first child.

D: Did you have any doubts about starting a family?
P: (long pause) No.
D: Were you keener or was your wife keener on starting a family?
P: My wife was keener.
D: And what did you say at the time: We haven't enough cash in the bank, or not been married long enough or ...
P: No, no, I didn't express an opinion.
D: But you may have had reservations?
P: I can't recall any.
D: No, but you had reservations as soon as the first child was born?
P: Yes.
D: You felt in the cold?
P: Yes.
D: It hit you?
P: It did – my wife said: If you want affection now, you'll have to find somebody else.
D: Do you remember what you felt?
P: (Long pause) I felt I did not know how she could do it to me. ["giving-up response"]

Another woman [7], who had a relapse of MS when her daughter was about to have her second child, said: "Sad", when asked what she felt. Pressed at ensuing interviews to think why she had felt sad, she said eventually: "Poor Jason".
D: Why poor Jason?
P: Because he will be so hurt.

Jason was 6 and the first grandchild. The patient was identifying with Jason because both she and her sister, who also had MS, had been similarly displaced from their mother's affection by the three younger brothers who followed.

Patients with a hang-up about having a baby may consciously want one, while subconsciously finding all sorts of excuses for putting it off. In one example from personal experience [6] psychological management enabled her to overcome her fears of being displaced and then to have two children without relapse of her MS.

Because MS patients identify so strongly, birth of a baby to a sister or friend may provoke an attack [6, 7]. Mei Tal et al. [12] describe one patient whose twin sister had just had a baby.

Christenings are commonly provocative for women with a hang-up about having a baby. During psychological management they should be warned of the threat that this can pose for them, and helped to express their feelings about it. If necessary they should refuse to be a godmother until psychotherapy has helped them resolve their problem.

When the Doctors's Advice May Be Harmful. Physicians' and neurologists' advice to MS patients not to have children or to be sterilised can be as dangerous for them as having a child, because without children many fear for the durability of their marriage. Some suffer terrifying fantasies of a spouse's infidelity even if he or she is out for an hour or two. It is therefore not uncommon for a relapse to occur within a day or two of news of a relative's or close friend's marriage breaking up, or of being made privy to someone else's infidelity. They may identify with the deserted spouse, but in therapy some reveal that they identified with one of the deserted children.

MS patients should not be told to avoid having children or told that they should be sterilised without psychotherapeutic help to reach such a decision as free as possible of unconscious hang-ups about babies. Many unfortunate women deeply regret accepting such advice, given in good faith but in ignorance of the consequences.

9.2.5 Psychological Management

Outcome. Experience over the past 17 years has shown that psychodynamically orientated psychotherapy/management has helped approximately 5 out of 10 patients materially, with long remissions and greatly reduced number, severity and duration of attacks, compared with the previous course of the disease. Another two probably can be helped, leaving approximately three of the ten who deteriorate despite every attempt to help them. Usually, the reasons are lack of sufficient *ego strength* [17], or because the domestic situation is so overwhelmingly unfavourable that the patient has almost no chance of obtaining the necessary minimum of emotional independence (the "Lorna Doone syndrome" [6]). Sadly, such patients are soon symbolically back to toddling, and then further back to nappies and incontinence of bladder and bowel [14]. Therefore, advanced disease not only creates physical dependence but all too often loss of any degree of emotional independence, always so hard won in MS. Thus a vicious circle develops with relatives and care givers engulfing the patient because of understandable anxiety, guilt and consequent overconcern. Such patients deteriorate rapidly. The prognostic figures are, of course, approximate and are offered only as guidance pending long-term trials which will require matched controls.

Assessing Suitability for Psychotherapy and/or Psychological Management. From what has been said the chances of success in advanced cases are less good than in those seen early, and we feel that all in the last category should be offered psychological management. Assessment of likely success can usually be made after four interviews, when some idea of the patient's ego strength [7] should have been gained, and also the amount of help likely to be forthcoming from a co-therapist such as a spouse, partner, fiancé(e) or occasionally a sibling.

Couple Therapy. In MS, as in IBD with its comparable psychopathology, couple therapy, where possible, does better than individual psychotherapy. Case histories illustrating this may be found in Paulley [6]. The aim of couple therapy is to give the potential co-therapist a positive role rather than the one usually adopted, for understandable reasons, of being puzzled, frightened, guilty and overconcerned, all too much like the original engulfing parent, and very counter-productive. Unhelpful collusion and manipulation by patient and spouse, which are unconscious replays of the earlier parent-child relationship, can be pointed out in such sessions and alternative paradigms explored. The co-therapist learns with the patient to anticipate separation or engulfment threats before they occur, and thereby they may jointly succeed in forestalling them. The co-therapist may therefore be likened to a lightning conductor or defuser of bombs!

Essentials. A doctor or therapist needs some knowledge of the psychopathogenesis of MS before embarking on psychological management. This is why earlier sections have been presented in some detail. With an appreciation of these points any doctor can undertake psychological management in MS with an expectation of some success in 50% of cases, but without it the doctor is likely to spend much time making little headway. Even someone with an orthodox training in psychotherapy may find the training of limited value in MS management because most of these very dependent people fail to move [18, 19] with orthodox psychotherapy.

Facilitations. In taking a history from any patient with a disorder suspected to have a large psychosomatic determinant, the kind of facilitations described in Chap. 5 are necessary because these people habitually bottle up their feelings, and none more so than patients with MS. Just as in other psychosomatic disorders it is necessary for a doctor to be aware of *typicality* of *attitudes* and *coping mechanisms* and those stressful events which are *typically* provocative.

One technique which should be tried in a patient who says: "What you say is very interesting but ...", is to say: "Perhaps if I tell you what caused an attack in a patient I saw last week, it may help you to understand". It may be necessary to quote from two or three case histories. It is also worth adding that patients sometimes feel that something is too trivial to mention, although the usual reason is that it is too frightening.

For example,

Mrs. T. V., aged 30, whose husband said she and her mother were like sisters and never apart, presented with retrobulbar neuritis and was asked if she had had any shocks or bad news prior to the attack. At first she could not think of any, but after being given a few examples the interview proceeded:
P: I know I listen to our neighbour; she has just lost her father.
D: Has she?

P: Mmm, I suppose it sort of makes you think sometimes, you know, it could happen to my father.

D: I know, when did it happen? How long ago?

P: Last week, last Wednesday I think, he died.

D: But you felt all that in your bones?

P: (pause) Well, I kept imagining it was my father, you know what I mean.

D: (rewarding patient by shaking hands) I think you did.

P: I often do, and think what would you do then, you know, I run off and do all things like that.

D: You began to get inside the other woman's shoes?

P: Most probably.

D: You don't remember which day you heard about it?

P: Well, he had been ill for about a fortnight, he was in hospital, I think it was last Wednesday he died.

D: That was 1–2 days before your eye trouble. Do you remember what you *felt* when the news was broken?

P: Mmm, well, I felt a little bit sad, I felt, as you say, unconsciously it was my father and that, but seeing he is an older man – although (hurriedly) he is very well and not feeling ill or anything.

D: Surely.

P: I've always been fairly close to him as far back as I can remember.

D: Yes.

P: I always got on well with him.

D: I understand.

Having been told a story, patients may be asked to say how they would have felt and reacted had they been in the same position as the patient in the story, and whether anything like that had happened to them. To help them, it is often necessary to give examples of separation and engulfment threats not only to themselves but also to those with whom they may identify, e.g. friends' marriages breaking up, not forgetting pets being injured or dying.

Because these sensitive people, just as those with IBD, often need several interviews before they are able to trust a doctor or therapist, it is necessary to return time and again to the question, What did you *actually feel* when this thing happened? Patients eventually reply with such terms as "horror", "cold", "frozen", "empty", "hopeless", "defeated" – "Defighted," said one – and these may be accompanied by a sigh, epitomising the giving-up response.

Duration. Before embarking on psychological management patients and close relatives wish to know how long it will take and how often they will need to attend. The answer to the first question is not less than 2 years and possibly 3–5 years. Contrary to most teaching of orthodox psychotherapy we have found that in psychosomatic disorders, including MS, the passage of time is probably more important to the patients' ability to change their coping mechanisms than frequency of attendance or intensity of therapy.

Initially, frequency of interviews will depend on the severity of the case and the patient's reactions at the first interview. The space between the first and second interviews should not be more than 3 weeks, and should be only a few days if much material has emerged and there is a need to hear a spouse's or partner's feelings about the patient's alarming symptoms. Alternatively, if nothing has come out of the first interview it is essential to have an early joint interview, with the spouse to obtain help in identifying the provocative event. For example, a woman hiding her sensitivity behind a flat mask had been unable to recall any provocative stress until her husband, after being given an idea of what we were looking for, reminded her that her paraesthetic legs had come on while walking across a speedway stadium at which her younger son was about to race for the first time. She had a terrifying fantasy of him being killed.

After the initial interview the patient, and not the doctor or spouse, should decide the date of the next session. Patients typically turn to spouses to answer, just as a child would turn to its parents. It is by such means that patients can be encouraged towards greater emotional independence. By 6 months, according to progress, interviews may be 1–2 monthly and after a year, 3 monthly. In the event of relapse, however, the patient and co-therapist, if there is one, should be seen without delay, so that the provocative emotional event and its intrapsychic meaning can be brought into consciousness where there will be a good chance of the patient being able to cope with it in an adult way.

As in all forms of psychological management, the patient must be held long enough in the therapeutic relationship for psychological change to take place. With their extreme childlike dependency patients with MS, just as with UC, require their doctor to be initially more supportive than is regarded as wise in orthodox psychotherapy. However, without this avuncular approach patients either drop out of therapy or relapse symptomatically (retreat into illness). However, it is essential that such support is not felt by the patient as engulfment.

One other caveat: patients always ask how you feel about other forms of treatment, such as the Russian vaccine, diets, hyperbaric oxygen and spiritual healing. It is necessary, if the doctor is not to engulf or put down the patient, to say that there are no objections to any additional treatment, provided it is not seen as alternative but as additional to the psychological work. The patient must be helped to see that they will be tempted to seize on such treatments in preference to the psychological work which is harder and often painful. Without such insight the doctor will fail to hold the patient, or the patient will only pay lip service without really working, just to keep the doctor happy, and thus avoid the risk of separation.

Continuing Management: Learning to Fight in Place of Giving up. Having helped patients to recognise potential future threats, and thereby perhaps forestall some of them, especially with the help of a co-therapist, it is also essential through the transference to help them change their habitual coping response of giving-up to one of fighting; in other words, they have to learn to fight. As this has always been difficult for them because of fear of withdrawal/separation from key figures, they may not succeed for some time and then only partially. Perseverance is necessary.

For example, Mrs. E. Q's husband telephoned one day to say that his wife was in a terrible state. The conversation then went as follows:

D: What has been happening?

H: Peter has thrown up his university career and come home.

D: How has that affected Eileen?

H: She has got the most terrible migraine.

D: Good.

H: What do you mean good?

D: Well, it means she is angry and uptight instead of feeling hopeless and defeated as she did when Peter was breathalysed and taken to court. Then she had an episode of MS, but this time she has changed her response – better migraine than MS.

9.2.5.1 Termination

The process of termination is as described in Chap 5. Successful negotiation of this phase is of particular therapeutic importance in MS because of the basic psychopathogenesis of separation/engulfment threats, which are always involved in transference and countertransference and which necessitate repeated interpretation. For example, from the end of the first year onwards, patients should be asked how they feel about continuing and for how long, and encouraged to express any feelings they have about the doctor being just another engulfing person. This is usually seen as a separation threat, and the reply will be: "It sounds as if you want to get rid of me." By such means the patient is helped by degrees to cope with the separation threat of termination for months or years beforehand, and often for the first time in their lives they achieve it without a return of their old coping device of going back "in" again – *engulfment*.

After mutual agreement on termination it is wise in this disorder for the doctor to assure the patient that the door will always be open if the need to come back is felt.

Some doctors may feel that they will not have the time for the kind of management described, but the amount of time spent on a case may amount to no more than 10 h over 10 years [7] which is what many neurologists would spend in repeated neurological examinations, carrying out tests and pursuing various treatments. (Another case took up 15 h over 3 years and another, 13 h over 3 $^1/_2$ years.) Similarly, MS patients, because of chronicity or frequent relapses, occupy comparable amounts of a GP's time. Once again it is not *either* psychological management *or* standard treatment; both may be pursued simultaneously in the same session.

Associations and Societies. Most MS patients join groups for the obvious reasons of obtaining help and information and the wish to support research. However, a few are fearful of attending meetings at which very disabled people may be present, and seek their doctor's opinion about it. One must be careful. By saying: "No", doctors may put themselves in the role of an "engulfing parent" as well as posing a possible threat if overconcerned relatives, friends and usually a health visitor are pressing the patient to join. On the other hand, the doctor should not say: "Yes", without first helping the patients express their unconscious feelings about meeting dedicated organisers and engulfing care givers who tend to infantilise the patients by doing too much for them or, worst of all, getting them into wheelchairs prematurely. Unfortunately, it is not rare for some patients to be prevailed upon to go to camps or on cruises before they are as disabled as their fellows with advanced disease, for whom such events are truly the highlight of their monotonous lives. Lastly, patients themselves can be tactless and often tend to engulf the new boy or girl. Doctors and care givers always need to be aware of MS patients' sensitivity and vulnerability to things which most people would not notice.

Exhaustion and Hyperventilation. Many patients with MS complain of exhaustion or light-headedness. Severe spasticity is one obvious reason, because of the sheer effort required in locomotion. However, the symptoms affect many patients who are not spastic and may occur early in the morning and at about 5 p.m. upon returning home from work. During the past 3 years we have found that several such patients are actually hyperventilating and can be helped by physiotherapy and management as described in Chap. 7. For many MS patients every new day is frightening and engenders feelings near panic. Fear of relapse and separation/engulfment threats are seldom out of their minds unless they are busily occupied. Returning home in the evening for many means either to loneliness or domestic separation or entrapment, and leads to evening hyperventilation.

Link Between Psyche and Soma. This is as yet unknown: the possibilities were discussed in 1985 [7]. Immunological competence is probably involved, and a small measure of inherited HLA disposition has been demonstrated. An infective agent may or may not be contributory, while the vascular hypothesis advanced by Putnam [20] has not been excluded.

9.3 Stroke

Summarising a recent review on the emotional aspects of cerebrovascular disease, Storey [21] wrote: "There is no doubt – as there never has been – that strokes can be precipitated immediately by major emotional turmoil." Such, too, has been our experience over many years as physicians on-take for hundreds of admissions with strokes.

One difficulty in evaluating earlier research on psychopathogenesis is that before CAT scans, diagnosis lacked precision. Unsuspected intracerebral haemorrhage would have accounted for some cases in any series diagnosed as cerebral thrombosis. Another problem is what Dunbar (see Chap. 1) termed combined or overlapping syndromes. In cerebrovascular disease this applies particularly to hypertension, IHD and diabetes. Several studies support a relationship between stroke and type A behaviour. Adler et al. [22] referred to it as "the pressured pattern". Carasso et al. [23] found that 85% of 384 successive stroke patients had type A personality and that there was also a high incidence of apparently precipitant life events.

9.3.1 Psychological Management

To date there is no evidence that any form of psychotherapy or psychological management has reduced the risk of strokes recurring. On the other hand medication such as soluble aspirin for TIAs due to carotid artery stenosis [24, 25] or moderate reduction of underlying hypertension [26] has been shown to do so.

Even so, physicians who would deny any relationship of emotions to disease tell their hypertensive and stroke patients to take it easy. Telling such patients not to strain themselves and not to worry is often counter productive in a group of people when achievement is an important part of their personality make-up. Instead, we would advise the type of psychological management outlined in the section on IHD, or if they are severely hypertensive, that advised in the section on hypertension.

9.4 Subarachnoid Haemorrhage

Storey [27, 28] showed that in 6 of 30 patients with this condition who had no angiographic evidence of aneurysm, an emotional precipitant had occurred immediately prior to the haemorrhage. In only 1 of 231 patients with evident aneurysms was such an episode described.

The same 30 patients had a high incidence of psychiatric disturbances before as well as after the haemorrhage. Penrose and Storey [29] reported a small prospective study in which relatives of the patients were interviewed before the results of angiography were known. They described more emotional turmoil and more significant life events in those who were later shown not to have aneurysms.

9.4.1 Psychological Management

Our experience has been in keeping with Storey's. For example, a young woman of 23 with three children had just been abandoned by her husband. She sought shelter in her mother's house. Her subarachnoid haemorrhage occurred 12 h later. Her blood pressure was slightly raised to 160/90. Another normotensive, middle-aged woman was staying with her mother by the sea. They had a quarrel immediately after which she went for a swim, was stricken by subarachnoid haemorrhage and had to be dragged from the sea.

Psychological management in such cases involved helping the patients to express their hostile dependent feelings without fear of condemnation or recrimination, and offering follow-up interviews until their inevitable fears that they would have to pay for their anger with a further haemorrhage had subsided or had been accepted. Whether such intervention is likely to reduce the relapse rate in this group will require further studies on patients so treated as compared with controls.

Psychological help would appear to have no place in preventing relapse in patients with aneurysms. However, such patients may need help because of somatopsychically induced fear and depression.

For the small number of patients whose subarachnoid haemorrhage is secondary to polyarteritis nodosa or giant cell arteritis, psychological management is very relevant and involves helping the patient to work through unresolved loss and mourning.

9.5 Idiopathic Parkinsonism

Neither author has any experience that psychological management in parkinsonism can halt or slow the progress of the disease. Nevertheless, the possibility exists, and it relates to evidence based on personality and attitude studies of these patients, of a premorbid disposition resulting from childhood experiences, coupled with a close temporal relationship of onset to severe emotional stress over 50 years. Todes [30] and Todes and Lees [31] have recently reviewed this work and wrote: "What is remarkable, reviewing these studies, is the surprising degree of uniformity of opinion." For earlier studies and reports on psychotherapy readers are referred to Jeliffe [32] and Booth [33].

The following case history is illustrative.

D. M., a single woman aged 46, had a brother 7 years younger who had been spoilt by herself and her parents. Her father, who himself suffered from parkinsonism, died suddenly of MI 5 years before her own symptoms began. She had been close to her father and felt bitter and guilty about his death. Like him, she said, she was sensitive and retiring but quick to take offence. She had no patience with people with "nerves", and kept herself busy. In her work she had to get things right.

Recent emotional stress: Her sister-in-law, who had always been jealous of her relationship with her brother, had begun to resent the affection given to a girl the patient and her friend had adopted instead of to the nephew and nieces. This became so bad that the patient and her brother decided they would have to stop seeing each other. She denied that her adopted child was causing trouble, but this was probably untrue as 2 years later the child was caught stealing from the patient and her companion.

The patient is a hardworking obsessional woman who denied that she had emotions until her father's death, after which guilt and bitterness troubled her. That was followed by the rift with her brother and sister-in-law, and recrimination with her companion over the management of this adopted child who began stealing, etc. Key words are inflexible, industrious, denial, suppressed anger, bitterness and guilt.

During investigation, X-rays of the skull and arteriography showed calcification and diffuse narrowing of left carotid syphon, and EEG scan showed epileptogenic peak activity in the left temporal lobe. Fasting lipids were normal. Father and daughter showed attitudes which are also those of hypertension and coronary disease. He died of MI and she has early atherosclerosis.

9.6 Guillain–Barré Syndrome

See Chap. 10.5 and illustrative case histories.

9.7 Myasthenia Gravis

This is now a recognised AI disorder. Our experience of many such cases is that their psychopathogenesis is *typical* for that group, and appropriate psychological management is as described in Chap 10.

References

1. Crisp AG, Kalucy RS, McGuinness B, et al. (1977) Some clinical, social and psychological characteristics in the general population. Postgrad Med J 53:691–697
2. Wolff HG (1948) Headache and other head pains. Oxford University Press, Oxford
3. Paulley JW, Haskell DA (1975) The treatment of migraine without drugs. Psychosom Res 19:367–374
4. Weiss E, English OS (1949) Psychosomatic medicine. Saunders, Philadelphia
5. Langworthy OR (1948) Relation of personality problems to onset and progress of multiple sclerosis. Arch Neurol Psychiatry 59:13–28
6. Paulley JW (1976/77) Psychological management of multiple sclerosis. An overview. Psychother Psychosom 27:26–40
7. Paulley JW (1985) Psychosomatic aspects in multiple sclerosis. In: Wise TN, Trimble MR (eds) Advances of psychosomatic medicine, vol 13. Karger, Basel, pp 85–110
8. Skynner R, Cleese J (1983) Families and how to survive them. Methuen, London
9. Erikson E (1950) Child and society. Norton, New York
10. Charcot JM (1877) Lectures on the diseases of the nervous system. New Sydenham Society, London, pp 194–195 (Transl. G. Sigerson)
11. Grinker RG, Ham GC, Robbins F (1950) Some psychodynamic factors in multiple sclerosis. Res Publ Assoc Nerv Ment Dis 28:456–459
12. Mei Tal V, Meyerowitz S, Engel GL (1969) The role of psychological process in a somatic disorder: multiple sclerosis Psychosom Med 32:67–86
13. Harrower MR (1950) The results of psychometric and personality tests in multiple sclerosis. Res Publ Assoc Nerv Ment Dis 28:461
14. Philippopoulos GG, Wittkower ED, Cousineau A (1958) The etiologic significance of emotional factors in onset and exacerbations of multiple sclerosis. Psychosom Med 20:458–474
15. Warren S, Green S, Warren KG (1982) Emotional stress and the development of multiple sclerosis: case-control evidence of a relationship. J Chronic Dis 35:821–831
16. Brown GW (1974) Methodological research on stressful life events. In: Dohrenwend BP, Dohrenwend BS (eds) Stressful life events. Wiley, New York.
17. Lake B (1985) Concept of ego strength. Br J Psychiatry 147:471–478
18. Nemiah JC (1973) Psychology and psychosomatic illness. Reflections on theory and research methodology. Psychother Psychosom 22:106–111
19. Sifneos PE (1973) The prevalence of 'alexithymic' characteristics in psychosomatic patients. Psychother Psychosom 22:255–262
20. Putnam JT (1936) Studies in multiple sclerosis V111. Etiologic factors in multiple sclerosis. Ann Intern Med 9:854–863
21. Storey P (1985) Emotional aspects of cerebro-vascular disease. Adv Psychosom Med 13:71–84
22. Adler R, MacRitchie K, Engel GL (1971) Psychological processes and ischaemic stroke (occlusive cerebro-vascular disease). Psychosom Med 33:1–29
23. Carasso R, Yehuda S, Ben-Uriah Y (1981) Personality type life events and sudden cerebro-vascular attack. Int J Neurosci 14:223–225
24. Jestico J, Harrison MJG, Marshall J (1978) Trial of aspirin during weaning patients with transient ischaemic attacks from anticoagulants. Br Med J 1:1188–1189
25. Herskovits E, Vasquez A, Famulari A, et al. (1981) Randomised trial of pentoxifylline versus acetylsalicylic acid versus dipyridamole in preventing transient ischaemic attacks. Lancet 1:966–968
26. Marhall J, Wilkinson MS (1971) The prognosis of carotid ischaemic attacks in patients with normal angiograms. Brain 94:395–402

27. Storey P (1969) The precipitation of subarachnoid haemorrhage. J Psychosom Res 13:175–182

28. Storey P (1972) Emotional disturbances before and after subarachnoid haemorrhage. In: Physiology, emotion and psychosomatic illness. Elsevier, Amsterdam (Ciba Foundation Symposium)

29. Penrose R, Storey P (1970) Emotional disturbance and subarachnoid haemorrhage. Psychother Psychosom 18:321–325

30. Todes CJ (1984) Idiopathic Parkinson's disease and depression. J Neurol Neurosurg Psychiatry 47:298–301

31. Todes CJ, Lees AJ (1985) The premorbid personality of patients with Parkinson's disease. J Neurol Neurosurg Psychiatry 48:97–100

32. Jeliffe SE (1940) The Parkinsonian body posture, some considerations on unconscious hostility. Psychoanal Rev 27:467–479

33. Booth G (1948) Psychodynamics in Parkinsonism. Psychosom Med 10:1–14

34. Barbellion WNP (pseudonym Cummings BF) (1948) Journal of a disappointed man. Penguin, Harmondsworth

10 Immune System: Disorders of Immunological Competence and Autoimmunity

In both humans and animals immunological disturbance has been shown to follow loss in its broadest sense, notably depression of immunological competence, typified by the infant bereft of a parent and predisposed to infections. Secondly, in humans pathologically prolonged mourning may precipitate distortion of the normal system for defence of self to an attack on self by antibodies and lymphocytes in the AI diseases [1].

Diminished Immunological Defence. Susceptibility to infections such as tuberculosis, pneumonia, herpes, etc., following loss by death or alienation has been recurrently reported in the psychosomatic literature since the 1930s [2–6]. Prior to that, it had been part of folklore ever since Job [7] was afflicted after love for his God turned to bottled-up anger and bitterness following the loss of his eldest son and flocks (see also Chap. 18).

Animal research has confirmed immunological deficiency following premature separation at 15 days [8], and studies [9, 10] have shown that in young rats, the stress of handling, or of infection, or of insufficient food results in changes in immunological competence, and that such altered patterns of response persist into adult life, at which point they may be *reactivated.* This parallels our experience in humans and is of particular significance in the psychological management of the AI disorders, i.e. unresolved loss or alienation of a key figure in childhood being reawakened later by the actuality, or the threat, of further losses (see transcripts). In man, depressed thymic-mediated immunity was found by Barthop et al. [11] in 26 bereaved spouses 5 weeks after their loss, but not at 2 weeks, and was 10-fold greater than in controls.

Psychoneuroimmunological Research. For key references to the role of the hypothalamus, see reviews by Solomon and Amkraut [12], Rogers et al. [13], Stein et al. [14], Ader [15] and Hofer [16].

Genetic Influences on Immune Responses. What is known of these has recently been summarised by Batchelor [17].

10.1 Rheumatoid Arthritis and Autoimmune Disease

As long ago as 1892 a very great physician, Osler [18], felt it probable that polyarthritis was nervous in origin, "based on such facts as the association ... with shock, worry and grief". Studies on the suspected relevance of loss, or anticipated loss, to the onset or relapse of RA and other AI diseases over the past 50 years are too numerous to quote, but references will be found in [13, 19–21]. We make an exception for the study by Meyerowitz et al. [22] on eight pairs of identical twins discordant for RA because it made possible an assessment of the relevance of environmental influence independent of heritable factors. Stressful situations which preceded disease in the affected sisters had not been experienced by their unaffected twin. The case histories provide ample evidence of the frequent occurrence of loss and/or alienation, but at the time (1963) the authors seemed less aware of the pathogenic implications than they might have been today. For example, in one set of twins it is stated: "Her brother 2 years older, drowned on the fishing boat in December and she was unable to return for the funeral", but no comment is made on what she felt about it. Another study by Cormier and Wittkower [23] on the psychological aspects of RA was notable because it used patients' siblings as controls.

For previous reports on the psychopathology of SLE the following are recommended: McLary et al. [24] and Otto and McKay [25]; and for thyrotoxicosis, Morillo and Gardner [26].

Typicality. Between 1930 and 1960 the reports quoted above from many countries were sufficiently consistent for a *typical* profile of personality traits and coping mechanisms for RA to be drawn. This was and remains an important step in enabling doctors faced with a patient with one of these dangerous or crippling disorders to channel their enquiries into significant areas, and in so doing initiate effective psychological management from the first interview onwards.

Evidence for a psychopathology *typical* not only for RA but for all other AI disorders which he had encountered to date was advanced by th J.W.P. in 1982 [1]. To support this claim, case histories from a wide range of AI diseases are included at the end of this section. The opportunity for one physician to have clinical charge of such large numbers of patients with AI disease is unlikely to recur because of increasing specialisation.

10.1.1 Typical Coping Responses and Attitudes

Halliday [27] was one of the first to recognise that patients with RA were typically stiff upper-lipped, enduring and inclined to martyrdom. Himself a Scot from Glasgow he used the local word *thole* (= to suffer and endure) to describe it. Subconsciously, patients with RA and AI disease often see their illness as the cross they must bear in reparation for guilty feelings of anger and bitterness over "lost" key figures.

Alienation. In the psychopathogenesis of RA and AI diseases (and of disease "phobias"), loss by alienation is usually regarded as equivalent to loss by death, separation or divorce. Some reports, however, have suggested that feelings of alienation from figures *still alive* may engender greater bitterness and be especially relevant in RA. Our own experience tends to support this, and is illustrated by the transcripts of Mrs. F. R., Miss. H. W., Mrs. N. I., and Mrs. E. I.. Further studies of sufficient numbers of patients and controls will be required to validate the observation.

Bitterness, Self-Pity and Martyrdom. Such passive-aggressive feelings, described by Halliday, are *typically* concealed until the sufferers are helped to recognise and express them, sometimes many years later (see transcript Mr. B. W.) These coping responses originate in childhood and arise from double feelings (ambivalence) for a significant figure; they may then be compounded either by loss, death, separation or alienation from such a person. Alienated key figures, although still alive, are as if dead to the patient. Common causes of alienation are a harsh or rigid upbringing or preference supposedly being given to a sibling or siblings (see transcript Mrs. F. R.)

Many RA sufferers have been "little mother" to the family and have felt exploited in contrast to their siblings, who could get away with serious misdemeanours and are regarded by the patients as having being spoilt and indulged (see transcripts Mr. E. I., Mrs. K. K., Mrs. F. R.). Mrs. E. I. is *typical*, an only girl whose mother was jealous of her closeness to her father, and who idolised her four brothers. Mrs. K. G.'s double feelings for her mother stemmed from being the exploited eldest girl, and her envy for her younger sister developed into bitterness and hatred after her mother's death in the car the sister was driving.

The failure of patients with RA and AI disease to express and then resolve their feelings of loss may in part be due to their inability to express feelings generally. That characteristic they share with sufferers from other psychosomatic disorders (Super-stability, Chap. 2).

Provocative Life Events. Cobb et al. [20] and Halliday [27] noted that RA often developed shortly after deaths of key figures. Life events research, however, has also shown that other stresses such as redundancy, retirement, injury or illness are reported by many patients in the year before onset [28]. Many case histories show that these other events operate by preventing sufferers from using their *typical* compensatory coping mechanism of *hyperactivity* at work or games to keep at bay unresolved feelings of mourning and feelings of loss or alienation going back to childhood [22, 29, 30]. Mrs. F. R. is a classic example. The electric shock appeared to cause her RA but her own testimony shows that it was her subsequent *inactivity* which allowed all her bitter feelings to surface. Mr. B. W. whose father had died when he was 14 had never got over his death, but his work as a signalman enabled him to keep feelings of bitterness and guilt at bay until the loss of a final surrogate, his dog, a few months after his retirement. He was left without his compensatory coping mechanism of work. For Miss H. Q. with juvenile arthritis whose alienation from her mother was all too evident, any compensatory activity was clearly discouraged, her tennis racquet and bicycle sold, and the possibility of keeping a dog heavily sanctioned.

Importance of Primary Loss in Childhood. For a bereaved child, mourning can never have been easy, but it has become more difficult in Western societies as death has increasingly become a taboo subject. Even symbols of adult mourning such as black arm bands have become rare, and in southern England rituals such as funeral teas less common. Whereas children in orthodox Jewish families are fully involved in the ritual of mourning, most children in Westernised societies are expected to go to school the next day where they too often suffer the pain of being avoided by their friends. Even very young children try to be helpful by doing the washing up and shopping and not to make demands on the bereaved parent or sibling by weeping. So the pattern of using activity to keep grief at bay is learned early as a coping mechanism. At the same time they learn to suppress any ambivalent (double) feelings for the deceased, and their guilt finds no outlet in tears. Such children later recall their feelings of anger at mother or father dying "on them" and suffer feelings of badness (guilt) as a result (Mrs. Q. L., Mrs. P. E.). Many remember feelings of resentment that school friends had a mother/father and they did not.

Summary of Psychopathology. Patients with RA and AI diseases experience largely subconscious feelings of guilt, remorse and self-blame over lost or alienated key figures. Frequently, the primary loss has occurred in childhood or adolescence. The unresolved (pathological) mourning which ensues may then be kept at bay for many years by their *typical* coping mechanism of using hyperactivity at games or work as a "drug".

The onset of RA or AI disease is later precipitated by loss or anticipated loss of surrogate key figures, which then reawakens guilt and bitterness for the primary lost figures, *or* when the compensatory coping mechanism of activity is blocked by such life events as immobilisation due to injury, redundancy, retirement, or a golfing companion moving away.

10.1.2 Psychological Management

Much has been written about grief therapy [31–33] for pathological mourning in patients referred with a psychiatric disorder such as depression, hypomania or a phobia, but very little about that for patients with the same psychopathology who develop psychosomatic disorders, notably AI diseases, RA, hyperventilation or disease phobias for cancer, brain tumour, MS, heart disease, AIDS, etc. This is because clinicians are generally unaware of the relevance of unresolved loss and mourning, and that appropriate psychological management can promote remission or a lessened requirement for drugs with dangerous side effects.

The First Interview: The First Step in Psychological Management. A doctor seeing a patient with one of the above disorders needs an index of suspicion that pathological mourning may be present. For this reason the family history should not be hurried, and facilitations or tin-opening questions may be required, for example: "Are your parents alive and well?", or "How many brothers and sisters do you have?", or "Where do you come in the family?" or if the patient is the eldest girl, the question: "Perhaps you were little mother?" often uncovers the cause of envy and bitterness. A useful open-ended question is: "Do you think you are more like you mother's side or your father's side of the family?" A revealing answer was given by Mrs. E. I.: "Mother always says that all my faults were father's." See the transcript of Mrs. E. I. also for a reason for her difficulty with her mother: "Perhaps she was jealous of your special place with father?"

The ages at death of deceased family members should be noted because some patients with unresolved feelings of loss do not take ill until they approach the same age, fearing they must pay by dying in the same year. "I see you are about the same age as your father was when he died," is usually enough to uncover such feelings. *Superstable* patients with psychosomatic disorders speak of their troubles unemotionally, including family bereavements, yet may still harbour profound feelings of unresolved loss which only a doctor alert for non-verbal clues may detect.

At the first interview it is important that all suggestions by the doctor be phrased in a neutral tone. This enables an easy withdrawal following a patient's denial. Too early an interpretation only tends to reinforce a patient's resistance.

Importance of Observing. Clinicians writing notes and not looking at the patient may miss clues such as suddenly averted eyes, a quivering lip or change in the tone of voice as the patient answers about deaths or alienations in the family. If any of these are observed, a useful remark is: "I am so sorry, it seems that you still feel it very much, although it is some time ago." This permits further emotional release and often tears, and a helpful facilitating remark is: "Take your time, tell me about it when you are ready." It is also advisable for doctors to offer some comfort rather than behave like embarrassed owls. A hand on the arm or an arm round the patient's shoulders will tell the patient that the doctor is human, which may enable a patient to speak sooner rather than later of guilt over ambivalent feelings for the deceased.

When no sign of emotion has been expressed verbally or non-verbally on taking the family history along the lines suggested, it should not be assumed that pathological mourning or loss is not present. However, if present, the following question will invariably uncover it: "You have been unfortunate to have lost people close to you, I wonder if any of them are ever much in your thoughts, and not just at anniversaries?" The reply will be: "My mother/father/sister/etc. is always there, never a day passes without thinking of him/her" (e.g. transcripts Mrs. K. G., Mr. B. W.), and it is usually accompanied by tears or other display of emotion. It is also our experience that if such a statement is not accompanied by emotional release it is a signal that resolution of prolonged mourning may be difficult or unsuccessful.

Recent losses or anticipated losses of surrogates who stand for a *primary* figure lost in childhood are common precipitants of AI disease. The importance of primary loss and inadequate mourning in childhood has already been discussed.

Anticipated Loss. This may be as relevant as actual loss, so that when a patient with an AI disorder (or a phobia) has answered negatively about recent losses or alienation of relatives or friends, the following question should be put: "Do you have any reason to fear the loss of anyone close to you?" A patient recently revealed that she was perpetually in fear of losing her husband because he ate all the wrong things, smoked, worked too hard, and was always flying. She had not expressed these fears to anyone in case by doing so she might make them happen.

The patient, an only child, had not suffered childhood bereavement, but as a teenager had become increasingly alienated from her possessive and rejecting mother. She had married unwillingly a childhood friend who was her parents' choice. The marriage failed and she had felt guilty ever since. "What have I done to my husband and to one of the children who was upset?" At about the same time two men she knew died, one in an accident, the other, the husband of her greatest friend, of a heart attack. She felt very guilty because she found herself: "Not as sad as I should have been." This related to her own unhappy marriage and guilty satisfaction that her friend, whose marriage had been happy, was now unhappy too. The reason for her fears that her second husband would die was now evident, i.e. reparation for her own wicked thoughts.

These patients have strong ambivalent feelings for the spouse, sibling or child they fear is going to die and leave them, but in our experience there has always been a primary loss or alienation in childhood (see transcripts Mr. T. A., Miss A. M., Miss E. V.). When a surrogate's illness is especially protracted and demanding, the patient may pray that God will "taken them" (Mrs. E. I.). Such prayers engender guilt, especially if the surrogate recovers.

Value of Joint Interviews. Unconscious ambivalence can often be uncovered in joint interviews, e.g. "I adored my father." Husband replies: "But he used to thrash you with his tongue." This is illustrated by transcripts Mrs. Q. L., Mrs. L. V., and Mrs. D. X.

Subsequent Intervies: "Working Through". At each interview patients must be led back to the day of the death, how they heard about it, what they felt, whether they were able to speak to the deceased before death, whether they saw the person after death – this is particularly important in stillbirths and abortions (transcript Mrs. P. E.) – whether they wept, and for how long (transcripts Mr. B. W., Mrs. K. K., Mrs. E. I.), and if not, why not? If a patient says, like Mrs. N. I.: "Do you want me to go through all this again?" a suggested reply would be: "You know it does not do you any good to bury it". Ramsay [32] found it useful to say to the patient: "Your mother/father/brother/etc. is sitting here now. What would you like to say to her/him? What would your first words be?"

   In this way patients are enabled to go through the normal stages of acute mourning, which for various reasons they were unable to do at the time of their loss (see transcripts Mrs. P. E., Mrs. E. I.).

Acceptance of Feelings of Guilt. A doctor, accepting without judging the patient's anger and guilt over a lost or alienated key figure(s), may be the first person to do so, and comes to be seen in any ensuing transference (see Chap. 4) as the non-condemning, caring parent the patient may subconsciously have always wished for. Such a therapeutic alliance has great potential. The way the phase of termination of psychological management is handled (see Chap. 5) is especially important in patients whose psychopathology centres on guilt and bitterness over unresolved loss when it is about to be replayed by the loss of the doctor.

   After three or four interviews happy memories may begin to balance the bad ones and ultimately take priority. It is then time to ask the patient how long they think the sessions should continue and at what intervals. In other words, the patient should be introduced gradually to the prospect of termination and feelings they may have of being "abandoned" once again.

Is Orthodox Grief Therapy Suited to Psychosomatic Patients? The valuable techniques described by Worden [31], Ramsay [32] and Parkers [33] for the treatment of psychoneurotic or behavioural reactions of grief are also applicable to patients with psychosomatic disorders and may be learned by non-psychiatrically trained doctors. However, in the management of psychosomatic disorders it is probably better that the patient's grief therapist and orthodox doctor be the same person. The doctor who takes care of these *superstable* people's physical complaints is better placed to introduce them to the possibility that their emotions may be relevant to the onset and course of their disease.

All psychosomatic patients need to see the relevance of their somatic disorder to their emotional feelings and none more so than in the AI diseases. Unless doctors accept the relevance themselves, the patients are unlikely to accept it from anyone else, e.g. a lay therapist.

Second, because termination of drugs or other treatment of the somatic aspect of the disorder is rarely possible in less than 2 years, yet needs to be conducted as sensitively as the psychological management, it is difficult to separate the two. Most orthodox grief therapies require the patient to make a "contract" to attend for 10 weekly sessions before termination. Because somatic management may take longer, a splitting of therapists becomes as serious risk.

How Long Shall I Have to See You? Experience has shown that resolution of the worst pathological mourning can be achieved in as little as four interviews over 3 months, but it usually takes 6–8 interviews over 6–12 months, and in the worst cases, 2–3 years. As orthodox grief therapy sessions often take 2–3 hours, the total time for management for a psychosomatic patient on the lines suggested may in the end be less. We have found that in psychosomatic disorders the passage of time is often more important than the intensity or frequency of interviews.

When Does One Know That the Worst Is Over? Remarks such as in the transcript of Mrs. D. X.: "The sadness is shifting – I am easier and not so guilty as I was ... My mother is no longer so much in my thoughts as she was", and "I was able to give my granddaughter a doll in her cot and for the first time I did not think of the dolls I gave my two children in their coffins 12 years ago" (see Chap. 9, p. 174, Paulley [6]) or the girl who stopped having nightmares of her parents dying (see transcript Miss A. M.) or the dream of Mrs. N. I., or the chance meeting of the man with temporal arteritis with someone the same age and the "spitting image of my dead father" (see transcipt Mr. E. N.) give indications of progress.

10.1.2.1 Previous Reports

These have been few, and studies on outcome even rarer. Robinson [34] described benefit in 25% of 43 patients with RA over 5 years by casework done by social workers in a medical setting. He found the onset of RA in many instances associated with loss of support such as (a) death of spouse, (b) separation from spouse, (c) prolonged separation from family and (d) leaving home to become established.

Ross, Browning and Kaplan [29] provide 13 points of counsel on the practical principles of psychological management of RA. Most of these points, such as timing of visits, doctors' holidays and that doctors should not stop drug treatment and cut themselves off from the patient at the same time, are covered in Chaps 4 and 5.

Cormier and Wittkower [23] compared 25 RA patients with 18 siblings and stressed that understanding of the emotional problems underlying the illness by all members of the therapeutic team seemed to enhance the prospects of successful treatment, and that "intensive psychotherapy was indicated where emotional problems were found". Baker [35], a psychotherapist, has recently described his work on psychological management in a department of rheumatology.

All these studies concern RA. There have been none on the management of other AI disease.

10.1.3 Transcripts and Case Histories

The requirements of space prevents inclusion of more than one or two examples of the less common conditions, and for the same reason some disorders have been omitted altogether. These include *typical* case histories of relapsing polychondritis, Wegener's granulomatosis, myasthenia gravis, retroperitoneal fibrosis and progressive hepatitis. In other recognised AI diseases such as pernicious anaemia, Addison's disease and vitiligo, although psychopathology is *typical,* psychological management is usually irrelevant because the somatic component is irreversible by the time of diagnosis. Our experience of each of the more common disorders, RA, thyroiditis and giant cell (T) arteritis [36, 37], amounts to hundreds over 35 years; in those less common, such as MCT disease, it is numbered in fives or tens.

Mrs. F. R. was one of three children. Onset of RA occurred 3 days after an electric shock. She was 5 when she saw her sister, 18 months older, killed by a bus.

P: We were like twins – I would not talk for 6 months, and my mother had four doctors to see me. If my mother mentioned her, I did not want to hear and went out. I visited her grave every Sunday – Mother never really got over it. She always seemed to prefer my younger sister to me.

Transcript of interview *2 months after onset.*

P: My sister has been down here with my mother, she was pushing her baby, we couldn't all be together on the pavement, they were talking about the children – I felt left out of it, I felt nobody bothered to walk beside me to talk to me – they were either behind or in front.

D: Who are you referring to chiefly?

P: Well, mostly my mother – I went straight to my bedroom and broke down, I was so depressed. My husband came up to me, and he said: "We'll try and talk to your mother," but I thought I didn't want to – because I didn't think she would understand. She thinks I'm jealous of my sister, which I'm not, I know she gives my sister ten times more than what she gives me, but she is rather sly. My mother sent her £50, I never ask my mother for money, My sister practically lives off my mother. ...

The night we got married we didn't go on a honeymoon because my husband was on short leave ... we slept at mum's that night – and in the morning my father brought us up a cup of tea – but when I came down stairs she said: "To think lying in bed with a man like that", you know – and I felt I had done something bad.

[Sweets and money are clearly symbolic of love]

P: When my mother is with us, the first fortnight she can't do enough for us. After that she gets rather sly – she hides her sweets away – and will take her purse to bed with her every night and that – made me think she fears I'll take her money.

(When she married the patient felt at last one up on her sister, but when her sister married 2 years before onset of RA, this compensation was lost.)

P: I told you when we had that terrible "bust up" with mother, I didn't shout and bawl, I just said I knew she thought my sister did come first. She said: "You've always been jealous," and I said, "I've got nothing to be jealous of." *Before my sister was married I had no need for jealousy, I had two lovely children, a good husband and a good home, and I was quite contented with that. I mean – my sister had nothing* ... I didn't want to be alone in the bedroom and I kept thinking to myself, I hope by husband comes up to talk to me.

D: Was that the longest you'd been in bed with anything?

P: No, I was in bed with a bad flu 18 months ago, that got me very depressed.

D: What sort of things were you thinking about then?

P: Well, if my husband went anywhere – I didn't want him to go – I would say anything to keep him in – and I got right nasty. The children were at school – no one came to see me – and I just laid in bed, fed up reading books and knitting, just didn't want to do nothing – the house was so quiet even with the wireless ...

D: But normally? (She explains how activity had been her "drug".)

P: I like being out a lot, I take the children out and in the summer we're always on the beach – never really an indoor type, I can't sit down, well – that's why I feel it so much now, I think – I used to go dancing a lot with my husband, I just like being jolly, it's just that I like being active ...

Subsequent Course. The patient needed low dosage corticotrophin IM for 2 years. The transcript shows how she was enabled for the first time to express her long-standing, ambivalent feelings for her mother and sister, and to recognise how she had always used hyperactivity to keep these feelings at bay. She gradually saw that the electric shock had not *caused* her RA, but by putting her to bed allowed guilt and bitterness to surface. Despite her mother's and sister's deaths, which without psychological help would probably have exacerbated her RA, she was in full remission in 1972, 10 years after onset. She recently returned with back pain due to intervertebral disc degeneration of 12 months' duration, promoted by a quite different life situation to that of her RA (see Chap. 12 transcript Mrs. F. R.).

(Therapy time 12 h over 15 years).

Mr. T. A., a man of 71, was admitted to hospital with a 6 weeks history of severe RA. On a ward round he averted his eyes when saying that his mother had died 25 years previously, and that he had never got over it. He replied negatively to questions about recent losses of relatives, friends or pets, but when asked if his wife was well, he said that she had survived a severe MI only 4 months before. Later in private he accepted that unresolved double feelings for his mother had been reawakened by the threatened loss of his wife. Anticipation of being abandoned once more aroused feelings of guilt and bitterness. He was helped to express anger, previously unconscious, as well as his love for his mother. At the first two interviews he wept a great deal and came to terms with the likely loss of his wife. His RA was in remission at 6 months, and medication was tailed off. His wife suffered two further MIs without his RA relapsing.

(Therapy time 6 h in hospital and at clinic).

Mrs. P. E., aged 56, presented with recent peripheral neuropathy, a high ESR and leucocytosis. Nerve and liver biopsy confirmed PAN. The eldest of three, she was 5 when her mother became bedridden with tuberculosis in a tenement in a northern city. From the age of 5–7 she shopped and cooked and looked after her mother and younger brother and sister. She was 7 when her mother died and was too busy supporting her father and siblings to weep. This continued until she left home to marry. She remembers feeling angry and bitter at school and envious of children with mothers, who had not been robbed of their childhood by early responsibility.

Her marriage had been happy except that she felt that her husband was hard on the children. She overindulged them to compensate for the lack of love in her own early life, and he disapproved. When 17 her daughter rebelled and became pregnant by a married man. She feared her husband would throw her daughter out of the house, so she pressed her to have a secret abortion. PAN began within a few months of this. Her grief had to be kept from her husband, and she wept bitterly as she told the story. She expressed guilt over her "murdered" grandchild, the last of a series of "lost" surrogates leading back to the long suppressed, unresolved mourning for her mother, kept down for 50 years by toil, first for her father and siblings, and then for children who now no longer needed her in the same way. Symptoms remitted with psychological management for unexpressed grief and corticotrophin. Because the patient left the area, follow-up was restricted.

Mrs. D. X., a woman of 32, developed MCT disease 1 year after the death of her mother, with ANF 1/400 speckled pattern, extractable antigens Anti-RNP and anti-SM +. Ambivalent feelings for her possessive, strict and pious mother had been heightened when an aunt told her that the patient was 3 before her mother married. She felt hurt that her mother had confided this to her sister, but not to her. Mother had tried to stop her from marrying and then grieved because she moved away (admitted to be partly an escape). During a quarrel with her mother 8 months before her death, she had slammed the telephone receiver down. As a result she had not been told until too late that her mother was dying. She rushed to the hospital, but her mother was moribund and too drugged to communicate. She was told by her sister at the funeral that if she wept, she would only be thinking of herself and not her mother's suffering. Her husband said he thought she was ill because of her mother's death, but she angrily denied it. At consultation she wept when asked if her mother was much in her thoughts and said: "I don't think I shall ever accept my mother's death"; she nodded her head when asked if she knew the expression "God does not pay his debts in money." For years she had been angry with her mother for the latter's deceit and hostility to her husband, and this was enhanced by the telephone quarrel and her inability to make peace with her mother before she died.

Seen a few days later with her husband she said that they had talked about the first interview and wept a good deal, and she could now allow her husband to comfort her. A month later she said: "The sadness is shifting – mother is not as much in my mind but I am easier and not so guilty as I was." She was returned to her doctor after two more interviews; 3 years later he reported that her symptoms are minimal, that the ESR has been near normal for 2 years, immunosuppressives and ACTH were reduced to 5 units on alternate days.

(Therapy time 6 h over 9 months).

Mrs. Q. L., a married woman aged 49, had lost her mother in infancy. She recalled feelings of loss and anger at this deprivation as a child, and these were reawakened just prior to onset of RA by anticipation of her father's death and the inability to be with him because of the demands of her family. Second, she had felt alienated from her husband for some time. He was annoyed at the demands made on her by a disabled son, a cross she bore to assuage deeply repressed double feelings for her mother. Hardworking, active, tomboyish, a games player, the loss of these compensatory activities allowed feelings of bitterness over deprivation of a mother's love to come to the surface. At the same time she felt distanced from her husband and was torn with guilt at not being with her father whose death was imminent.

Psychological management involved couple therapy during which she was helped to weep for her mother and anticipated loss of her father and express her feelings of guilt and bitterness to her key figures including her husband and disabled son. In couple therapy he was helped to accept his wife's pain and tears. Her RA remitted after 9 months as happier feelings for mother, father, son and husband began to supersede bad ones. Anti-inflammatory drugs were stopped without relapse. She is an example of repressed early loss, anticipated loss and alienation when her usual compensation of hyperactivity was blocked by increasing family demands.

(Therapy time 7 h).

A woman of 32 first developed scleroderma with lung involvement when her husband went away to work and did not return, making excuses to cover up that he was living with someone else. With low dose corticosteroids and family support her disease progressed only slowly for 30 years at which time her colon became obstructed due to visceral sclerosis. Psychological management was not pursued.

Two younger married women developed rapidly progressive scleroderma and visceral sclerosis and were dead within 3 years of onset. Both had left home to marry to escape from possessive but rejecting mothers. In one the onset followed within months of her husband's infidelity which he flaunted in front of her friends. In the other it started after the husband left a note on the mantelpiece saying that he had left and she should not try to find him. Her distress was increased when he would occasionally turn up to see the children but would give no explanation of his behaviour. Both women felt martyred and bitter, a replay of their childhood feelings.

Psychological management was attempted, but events and rapidly advancing disease prevented the patients from attending.

Mrs. J. N. (dermatomyositis), married with three children, had seven brothers; a twin sister had died at birth. As a schoolgirl she realised that because her parents had arthritis, her brothers expected her to stay at home to look after them. Cleverer than average at school she said: "I dare not let myself risk thinking about a career becauses I knew it would be impossible." Her parents and brothers had tried to drive her boyfriend away; she was only allowed to meet him for 1 h on Tuesdays and 2 h on Saturdays and had to take legal action against her parents in order to marry. After marriage her parents or brothers summoned her to travel 30 miles to do trivial things for them. Mother was cold to her; her father, who had leaned on her, had died 9 months before onset of dermatomyositis symptoms, and there was trouble over the will. "I never could cry ... I have never got over my father's death and have recently seen him over my bed – the other night he put his arms round my neck and said he was going to take me with him – that frightens me ... I am scared stiff of being on my own." The patient required corticosteroids and immunosuppressive in reducing dosage and made good progress after a relapse at the anniversary of her father's death. She later had a relapse at Christmas when she took two wreaths to her parents' grave.

The patient relapsed severely after her therapist retired and spent the next 3 years being referred to various centres and to physicians, neurologists, rheumatologists, dermatologists and ultimately to a psychiatrist for alleged hysteria. The fact that no effort was made to arrange for continued help with the unresolved mourning which was fully documented in her notes and in letters to her doctor, reflects a pressing need for better appreciation of the management of psychosomatic disorders in general and AI disorders in particular.

(Therapy time 8 h over 18 months).

Miss A. M., single, aged 19, with SLE, Raynaud's for 12 months, polyarthritis in knees, hands and proximal interphalangeal joints of 2 years' duration, lack of energy, no sunlight sensitivity, but drug rashes and on examination atrophy of the finger pulps. She is the middle of three girls; the youngest is 3 years younger, eldest is 2 years older.

P: I don't show anger, my elder sister has always said what she thinks. A friend of hers died 3 years ago – it upset me – I didn't know her but it hit me – I felt for her family – an awful waste.

Asked if she had dreamt about her, the patient said she had been having a recurrent nightmare every 2 weeks for 2 years in which her father and mother were killed, but she had told no one about this.

P: I am very attached to home, yet I couldn't live with my parents although I am very close to them.

Later interview:

P: I wonder how I am going to get by without Mum and Dad. ... When I was 13 it worried me that my sister was cleverer. I squirmed when she was "pushy". Between 13–15 I was very annoyed with her. ... My sister was very upset when her friend died. ... I used to brood about her and I felt I just wasn't a Christian ... I felt guilty about her.

D: When the friend died perhaps you felt you had to pay for your angry feelings by losing your mother and father?

P: Yes, I felt guilty.

At the next interview 2 months later she said she had had no more nightmares, and these did not return. Polyarthritis subsided, termination of interviews was mutually agreed after 12 months, and after 2 years immunosuppressives were tailed off by her doctor. She became increasingly independent of her family. This is a example of a complex psychopathology in which the cause of guilt was not at once apparent. The key was her answer to the question whether there had been any deaths among her friends and relatives. She felt she had not lived up to her Christian beliefs and feared she would have to pay by losing those she loved most. Fears of anticipated loss were expressed in her nightmares.

(Therapy time 7 h over 1 year).

Miss H. Q., aged 19, had had juvenile rheumatoid arthritis since age 14. The following interview with mother (M) reveals intense ambivalence.

M: My mother and I were like sisters – I was never one to show my emotions – I still feel if I had cried instead of keeping them down here, it wouldn't have affected her (daughter's) nervous system so much. Up to the age of 5 she was a beautiful little thing, but she never wanted to mix. When she went to school she wasn't a child to create a fuss, and the teachers said that she is such a *good* child.

(Money and material things now seem more important than demonstrated affection.)

M: She has never gone without anything. I said today: "Why don't you put that pretty suit on?" She couldn't be bothered. She's got 14 pairs of beautiful shoes, every suit we buy her, there are coats I had cleaned, still in the cellophane. I bought her new shoes last week, I said: "Why don't you wear them? When are you going to wear them?" "I will," she said, and I said: "I hope so." I put her money in the money savings club, her pocket money I divided for her, Uncle Ben gives her pocket money, Auntie Tina gives her money, I give her money, her Dad gives her money. She's a damned sight better off than if she were working. I don't begrudge it, but it's a big disappointment.

(Now the patient is set some sums.)

M: In the lowest grade of shop work one has to be able to do some arithmetic. I said, "Carry on with some of that; you wouldn't do it at school, you've got nothing else to do." So I set her seventy-four sums. I said: "You do those by the time I come home." She said: "I hate doing them," and I said: "You do it."

D: She's fond of animals?

M: Always animals, as you know I would have loved her to have a dog, but I said to her: "If I got you a good one you realise that I wouldn't take it out after cooking dinner every night, and if you were cruel to that animal by letting it stay indoors instead of feeding it properly, I should get rid of it."

As the patient's condition worsened, including high fever despite all treatment, insensitivity reached its climax when it was stated in front of her that her bicycle and tennis racquet had been sold. Her father had hoped for a boy and gave her a cricket bat when she was 13! When the girl was seen with her mother, she was unable to say anything but sat cowed, sad and sour. Attempts to see her alone were blocked; her mother said it upset her. Psychopathology, harshness and intense ambivalence were evident, she was possibly rejected for not being a boy. She died within 6 months of this interview.

Mrs. J. O. This widow with polymyositis had lost her mother when she was 2: "a grievous memory". At school she felt it unfair that her friends had mothers. Her father married her mother's sister, an austere woman, and she felt alienated from her. Her early loss was reactivated by her husband's death after a tragic illness from cancer 2 years before onset of her disease; she was unable to weep and said she had always been a person to get on with things. Then her cat died, and she was dreading her retirement due in a few months because it would rob her of work which she had always used like a drug to keep the feelings of loss at bay.

Mrs. J. K. A married woman of 34 with SLE, fostered at 6 weeks of age and had never known her parents. "How could they have abandoned me?" She said she had never got over her foster father's death 10 years previously while she was abroad on her honeymoon; he had known he was dying but kept it from her. Her foster mother had been possessive and had never forgiven the patient's husband for taking her away and was forever accusing the patient on the telephone of neglecting her. The patient's feelings became murderous: "My husband had to pull me off her not long ago." He said he had noted that her personality changed every May – the anniversary of her father's death. After psychological management for the first time she was able to assert herself during a visit by her mother. Then her GP telephoned to say that she had spent 2 months in Brighton nursing her mother who had died from cancer 2 weeks previously. The strength of her love for her mother had surprised her, and she now readily accepted that in the past her repressed anger had blocked it: "Do you know in the last 2 months I've grown up." She added that a week before her mother died, she felt accepted by her as an adult for the first time. She had said, "Janie, hold me tight." She needed further help at the first Christmas after her mother's death and at the first anniversary. Her SLE remained controlled on low dose corticosteroid and azathioprine.

Mrs. J. T. has had Sjögren's syndrome for 2 years and Hashimoto's thyroiditis for 5 years. Now a woman of 60, at 18 she had lost a sister to whom she was very close, from aortic dissection, and then her first husband 10 years prior to presentation, from malignant hypertension. Just before onset of Sjögren's syndrome the dog which had been a puppy when her first husband was alive and thus her last link with him went missing. "I couldn't cry – it was like losing a child." Her second marriage was unhappy, and she was bitter because she was sure that her second husband and his son had killed the dog.

With psychological management her bitterness lifted and also her anger with her second husband so that when he became ill and died, she coped well and remained fit.

Mrs. K. V. presented in October 1973 with RA of 18 months' duration. It had come on a few months after her first child had been born with an imperforate oesophagus, which had required surgery in London. During the pregnancy her mother-in-law, with whom she had lived for 4 years, died. "I fear that if I had another child it may also be abnormal because she will make me pay for my dislike of her. God doesn't pay his debts in money, you know." She felt her difficult labour and the near death of her baby was retribution for her feelings for her mother-in-law. Over the next 2.5 years and nine interviews, mainly together with her husband, she was helped to recognise and then accept her guilt, and that she was in fact mourning the second baby she dared not have: the RA became less and less troublesome. At the seventh interview it was suggested that she must have known her mother-in-law very well having lived with her so long.

P: Sometimes I feel she is disapproving of the way I bring up my child.
D: It sounds almost as if she were still there?
P: She is, she's at the top of the stairs wearing her old red cardigan and stripy dress, she's always there, but when I go up, she's gone.

At the end of the interview she said she was moving to a new house and felt happy at the thought of leaving her mother-in-law's ghost behind her.

Within a few months she was pregnant, and the following letter was written to her GP after the final interview in 1976:

> I saw your patient with her husband this morning, and she brought her new baby with her. She is clearly delighted with it but admitted to being on tenterhooks throughout the pregnancy in case it was not all right, in other words, fear of retribution was still "bugging" her. I have never seen her look more cheerful and outgoing, and she no longer seems to be troubled about her brother-in-law's behaviour, and there certainly has been no sign of her mother-in-law at the top of the stairs. We discussed whether she need come and see me again, and decided that it was no longer necessary unless she relapsed or if you felt it would be usefeul. I am returning

her to your care. Thank you very much for allowing me to share in her therapy over the last 4 years; I have learned a lot from her.

Mrs. E. I., aged 54, had had rheumatoid arthritis for 3 months. She has four children, and a fifth adopted. Transcript of first interview typically features unresolved loss, double feelings and bitterness.

D: (Pointing to ankle) This is a bit puffy isn't it?
P: They both are at night-time.
D: Does it hurt you there when I press it?
P: Not particularly, no. [Standard medical history omitted to save space]
D: Are you one of a large family?
P: I'm the eldest of four.
D: Who was the next in age?
P: My brother – they were all brothers – there's 8 years between me and my youngest brother.
D: Are your mother and father alive?
P: My father's dead, my mother's alive.
D: I see, when did you lose your father?
P: About 10 years ago.
D: Was it a shock to you, or had he been ill long?
P: He had fall while working and fractured his skull and spent the last 3 years in the mental hospital.
D: Oh dear, that's sad.
P: It was a great strain.
D: Do you think you were like you father's side of the family or your mother's side in temperament?
P: Oh father's I should think, well, mother says all my faults are father's. (wry smile)
D: What does she consider faults in you?
P: Well, she thinks I'm a bit stupid – a bit soft – she doesn't agree with pills and doctors.
D: I see.
P: We're rather a close family, we all live in the same town.
D: But you meet your brothers at your mother's?
P: They go in the evenings, I go during the day. They send for me when they need me. (wry smile)
D: That sounds as though you've always been the one they turn to?
P: Yes, always.
D: When did that start do you think?
P: Always has – because I was the only girl I expect.
D: As you were the only girl your mother might save expected you to help bring up your brothers, I mean this often happens to the older girls in the family (little mother).
P: I don't know, I was father's girl, the boys were mother's.
D: Do you think your mother may have been a bit jealous of your relationship with your father, I mean sometimes –?
P: She could possibly have been.
D: She didn't show it?
P: No ...
D: Perhaps you were jealous of her relationship with your brothers?
P: Possibly, I always thought I was the odd one out.
D: Did you? Perhaps you were cleverer at school?
P: No, I always thought mother thought more of the boys than she did of me, you know.
D: Did you confide in your mother?
P: No, you couldn't ...

D: Not easy? Could you talk to father?
P: Yes. (pause)
D: Have you any children?
P: Yes, I have four – two boys and two girls – and ten grandchildren.
D: You are doing well!
P: Nearly eleven! (pause) I have one foster boy.
D: You personally have a foster child?
P: Yes.
D: How long have you had him?
P: He's 16, I had him when he was 2.
D: Mm, is he any problem?
P: Yes – he has been a great problem – he had to go to a special school; he left school a few months ago and has no work.
D: Does that raise difficulties for you and your husband?
P: A bit – my husband doesn't understand him – he's set in his ways – he's older than I am …
D: Mm, when did boy leave his special school?
P: Oh, February.
D: So there may be a bit of tension for you at home?
P: Quite a bit I should say.
D: Sometimes we find people don't just take ill by accident. If I were to say that possibly the rheumatism came on because of these tensions and emotional feelings, would you be surprised?
P: No.
D: You wouldn't
P: No.
D: The reason we need to understand it, is that by understanding it and helping you to as well, the rheumatism may settle down and in the end you may be able to get rid of or reduce the pills you have to take, whereas if we leave the problems unresolved, they may continue to work on you.
P: Yes.
D: How long have you been a bad sleeper?
P: Not as a child, but now years and years actually.
D: Do you think you get depressed at all?
P: Yes.
D: How long have you been depressed?
P: … just this year, just previous to this trouble, I got so I felt I couldn't cope – it's very unlike me.
D: Perhaps you felt that something was getting on top of you? Do you know why? Have you lost anybody, or has anybody you are very close to been ill this year? Or have you lost any pets or relatives?
P: I was very concerned about Jamie coming home, I didn't know whether to say no, but it's his home.
D: But you couldn't do much about it. What about your brothers who turn to you?
P: Well, that's what you are there for isn't (sadly) I wouldn't like to think they turned to anyone else. I am worried about my eldest brother who is closest to me since my father died.
D: But you still think about him sometimes?
P: Yes.
D: How often?
P: Oh – when I wish he was here, especially for the children. (Tears)
D: Mm, do you think about him at anniversary times? Christmas times?
P: Yes – you do, don't you? (Tears)
D: Maybe you didn't cry enough when he died? Do you think so? (Doctor comforts patient)
P: Sorry (apologies for tears).

D: It's all right, I just wondered.

D: My father died on a Tuesday, my daughter was getting married on the Saturday – I couldn't cry.

D: You couldn't cry could you – you had to be brave then for her.

P: You have to be sometimes – I'm not being very brave at the moment.

D: No, but it's better for you to show your feelings now than not. If you do cry at home, is your husband a person who can tolerate your tears?

P: Oh, I wouldn't let him see – he's not the type.

D: He wouldn't like them?

P: Oh, he wouldn't understand.

D: He knew you were close to your father?

P: Yes.

D: Did he understand that?

P: Yes.

D: Do your daughters understand how close you were to him?

P: They were too – particularly the one that was getting married.

D: During your father's long illness you must have had a lot of distress – I mean at times you must have wished it would come to an end, I imagine?

P: Yes, many many times.

D: Did that worry you when you had these feelings?

P: Well, you do ask God sometimes.

D: You didn't get any answer unfortunately. But you may have prayed sometimes too for God to take him?

P: Oh yes …

(Treated with corticotrophin and outpatient psychological management, 10 h over 9 years).

The improvement lasted 2 years until the foster son got into trouble with the police and was still out of work. She then developed polyarteritis and neuropathy when the corticotrophin was suddenly stopped by a psychiatrist who gave her antidepressants. Eventually she was admitted as an emergency, severely ill and unable to walk. Psychotherapy was resumed plus low dose corticotrophin, and the polyarteritis remitted. Her foster son married, and she experienced both relief and feelings of loss. She was seen together with her elder daughter who later proved to be a valuable co-therapist. Five years later on a telephone follow-up she said she was well.

Mr. B. W., aged 63, retired 6 months from being a railwayman, never having been off work. He presented with acute RA of 6 weeks duration following his dog being put down and having to hold it while the vet injected it [1].

Initial interview:

P: And then I've got this awful pain in the knee, and it just didn't go.

D: And that was 6 weeks ago?

P: Yes, I went to the doctor and while I was seeing him, the wrists and hands started playing up.

D: And it is particularly the wrist and also these joints here? (standard medical history taken.)

P: Dad died in 1931.

D: You were only 14?

P: I was the bread-winner then.

D: And you lost your brother too?

P: I never saw him from the day he went into hospital.

D: But that was grievous?

P: If you cut one, the others bled, you know.

D: I do understand. And then of course, almost at once, you lost your father?

P: Yes.

D: Maybe your biggest loss recently has been this dog?

P: Yes, and I rather went in the deep end with old Dill (tears) ... My wife had a job, and unfortunately the dog and I were left to our own resources. My love for him seemed to be reciprocated.

D: Perhaps that is something you felt very much?

P: (In tears)

D: It's all right. You may have felt it. You take your time and tell me what you felt.

P: The biggest feeling I had was, never again.

Later:

D: So if a parent is not very demonstrative, the baby soon gives up smiling. You mother may have been very busy?

P: Oh God! Excuse me. (Rises in pain)

D: That's all right. Would you like to go for a walk?

P: Yes, if you don't mind.

D: Please go around, and have a walk round the room ... I would suggest that when your father died, you probably couldn't weep?

P: My mother woke me up at 1 o'clock in the morning and said that a policeman had come from the hospital and that father had died, so I laid in bed until 5 o'clock. Then my mother came to see me again and she said, "It's 5 o'clock," so I had to get up for work, and I went. You know, it was hard times, doctor, they were hard times.

D: So he is very much around for you in your thoughts?

P: He is always with me. It is almost as if he is alive.

D: Sit you down a second if you can manage it.

P: (in tears) Yes, it's almost as if he is alive, but I don't think I could sleep in a dark room alone.

D: No?

P: I feel that he would come and stand beside my bed in the dark.

D: Yes, you are frightened of what he might ...?

P: Walking corpses, and I don't think he would hurt me, but ...

D: No, but you are just a little bit frightened?

P: Oh, terrified. Oh yes.

Psychological management combined with standard treatment resulted in improvement, A temporary relapse occurred when a woman came to the door and, seeing the rheumatoid deformity of his hands, told him her husband had had it, and as a result had been in the churchyard for the past 2 years.

Mrs. K. G., aged 50, developed Sjögren's syndrome in 1972, only months after her mother was killed. In 1979 she presented with thyroiditis shortly after her father's remarriage, which she saw as an insult to her mother and constituted a further loss [1].

D: That might have come on really quite soon after your mother's death, I think?

P: It did actually. That is when I got the ulcers in the eyes, and that was after my mother died actually. Yes.

D: Perhaps a few months afterwards?

P: Yes, and I had to come up to the hospital. She had had an accident. My young sister was driving the car and when we got there, she had already gone, and I suppose for a little while you feel a bit bitter. I did towards her. It was silly really, because it wasn't ...

D: No, it was understandable.

P: It wasn't her fault, you know.

D: No, but you feel it.

P: I did. I was bitter towards her for a little while.

D: Could you cry at the time?

P: Well, I remember breaking down and I would have cried and cried, and I don't think I have cried since.

D: You stopped?

P: I don't think I have cried since. I get a choking feeling (points to chest) but never any tears.

Four interviews and 7 months later:

P: I still think about my mum quite a lot.

D: How often?

P: Oh, I still do.

D: Can you say how often it is that she comes into your thoughts?

P: About every day. I was dreaming about her last night actually.

D: Did you?

P: Yes.

D: What was it about?

P: Well, I was doing all the work for her and she wasn't doing anything. I was getting on to her. It was terrible.

D: Is that what happened in your childhood because you were the eldest girl? Can you remember?

P: Yes. Yes. Yes.

D: Can you remember?

P: Yes. Well, I didn't get away with, so much as the others got away with, when they came along.

D: Can you remember what you felt at the time?

P: I used to get angry I think at the time. I used to say, "It's not fair, it's not fair." That's what I used to say.

D: Well, it wasn't fair really. What would you say to her if she was sitting here now? What would your first word be?

P: I am sorry.

D: And the second word?

P: I just love her.

D: Yes, that's right.

P: And although I was so close to my mother, I mean I really idolised her, you could never sort of get close enough to say those sorts of things, that I loved her. You don't think you'll ever get over it, but as I say, since I have been coming to you in February people have noticed how much better I am.

(The patient's ambivalent feelings for her mother stemmed from being the "little mother" and resenting it, with envy for her younger sisters.)

Mr. E. N., aged 52, had severe giant cell (temporal) arteritis. He was emaciated, initially confused and had a retinal infarct. Treatment included ACTH and then prednisone [1].

D: They are rather like snakes, aren't they?

P: What, here? (points to inflamed arteries).

D: Yes.

P: Yes, and funnily enough it goes down there, but then, all I thought was that I was having a stroke ...

D: I know.

P: And it became like lockjaw and I could hardly open my mouth, and then you can feel the continuation of the line you are talking about, going right under the cheek here (points to the thombosed facial artery)

D: Yes, I'm sure you can; have you any children by your marriage?

P: By this one, no.

D: By your first marriage?

P: Yes.

D: Are they boys, girls, what are they?

P: One boy, one girl.

D: Yes, how old are they now?

P: Elizabeth will be 21 now. Robin will be 19.

D: Do you see anything of them?

P: I've not seen them since 1958 (voice drops in sadness).

D: Why is that?

P: Circumstances really. As a matter of fact, my father and I became very close indeed over the last 12 months.

D: Yes?

P: And I hear my daughter is getting married (emotion breaks voice).

D: Did you? When did you hear that?

P: My father told me.

D: How did he know?

P: Because they have always kept in contact with each other.

D: Have they?

Joint interview with his third wife, 1 week later:

W: I know that after his father died, on a number of occasions he went to Felixstowe to the garden of his father's house and I didn't realise until be came back. He said: "I just felt I had to go." He felt nearer to him there, but he didn't want to take me with him.

D: Because he wanted to be alone.

P: I felt I wanted to go to try and get closer to his departing spirit, but he was too far off.

Convalescent, 3 months later (voice and manner now assertive):

P: Do you remember the elderly gentleman who came to the convalescent home on Friday, who was in the bed opposite me, Mr. D., aged 90? He has a very, very great resemblance and manner to my father. His grandson had a divorce not so long ago, and he said: "I still see his old wife and their children, but he doesn't know I do," and he said: "Do you know, I think I'm cheating." When he said that, I thought to myself, now I wonder if that is a fair comment about my father. Well, he was just kind of cheating a little bit, so I was wondering perhaps, if this may be part of the answer, perhaps Dad was just cheating a little bit, you know, without meaning to be in any way unkind.

Three months of psychological management of his pathological mourning for his father enabled him to finish his business with someone who had done what his father had done, and stood for him.

For further case histories of GC(T) arteritis the reader is referred to previous reports [36, 37]. These emphasised the need to check the ESR for 2–3 years after discontinuing psychological management and/or corticosteroids, because relapses of arteritic activity may be silent. Only by careful monitoring can relapses be averted, some of which are sudden and life-threatening, e.g. aortic dissection or myocardial infarction.

Mrs. N. I., aged 56, had RA since 1967, thyroiditis since 1968, SLE since 1976 and Sjögrens syndrome since 1978.

This dutiful daughter with strong ambivalent feelings and many AI diseases had been left by mother in a workhouse when she was 12; her father had left when she was 7, her brother had been killed in the war, her mother died in 1976, and her husband died in 1978 after 10 years of heart trouble [1].

P: The last time you wanted to talk about my mother.

D: Yes.

P: And I go home and I am in a state of emotional upheaval for days after.

D: Yes.

P: That's why in a way I wish you would drop it.

D: I know, but as it still upsets you so much it is better for you to talk about it ... (later in interview) Do you think about your mother these days at all?

P: Yes.

D: What odd thoughts have you got about her now?

P: Oh, I think I've got to accept the fact that there was something mental which I didn't recognise.

D: The last time you came you called her "and old humbug".

P: What, my mum? Oh, yes. The last thing she said was: "I have worked hard all my life," and she had never been out to work in her life at all.

D: Do you remember her kissing you?

P: No, I don't remember her kissing me.

D: Could you bring yourself to kiss her?

P: Yes, when I had to see her.

D: You did do?

P: Oh, yes.

D: And would she respond?

P: Oh, no. I just kissed her cheek.

D: Do you remember that day when she left you in the workhouse? What were your feelings?

P: Oh, yes. Oh, I was feeling dreadful. You are a one you know! If you keep on like this I shall be going all over this again.

D: I know. It isn't any good for you to bury it.

P: Do you believe in dreams?

D: Yes.

P: Since mum died (a few months previously) I dreamt that I was in a showroom, like the motor show might have been, and suddenly a sash window went up and it was Mum, young and lovely, because she was a nice-looking woman, mum with a beautiful-looking face and black hair. She waved and smiled, and her smile was radiant.

D: Now that is a nice story. That is a nice dream.

P: And her hair, it was so wavy, and her face was full of peace. Oh God, I thought, everything is all right. I think that is how the Holy Spirit comforts us.

D: All right, I agree with that.

The dream signifying resolution of her pathological mourning for her mother was her reward for the grief work which she had at times found so distressing.

When a patient with one AI disease later develops others, these follow a further loss, or threatened loss, of a surrogate. Mrs. K. G. and Mrs. N. I. are examples of this.

10.2 Infectious Mononucleosis

This disease is notable for false positive serological reactions and antibody formation against the patient's own red cells, platelets, etc. The EB virus is regarded as the likely primary antigenic agent, but there may be others. It is also a disease in which the number of people infected with the virus greatly exceeds the number who develop clinical disease, and in this respect it resembles Guillain-Barré syndrome, poliomyelitis, and tuberculosis. We have reported [38] that a combination of physical and emotional exhaustion usually precedes the onset of the disease, for example, in students before their final examinations with much burning of the midnight oil, associated at the same time with family or social dysharmony, or in a nurse on night duty who is running three love affairs simultaneously.

Children with infectious mononucleosis usually recover spontaneously and without the prolonged morbidity which is the curse of the disease in adolescents and young adults. The cause of the intense exhaustion affecting so many adults for months or years, and which may jeopardise their careers, is not known, is rarely discussed and deserves more attention than it receives.

The symptoms mimic states of anxiety which may follow head injuries or accompany virus or toxoplasmic encephalitis, and are characteristically intensified by attempts at mental concentration or physical effort. Even a telephone call or someone coming to the door is likely to cause palpitation, sweating, shaking and exhaustion. Hyperventilation may develop secondarily, but there is no reason to see it as primary.

Because of the parallels with encephalitis and the aftermath of head injury, subclinical encephalopathy is a possible cause. Meningoencephalitis is a recognised complication of severe infectious mononucleosis, but EEGs and CSF tests carried out in the state referred to, have always been normal, as have liver function tests.

This problem is worth mentioning because it seems to be an example of a true somatopsychic disorder and because it responds dramatically to 10 mg prednisone b.d.; this dosage is gradually reduced until the patient is off the drug in 6–8 weeks. Such a response lends some support to the encephalopathic hypothesis because a patient with an ordinary anxiety state or hyperventilation would not respond in this way, whereas encephalitics do.

Another reason is that these patients are so often wrongly diagnosed as neurotic by GPs, relatives and employers and therefore provide diagnostic and therapeutic challenges to anyone interested in psychosomatic medicine.

10.2.1 Psychological Management

Emotional stresses such as broken love affairs or behaviour causing parental displeasure are common precursors of infectious mononucleosis in the adolescent and young adult. These young patients will talk about such problems if the doctor is empathetic and suggests that they may have suffered recent stresses. It may then be helpful to ask the patient if he or she would like one or both parents to be brought into the discussion. The doctor, by acting as an honest broker, can in this way help to break down barriers that may have grown up between patient and parents. Protracted morbidity appears to be lessened if this is done.

10.3 Sarcoidosis

Histology points to an abnormal immunological response to an allergen or allergens, which may have some similarity to the outer coat of mycobacteria or to beryllium. Again physical exhaustion combined with emotional exhaustion precedes the disease. Crohn's disease, another disorder in which lymphoid hyperplasia [39] has been felt to reflect an aberrant or excessive immunological response [40], but has a different psychopathology.

10.4 Cancer and Malignancy: Psychosomatic Aspects

There is an extensive literature covering half a century suggesting that certain emotional stresses, including loss, may determine the onset of malignancy. More recently work has been done on predisposing personality traits, especially the lack of emotional expression in such patients [41–43]. In the past 10 years the main focus of such work has been to demonstrate the predisposing effect of the "giving-up response" in such patients and that psychological counselling designed to modify this attitude can delay or prevent relapses after treatment for breast cancer [44], a disorder in which psychoneuroendocrinology may also be influential. We do not have personal experience of the effect of psychological management but can testify that malignancy often follows closely on loss and pathological mourning as well as being an apparent hazard of immunosuppression.

10.5 Guillain-Barré Syndrome

Similar stresses to those described preceding the onset of infectious mononucleosis are usual in GBS. A number of viruses have been implicated in the pathogenesis, e.g. ECHO and swine influenza viruses. However, in the series of cases which followed swine influenza innoculation in the USA, the incidence, while much higher than normal, was still a small percentage of those innoculated.

This variable, immunological responsiveness is almost certainly genetically determined in some cases, while also related to emotional and physical exhaustion.

10.5.1 Case Histories

A woman aged 26 was engaged to be married, but her mentally defective brother resented it so much that he tried to murder her by throwing a small piano down the stairs on top of her. Until the wedding a few weeks later, she went to live with her fiancé's parents. She was still in their house when a year later she went into a long labour with an abnormal presentation. Forceps delivery was attempted but failed, a further forceps delivery was attempted under anaesthetic on arrival in hospital where her pulse was uncountable. She required Caesarean section to deliver a dead baby, and then remained for hours in shock requiring large amounts of hydrocortisone to restore her blood pressure. Although aware of the baby's death her family felt it better not to tell her that her father-in-law, of whom she was very fond, also died unexpectedly shortly after her admission to hospital. She was told 3 days later when her own condition was improving. Polyneuritic symptoms then developed, and GBS was confirmed. The patient had been withdrawn since admission, and this behaviour now increased. She would lie with her face to the wall and would not speak unless addressed. A black wooden cross appeared on her bedside table, and it was learned that she was about to be converted to an obscure religous sect by a man who was constantly sitting outside the ward. She presented every indication of giving up this life and following her baby and father-in-law.

Psychological management involved helping her to talk and weep, and by discouraging visits from the man trying to convert her. She became less withdrawn, the cross disappeared, and she began to fight to get better. Recovery was slow, but she was fit enough to go home to her husband in a specially equipped bungalow after a year.

This illustrates the combination of severe emotional stress and physical exhaustion preceding onset of polyneuropathy.

A fisherman's son of 15 heard that his father was missing at sea in bad weather. The boy, although unwell with a cold, persuaded the crew of another boat setting out to search to take him with them. He was 2 days at sea and suffered severe exposure as well as the grief of not finding his father. He developed GBS a few days later.

A waitress was left by her two employers in charge of their restaurant while they went on holiday for 5 weeks. She became exhausted doing her own work as well as management and accounts and often did not get to bed until 4 a.m. She became very worried about the responsibility and coping with the money. GBS developed at the time of her employers' return.

A man shortly to be married found himself in difficulty over raising enough money to buy the house. As a result he took a second job which involved little time for food, getting to bed at 2 a.m. and getting up again at 6 a.m. He developed GBS.

A married woman with two children was 5 months' pregnant. She had always driven herself hard at work and play. At the time of onset, she had suffered disappointment over a projected trip abroad with her husband. For some reason she felt more hurt than usual. Mild gastroenteritis preceded onset of GBS. She soon became totally paralysed and required tracheostomy and ventilation. ECHO 6 virus was isolated from her CSF. Psychological management involved encouraging her to show her feelings which she normally concealed. She was able to weep a little when her husband chose to go away on her birthday. She began to move a toe shortly after this, and a normal baby was delivered at term by Caesarian section.

Earlier she had been understandably worried that her baby would be paralysed too, but she was reassured when it was pointed out that the baby's vigorous movements proved that it was not affected, and she was able to listen to its normal heart sound. Its immunological reponse to the virus had not been the same as hers because half of its genes came from the father.

References

1. Paulley JW (1983) Pathological mourning: a key factor in the psychopathogenesis of autoimmune disorders. Psychother Psychosom 40:181–190
2. Day C (1951) The psychosomatic approach of pulmonary tuberculosis. Lancet 1:1025–1028
3. Kissen DM (1958) Emotional factors in pulmonary tuberculosis. Tavistock, London
4. Schmale AH (1958) The relation of separation and depression to disease. Psychosom Med 20:259–277
5. Imboden JB, Canter A, Cluff LE (1961) Convalescence from influenza. A study of the psychological and clinical determinants. Arch Intern Med 108:393–399
6. Yamada A, Jensen MM, Rasmussen AF (1964) Stress and susceptibility to viral infections. Proc Soc Exp Biol Med 116:677–680
7. Job 2:42
8. Keller SI, Ackerman SH, Schleiffer SJ et al. (1983) Effect on premature weaning on lymphocytic stimulation in the rat. Psychosom Med 45:75
9. Solomon GF, Levine S, Kraft JK (1968) Early experience and immunity. Nature 280:821–822
10. Dutz W, Kohout E, Rossipal E, Vessal K (1976) Infantile stress immune modulations and disease patterns. Pathol Ann 11:415–454
11. Barthrop RW, Luckhurst E, Kiloh L, Penny R (1977) Depressed lymphocyte function after bereavement. Lancet 2:834–836

12. Solomon GF, Amkraut AA (1972) Emotions, stress and immunity. Front Radia Ther Oncol 7:84–96
13. Rogers MP, Dubey D, Reich P (1979) The influence of the psyche and the brain on immunity and disease susceptibility. Psychosom Med 41:147–164
14. Stein M, Keller S, Scheifer S (1979) Role of the hypothalamus in mediating stress effects on the immune system. In: Stoll BA (ed) Mind and Cancer Prognosis. Wilay, London
15. Ader R (1980) Psychosomatic and psychoimmunologic research. Psychosom Med 42:307–321
16. Hofer M (1984) Relationships as regulators: a psychobiologic perspective on bereavement. Psychosom Med 46:183–197
17. Batchelor JR (1984) Genetic role in autoimmunity. Triangle 23:77–84
18. Osler W (1892) The principles and practice of medicine. Appleton, New York
19. Ellman P, Mitchell SD (1936) The psychological aspects of chronic rheumatic joint disease. In: Buckley CW (ed) Reports on chronic rheumatoid disease. MacMillan, New York
20. Cobb S, Bauer W, Whiting I (1939) Environmental factors in rheumatoid arthritis: study of relationship between onset and exacerbations of arthritis and emotional or environmental factors. J Am Med Assoc 113:668–670
21. Solomon GF, Moos RH (1976) Psychophysiological aspects of rheumatoid arthritis. In: Hill OW (ed) Modern trends in psychosomatic medicine 2. Butterworths, London, pp 189–215
22. Meyerowitz S, Jacox RF, Hess DW (1968) Monozygotic twins, discordant for rheumatoid arthritis. Clinical and psychological study of 8 sets. Arthritis Rheum 11:1–21
23. Cormier BM, Wittkower ED (1957) Psychological aspects of rheumatoid arthritis. Can Med Assoc J 77:533–541
24. McLary AR, Meyer E, Weitzman EL (1954) Observations on the role of depression in some patients with disseminated Lupus Erythematosus. Psychosom Med 4:311–321
25. Otto R, Mackay R (1967) Psycho-social and emotional disturbance in systemic Lupus Erythematosus. Med J Aust 2:488–493
26. Morillo E, Gardner LE (1979) Bereavement as an antecedent factor in thyrotoxicosis of childhood. Psychosom Med 41:545–556
27. Halliday JL (1942) Psychological aspects of rheumatoid arthritis. Proc Soc Med 35:455–457
28. Empire Rheumatism Council Report (1950) A controlled investigation and clinical features of rheumatoid arthritis. Br Med J 1:799–805
29. Ross WD, Browning JS, Kaplan SM (1961) Emotional aspects in medical management of rheumatoid arthritis. Acta Psychosomatica 4:9:39
30. Johnson A, Shapiro LB, Alexander F (1947) Preliminary report on a psychosomatic study of rheumatoid arthritis. Psychosom Med 9:295–300
31. Worden JW (1983) Grief counselling and grief therapy. Tavistock, London.
32. Ramsay RW (1979) Bereavement. In: Sjoden PO (ed) Trends in behaviour therapy. Academic, New York, pp 217–248
33. Parkes CM (1972) Bereavement studies of grief in adult life. New York International Universities Press, New York
34. Robinson CEG (1957) Emotional factors and rheumatoid arthritis. Can Med Assoc J 77:344–345
35. Baker GHB (1981) Psychological management. In: Clinics in rheumatic disease, vol 7, no 2. Saunders Philadelphia, pp 455–467
36. Paulley JW, Hughes JP (1960) Giant cell arteritis, or arteritis of the aged. Br Med J 11:1562–1567
37. Paulley JW (1980) Coronary ischaemia and occlusion in giant cell (temporal) arteritis. Acta Med Scan 208:257–263
38. Paulley JW, Hughes JP (1960) Steroid therapy in glandular fever. Postgrad Med J 36:553–556
39. Hadfied H (1939) The primary histologica lesion in regional ileitis. Lancet 2:773–775
40. Aluwihare APR (1971) Electron microscopy in Crohn's disease. Gut 12:509–518

41. Kissen DM (1964) Relationship between lung cancer, cigarette smoking, inhalation and personality. Br J Med Psychol 37:203–216
42. Greer S, Morris T (1975) Psychological attributes of women who develop breast cancer: a controlled study. J Psychosom Res 19:147
43. Morris T, Greer S, Pettingale W, Watson M (1981) Patterns of expression of anger and their psychological correlates in women with breast cancer. J Psychosom Res 25:111–117
44. Greer S (1983) Cancer and the mind. Br J Psychiatry 143:535–543

11 Endocrinological Disorders

11.1 General Considerations

There is probably no other area in human pathology where it is as difficult to distinguish between psychosomatic and somatopsychic mechanisms in the causation of symptoms as it is in the field of endocrine disorders. This is largely because most endocrine secretions are regulated from hypothalamic centres which, on the one hand, are functionally intercalated in the limbic system and thereby subject to either neuropsychological stimulation or inhibition (like with arousal, apprehension, anxiety, fear, depression, appetite for food or sexual gratification) and, on the other, are functionally modified by the specific hormonal effects of their altered secretory activity through a negative feedback mechanism.

Some of the intricate interactions between psychosomatic and somatopsychic mechanisms operative in endocrine disturbances are better recognized nowadays; others, however, are still controversial or insufficiently investigated. The effects of increased production of gonadal hormones on both body development and specific changes in behaviour during puberty and adolescence, for instance, are even prescientific common knowledge, as can be corroborated by any farmer who castrates a full-grown bull or stallion in order to get rid of its aggressiveness but not of its muscular strength. On the other hand, there is no scientific consensus on the question of whether "idiopathically" delayed puberty can be caused by psychogenic inhibition of the episodic secretion of hypothalamic gonadotrophin releasing hormone (initiated by a still obscure stimulus) which normally marks the onset of the characterisitc developments of puberty [1]. Yet there are indications that in women with unexplained secondary amenorrhoea, increased and persistent opioid activity in the hypothalamus might be responsible for the reduced pulse frequency of gonadotrophin releasing hormone secretion [2], which has been shown to be probably the directly underlying functional disturbance in this endocrine disorder of "unknown etiology" (Chap. 16). If these findings were to be confirmed, they could shed a new light on the causative mechanism of the amenorrhoea in women with anorexia nervosa, or inmates of concentration camps, or those subjected to less extreme but also stressful life situations, other than the loss of body weight to which the amenorrhoea is usually attributed.

This is, however, not the place to expand on the pathological mechanisms in endocrinological disease. The authors only want to emphasize that, especially with endocrine disorders, the psychological approach to and management of the patient depend greatly on both the correct diagnosis of the somatic pathology and the proper use of specific medical (and sometimes also surgical) interventions aimed at an adequate restoration of the patient's disturbed metabolic equilibrium. Until the metabolism has reached a reasonable physiological steady state, the patient needs reassurance and support rather than any deeper exploration of his or her psychological or psychosocial situation; in view of the emotionally or even mentally disturbing effects of the actual hormonal imbalance, this would be likely to lead to misapprehensions anyway. But if the patient, in spite of a satisfactorily restored hormonal and metabolic equilibrium, remains emotionally disturbed, the doctor or clinician should not hesitate to try and get the patient's cooperation in discussing his or her personal emotional problems.

Another important aspect of the management of patients with endocrine disorders is, that many require long-term or even life-long hormone substitution treatment. In order to further the patient's cooperation in maintaining this treatment properly and consistently, adequate information should be given concerning the effects and side effects of the medication, and especially the symptoms that may occur if either too much or too little of it is used. And since hormonal imbalance often leads to changes in mood or emotional susceptibility (like lethargy, depression, anxiety, irritability, obstinacy or obstrusive hyperactivity), which are usually noticed first by the patient's direct entourage, it is advisable to teach both the patients and their partner (or in the case of a junior, the parents) that these changes – if not otherwise explicable – may represent the symptoms of a deficient hormonal equilibrium, requiring medical advice.

11.2 Diabetes Mellitus

For all the scientific research done in the last decades into its epidemiological, endocrinological, immunological, virological and genetic aspects, the aetiology of diabetes mellitus is still obscure. Oddly enough, however, systematic investigations into the possibility of psychological or psychosocial factors contributing to the cause of diabetes are conspicuously scarce, despite an impressive number of well-documented observations suggesting that some kind of emotional stress situation may have a strong impact on the course of the disease [3, 4] (see Sect. 11.2.4). It seems as if the very concept of some psychogenic contribution to causing the organic defect that produces the diabetic state is too much contrary to the 20th-century medical paradigms to be considered a serious hypothesis worthy of testing.

Yet recent findings from immunological research may promise a further elucidation of a possible psychosomatic determinant in the causation of Type 1 diabetes [5] (see Sect. 11.2.4). The mechanism of endocrine autoimmunity is still unexplained. The strong HLA association on the one hand and the alleged noxious effect of antiviral antibodies on the other with regard to the causation of Type 1 diabetes mellitus are still subject to much debate [6]. At present the available evidence suggests, however, that the formation of islet cell antibodies can be triggered by a multiplicity of environmental agents leaving room for a contributory effect of psychogenic factors, e.g. emotional stress.

However, among doctors, nurses and other health care professionals, the psychological management of diabetic patients is gaining more and more attention, especially since it is coming to be scientifically recognized that the most disabling sequels to the disease, viz. the neurological (peripheral and autonomic neuropathy) and microvascular (nephropathy and retinopathy) so-called late complications, are essentially caused by a longstanding hyperglycaemia, and are consequently due to insufficient or inconsistent treatment of the diabetic state. Since adequate treatment of diabetes mellitus can only be accomplished with the patient's active cooperation, it follows that the impending threat of the late complications and the attendant suffering, disability and socioeconomic consequences can only be averted if an optimum working alliance between the doctor and the patient is established right from the beginning of the treatment.

Now, one of the difficulties at the start of the doctor-patient cooperation in the treatment of diabetes mellitus arises from the following situation, peculiar to this disease. After the first symptoms of ketosis and/or hyperglycaemia have been dealt with effectively, the patient is usually feeling fine. But then the patient is confronted with a set of rules about diet, expenditure of energy, and mostly also the use of tablets or injections, which are to be observed for the rest of his or her life. However, even constant adherence to these rules of the treatment, which quite often necessitate a drastic change in the patient's way of life, will nevertheless not be rewarded with a cure of the diabetes, but at best only reduce the risk of future complications. To many young people, therefore, the required restrictions in their freedom of choice, which also interfere with their social life, obviously seem too high a price to pay for benefits too remote and indistinct to be visualized. "I want to live *now*, to hell with what may come later!" is a slogan often heard from them. On the other hand, elderly people who get diabetes, especially when they do not require insulin injections, often tend to ignore or minimize the seriousness of its long-term consequences: "Oh, I just got a little diabetes; nothing to worry about" or "Why bother, at my age?" Unfortunately, such ill-advised attitudes sometimes seem to be fostered by otherwise well-intentioned "reassurances" the patients are getting from their doctors!

In addition, practically every diabetic patient sooner or later finds out that if they tamper with the rules of the treatment occasionally, they do not get immediate "punishment" in the form of unpleasant sensations such as pain, dyspnea or muscular weakness, as usually occurs in other chronic diseases. As a result, many diabetic patients before long become less willing to accept the rules of their treatment, and sometimes only adhere to them for a short period just prior to their next appointment with the diabetologist.

Therefore, it has to be acknowledged that the rules and regulations of the treatment, to which the diabetic patient should adhere in order to prevent the development of both acute and late complications, require so much knowledge, skill and persistent motivation that it is rather inhumane to expect somebody to accomplish this task on his own. Yet only in recent years doctors seem to begin to realise that optimum treatment of diabetes requires first of all education of the patient [7], and that adequate education is a long-term endeavour which cannot be accomplished without the patient's active cooperation. Unfortunately, many doctors still seem to feel that they lack the time, the competence or the motivation to shoulder the responsibility for this most essential aspect of diabetes management themselves, and tend to dismiss it as none of their business or to delegate it to nurses, dietitians or, more recently, specially trained diabetes educators. It remains to be seen, however, whether the delegation of a task which most patients would expect their diabetologist to perform, contributes to their motivation to cooperate consistently in the treatment, which after all is the very purpose of the education. It seems appropriate, therefore, to consider what capacities, skills and attitudes are required to function effectively as a diabetes educator.

11.2.1 The Education of Diabetes Educators

A primary requisite for a diabetes educator is of course an adequate knowledge of diabetes and its treatment. But equally important is a comprehensive understanding of the various psychological and psychosocial difficulties a patient may have to cope with, both because of the diabetes and because of his or her personal life situation. This requires an ability to listen and become familiar with the patient's personal circumstances, views, relationships and social life, in order to be able to define and agree upon the objectives of the education with the patient, according to his or her potential faculties, needs and expectations. This approach appears to further the establishment of a working alliance in which the patient may acquire sufficient knowledge, skills and motivation to manage the diabetes in an optimum way.

Many diabetic patients still complain that, when the doctor first told them the diagnosis, he went on at once to explain the symptoms of the disease, the diet and the prescription of insulin or tablets they required, giving them no opportunity whatever to recover from the emotional shock and to realise what having diabetes would mean to them. As a consequence they never remembered one single word of his medical monologue, since they were too engrossed in a turmoil of feelings and worries at the time.

Such complaints only emphasize the futility of trying to pass on any technical information about diabetes and its treatment to a patient who, for some reason, is not ready to listen and take it in. Therefore, the doctor who has to break the news of the diagnosis should enable the patient to collect his or her thoughts, for example by asking the simple question: "What do you think this message means to you?" and giving the patient time to express his or her feelings, fears and apprehensions. Such an approach usually furthers the patient's receptiveness to a few essential items of information about the disease and the consequences of its treatment. In addition it serves to underline the doctor's interest in both the patient's physical and emotional comfort, which sets the tune for their future relationship and cooperation.

Another aspect of patient education and management, which often seems to be neglected, is that with their efforts to adjust and adhere to the rules of their treatment, patients need explicit encouragement and reinforcement when doing well, rather than only disapproval or rebuke when they fail to do so, or seem to be cheating. The latter situations require even more attention and care on the part of the educator, in order to find out and discuss the underlying causes with the patient. Occasionally some misunderstanding between patient and doctor, which can usually be solved by talking it over openly. More often, however, it concerns conflicts or problems at work or in the family situation which appear to be interfering with the patient's motivation to maintain the diabetes regulation routine. Lending an ear to their emotional troubles often suffices to help the patients to sort out these problems on their own, but sometimes more profound counselling is required, especially when the origin of the problems seems to reflect the patient's low self-esteem and a resulting helplessness or depression. In rare cases of persistent resistance or open refusal of the patient to cooperate in treatment, it is always more appropriate to increase the frequency and intensity of the consultations in order to strengthen the relationship, rather than to withdraw from an ostensibly uncooperative the patient, as unfortunately still happens. These patients want to experience over and over again that the doctor accepts them as a person in need, which essentially requires patience, tolerance and often persistence on the part of the diabetologist, rather than sophisticated psychological skill or technique. In the end it seems to serve the purpose better than refering the patient to a psychotherapist who may not have sufficient knowledge of diabetes and its treatment to inspire the patient to optimum regulation of the disease.

With children and adolescents it is essential to focus the diabetic's education from the start on self-reliance and on their own responsibility for the regulation of their metabolic condition. This often requires education of the parents as well [8]. Many parents, especially mothers, suffer feelings of inadequacy – if not guilt – and sorrow for having a diabetic child. They often feel insecure about handling the child's upbringing in accordance with the dietary restrictions which the treatment requires. Mainly beause of their emotional insecurity, some parents tend to become too protective towards the child, thereby interfering with its natural striving for independence. Others betray their feelings of concern, anxiety and grief to the child so often that eventually the child develops guilt feelings about having diabetes which causes its parents so much sorrow. Both types of parent-child interaction often seriously obstruct the child's acceptance of its having diabetes, and consequently its motivation to cooperate with the doctor in the treatment. Many juvenile or adolescent patients with a very unstable, so-called brittle diabetes appear to come from families in which the emotional interactions between the various members are seriously disturbed, which may or may not be caused by the diabetes. The work of Minuchin et al. [9, 10] on family therapy for anorexia nervosa is described in Chap. 17 and is also applicable to families with a brittle diabetic child; they have drawn attention to the deleterious effects of the "enmeshing" family situation upon the capacity of these patients to gain consistent control of their metabolic regulation. Significantly, Minuchin and his co-workers chose to dedicate their book, *Psychosomatic families* as follows: "To the first diabetic children, Karen, Patricia, Deborah, who forced us to look at the critical rôle of the family in psychosomatic disease."

Apart from the aspect of the family situation, however, it has to be considered that many patients who seem to be unable to use their knowledge of diabetes for the control of their metabolism have been taught the rules of their treatment by the usual one-sided intellectual, formal method. Since the introduction of glycosylated haemoglobin determinations, most diabetologists have recognized that even a number of patients whom they supposed to be in good control, only regulated their diabetes carefully during the week or few days prior to their appointment with the doctor, and lived in more or less severe states of maladjustment for the rest of the time. Confronted with this therapeutically alarming situation, implying the threat of late complications, the medical profession has to consider critically in what way the methods commonly in use for the education of diabetic patients can be improved. What may be needed for better results are new attitudes of both doctors and patients. Just as in the modern methods of teaching pupils and students, the newer forms of education of patients have to take into account both the intellectual and emotional aspects of what it means to have diabetes and to control one's metabolic equilibrium consistently for the rest of one's life [11].

11.2.2 The Group Approach

It is worth noting that in every culture an important part of the development of attitudes, motivations, skills and behaviour, especially those which prepare the individual for later social communication, takes place in groups. It seems, therefore, that a group – by which we mean a *limited number of people in close proximity who are sharing one or more goals* – provides the most "natural" setting for an educational communication in which intellectual and emotional aspects receive equal attention. Actually, in recent years several methods have been developed to make use of group processes for the regulation and the modification of attitudes and behaviour of the participants [12].

In 1974 Pelser et al. [13] started a pilot project on group discussions with diabetic patients. The main experiences and observations relevant to the patients' behaviour and motivation with regard to the control and acceptance of their diabetic condition can be summarized as follows:

1. In each group, the subjects which were discussed spontaneously were remarkably similar, and dealt equally with technical knowledge of diabetes, its complications and treatment, and with the emotional problems of the participants. Most of these problems were concerned with *ambivalent, interhuman relationships between the patients and key figures,* which in many cases included the diabetologist. Almost all patients had gone through far more periods of depression, despair and inner protest, and episodes of cheating and non-cooperation than they had admitted to anyone, least of all their doctors.

2. Several juvenile diabetic patients, feeling misunderstood as they were unable to discuss their emotional problems within the family, developed *different forms of protest behaviour,* e.g. refusing to adhere to their diet, going on sprees, shop-lifting, or running away from home. Others felt lonely or depressed and sometimes "forgot" to eat after having injected insulin, developing a severe hypoglycaemia as a result. At other times they indulged in bouts of eating sweets, in order to "feel better".

3. Sooner or later the *fear of late complications,* especially retinopathy, came up in the discussions and then inevitably the question was raised as to whether they could or could not be prevented. The affirmative response from the medical discussion leader repeatedly provoked very emotional discussions and opposition, especially from the younger group members. In their view, the requirement to maintain the blood sugar level within physiological limits based on a regular diet, the adjusted use of insulin, exercise and emotional stability would impose an unbearable burden on

them and only inflict guilt feelings as late complications would occur anyhow, no matter how hard they tried. In short, it became obvious that many patients, as long as they felt unhappy and inwardly hated their disease, could not possibly attain the equanimity and motivated concentration necessary to learn how to handle and control their metabolic regulation.

4. The group discussions with fellow patients gave the participants the opportunity to *exteriorize their feelings and talk freely* and at the same time deal with technical problems of diabetes, its complications and treatment. By discussing both the nature of these complications and the anxiety surrounding them, within the safe and supporting "togetherness" of the group, the patients were able to help each other to develop more rational attitudes than when these conditions and associated emotions had been either avoided or insufficiently expressed in the previous talks they had had with their doctors. In addition, the patients learned to talk more freely about their emotions in general as well with their doctors and spouses, which in a number of cases contributed to an improved relationship both within the family and with their diabetologist. It seemed as if this long-term group education also contributed to the patients' conscious acceptance of the disease and the rules for keeping it under control, because it combined discussion of the cognitive and emotional aspects of the problems of the disease, and provided mutual understanding and support.

11.2.3 Patients as Educators

After 15–18 months of weekly sessions, the participants unanimously expressed the opinion that the group discussions were more valuable than any form of instruction or guidance they had known before, with respect to the increase in knowledge about diabetes and the emotional support they had gained. They also agreed that this group approach was a superior form of education and should become available to all diabetic patients. When they realized that this would require a considerable number of group leaders with both sufficient knowledge of diabetes and experience in conducting group discussions, and that this combination of capacities is seldom found, most of them agreed to the suggestion of their former group leaders that they themselves could be trained to conduct group discussions with fellow patients.

Coincidentally, a small number of general practitioners and students of medicine and psychology had expressed interest in becoming involved in a training course for conducting group discussions like ours. We then suggested setting up a joint training course for doctors, students and patients, to which all prospective participants agreed. Three groups were formed, each consisting of six patients, two or three doctors and one or two students, which met weekly. Each group was conducted by the same instructor (J. J. Groen, H. E. Pelser or H. van Dis) [13] for seven consecutive sessions, which were followed by a meeting of the three groups. The instructors then switched groups for another seven consecutive sessions, and the procedure was repeated. Each session lasted for about 2 h: the first hour was taken up by a regular group discussion and was followed by a discussion of its group dynamic aspects. In later stages the participants took turns in functioning as group leader or observer in the discussions. In the general meetings the participants exchanged their experiences of the previous training period and together evaluated what they had learned. Two additional general meetings were inserted for formal lectures, one on the technical aspects of diabetes and one on group dynamics. Thus, the training course consisted of 26 weekly sessions. During the last session the participants discussed the question of who felt confident enough to act as a group leader or observer in a new discussion group with diabetic patients. It appeared that those patients who trusted themselves to fulfil one or either of these functions were also considered capable to do so both by their fellow group members and by the three instructors.

In the next phase of this project, these newly trained participants formed "duos" consisting of a group leader and an observer who started new discussion groups with diabetic patients. Nine groups were formed, comprising 73 diabetic patients. Four duos were diabetic patients, three duos consisted of a doctor and a patient, one duo consisted of two students and the last one was formed by one of the instructors (H. van Dis) and a student of psychology. Once a month these group leaders and observers met with one of the instructors for a supervision session to discuss their experiences and the problems raised in their respective groups. In this way, continuity and consistency of the group guidance were secured and the motivation of the participants maintained.

Remarkably, all new "tertiary" discussion groups, irrespective of whether they were conducted by two patients, a doctor and a patient, or two students, each of whom had completed the same training course, manifested both the same high attendance rate and the same degree of satisfaction expressed by participants about the increase in knowledge of diabetes and the moral support they had derived from the discussions as the original "primary" groups. In every tertiary group the participants committed themselves to attend the sessions regularly for the duration of 6 months. At the end of this period, however, most groups agreed to continue their weekly discussions for another 6 months, and some for even longer.

Another notable observation from this project was that the patients who functioned as group leaders and observers in the group education of their fellow patients were found to maintain better control of their diabetes than their peers from the primary discussion groups who had not been or were no longer active as group educators in diabetes. It seems, therefore, as if the motivation and its expression in active involvement with the education of fellow patients also strengthens the motivation to maintain an optimum regulation of one's own disease. This observation might provide an additional incentive to encourage diabetic patients to become actively involved in educating their fellow patients.

11.2.4 Future Considerations

Workers such as Dunbar and Daniels felt that emotional stress was a major factor in the pathogenesis of diabetes. In recent years this view has not found much support, partly because increasing knowledge has shown that diabetes is not a single disease entity but is made up of different forms such as late onset Type 1, Type 2, and diabetes secondary to endocrinological disorders such as acromegaly and Cushing's syndrome. However, a psychosomatic determinant may yet be shown to have a place in the causation of Type 1 diabetes, in which auto-antibodies against islet cells have been found in almost all newly diagnosed children [5]. In Chap. 10 we have already advanced evidence of such an aetiological determinant in all other autoimmune disorders we have studied, many of which are well recognised as having cross-associations of incidence with diabetes. From the viewpoint of any possible value of psychotherapeutic intervention in Type 1 diabetes it would clearly be necessary to identify individuals most at risk, and *before* clinical diabetes develops. Because either HLA-DR3 or HLA-DR4 are present in 95% of insulin-dependent diabetics [14], the possession of such markers in children who have first-degree diabetic relatives would be a necessary requirement in defining the "at-risk" group. Family disposition such as the possession of close relatives with disorders like thyroiditis, Addison's disease, and pernicious anaemia, with which crossed associations with diabetes are well known, could be added. In theory, therefore, a case could be made for attempting psychotherapeutic intervention, as described in Chap. 10, prior to the onset of clinical diabetes in an at-risk group with the factors mentioned, which also had rising titres of complement fixing islet cell antibodies (CF-ICAs).

Immunosuppressive drugs have already been tried [15] in newly diagnosed Type 1 diabetics, so far without much success. This is presumably because a high proportion of islet cells were already irretrievably damaged, and the extended use of these drugs for the at-risk group mentioned, would involve some ethical problems regarding their long-term side affects, an objection that would not apply to a non-invasive treatment such as psychotherapy or psychological management.

It is not yet known how many individuals whose islet cells have suffered an attack by antibodies recover without developing clinical diabetes; that some do was suggested by a study of 685 first-degree relatives of Type 1 diabetics, 20 of whom were found to have CF-ICAs at the time of testing [5]. Seven of these developed diabetes over 5 years but 12 of the original 20 lost their antibodies spontaneously; one continued to show them, but his glucose tolerance remained normal. Studies have also been done on identical twins where only one twin had diabetes [16], and we would refer to our comments on similar studies (Chap. 10) done in rheumatoid arthritis and multiple sclerosis in which some external factor such as infection or, as we have suggested, a particular form of psychological stress appeared to be critical. Bottazzo et al. [17] considered that complement-fixing islet cell antibodies could be regarded as possible monitors of active beta cell damage. However, it is now known that about 50% of Type 1 diabetics become antibody negative after some years.

11.2.5 Summary

Consistent maintenance of blood sugar levels to contribute to the prevention of late complications in diabetic patients can only be achieved with the active cooperation of an adequately informed and motivated patient. Consequently, more emphasis should be placed on patient education. For various reasons, most of which are connected with the emotional and psychosocial aspects of having diabetes and the consequences of its treatment on the patient's freedom of choice, only a minority of patients appears able to adhere to the rules of the treatment, despite having sufficient knowledge of diabetes. This observation indicates that critical reflections on the effectiveness of the methods commonly used in the education of these patients are required.

For psychological management or psychotherapy as described in Chap. 10 to have any potential in deferring or preventing Type 1 diabetes we need to know more about the duration and intensity of antibody attack on islet cells and about how many individuals may recover from such an attack spontaneously. Meanwhile, there would seem to be a case for a few small pilot studies to be done on the at-risk group we have described.

11.3 Dwarfism: Emotional Deprivation and Growth Retardation

The first report on growth retardation and emotional deprivation was that of Patton and Gardner in 1962 [18]. J.W.P.'s first appreciation of the condition occurred in 1966.

A girl of 16 was referred for investigation of possible hypopituitarism as a cause of her dwarfed stature and delayed menarche. All tests then available for hypopituitarism were normal. However, the more refined measurement of "pulse" discharges of growth hormone available today might have shown some abnormality. It was not until the patient returned to be given the results of the tests that some recognition dawned that there was something odd about the mother's attitude to her daughter, and vice versa. It was simply that the mother swept into the room with her daughter trailing behind, just as if she had been a 10-year-old child. At the same time it was immediately clear that she was intellectually a 16-year-old, despite her juvenile physical appearance. The thought then flashed through J.W.P.'s mind that this woman might always have treated this girl like this and that in some way her delayed growth and maturation had been the girl's unconscious response to try to fulfil her mother's need for her to remain a child. This seemed as possible as the more usual view that dwarfed children are inevitably treated as if much younger than their years. In an attempt to explore the idea further, the mother was asked if her husband would come with her for a special appointment, in order to hear what he had to say, and discuss the problems that the daughter's future might pose for them both. When the husband refused to come despite several friendly invitations, earlier suspicions that something unusual had been going on in the family increased. This was confirmed by the family doctor who, when asked, said he had always felt that there was something odd going on but had never been able to find out what it was.

The above case is in line with the report by Powell et al. [19], who wrote: "The majority of parents have been uncooperative and have continually failed to show up for appointments." These authors were studying a younger age group (3.3–11.5 years) and observed, as have others, that failure to improve the domestic environment results in recurrence of poor growth performance when the children return home after having made great improvement while in institutional care.

Since these early reports, much more has become known about what has been termed "the effects of emotional disturbance and deprivation on somatic growth", and readers needing more information are recommended to refer to a review of the subject by MacCarthy [20].

Most of the evidence suggests that growth retardation, at least in the younger patient, is quickly restored to normal by adequate feeding and removal from the emotionally adverse family environment. Some similarities to anorexia/bulimia nervosa (Chap. 17) are beginning to be noted, with only one child in a sibship being affected by an "enmeshing" family situation. Another similarity is a frequent history of scavenging, gorging, stealing of food – even cat's food, polydipsia, and occasional malabsorbtion with pale stools. However, all these pecularities soon subside with "catch-up" growth if the patient is removed from the family and admitted to hospital or another suitable institution.

Family Background: Common Features. The mothers of dwarfed children usually have severe personal problems and have suffered profound physical and emotional deprivation in their own childhoods. Yet because only one child in a sibship is affected, it has been postulated that the mother's pathogenic emotional response probably dates back to her first sight of the newborn baby. Conceivably, it may have been rejected while in utero. The fathers in another reported series drank excessively, had bad tempers or extramarital affairs, and generally spent little time at home.

It has also been suggested, as we have done for anorexia nervosa (Chap. 17) that immaturity in the fathers may be just as important to the psychopathology as in the mothers, who are commonly held to be totally responsible for the manipulative, collusory patterns of behaviour between themselves and the affected child.

Finally, one case described by MacCarthy somewhat resembles the girl mentioned at the beginning of this section. The patient was older than most in MacCarthy's series. Her foster mother had apparently wanted a little doll and had treated her as such, keeping her in nappies until she was 8 years old!

Psychological Management. The need for competent psychological management is clear enough and the Open Systems Model of family therapy as described by Minuchin et al. [10] and Russell et al. [21] would seem the most likely to succeed.

11.4 Idiopathic Hirsutism

Many authorities have listed idiopathic hirsutism as a psychosomatic disorder but surprisingly few studies have been published about its psychopathology [22], and even fewer about its psychological management. Experimental research has shown that androgen and prolactin secretion is partly related to emotional stress, and Strauss et al. [23] have reported on psychological factors determining hyperandrogenaemia.

An analytically orientated study of three cases seen weekly for 2 years was presented by D. Paulley to the Psychosomatic Research Society in London in 1963 (personal communication) and appears to be the most detailed account of the psychopathology and potential advantages and limitations of psychological management which has been offered to date.

Mary, aged 40, unmarried with an illegitimate son, had been jilted when engaged to be married and devoted her life to celibacy and care of her child. She had four brothers and she was the youngest child. She grew up a tomboy with a premium on boyish things. Her hirsutism appeared when she was 21, shortly after her father's sudden death and when she was in a state of pathological mourning and guilt over ambivalent feelings for him.

Jill, aged 29, was the youngest of a large family and started to grow excess hair and to menstruate irregulary after the sudden death of her first husband in a road accident. She had married again and had one child.

June, aged 26, was one of the younger members of a family of ten, who were mainly boys. Three of her siblings had died shortly after birth. Throughout her childhood her mother was recurrently ill as a result of childbirth or miscarriages and her elder sister Ruth was "little mother" to her. Her hair growth and menstrual irregularity began at her engagement to marry and hirsutism increased dramatically following Ruth's death from cancer shortly afterwards. This had special significance, as was revealed subsequently during therapy. She had been 4 years old when a sister had died, and said: "I am scared that she [mother] will kill one of mine … I had the power to kill hers [children]." Later, when regressed under hypnosis to the age of 4, she said in a childish voice: "I wished ever so hard – I knew I could get rid of *them* – I was magic – I wished and I wished and the baby went away. Mum keeps crying – I wish she would stop – she didn't want the baby, they never came back – I wasn't good magic – I wished ever so much I could put it right. Father brought one back in a box [coffin]."

The three women were meticulously made up, unusually so for country people, but all still had a dread of their unsightliness and being caught without their make-up: "It sticks out all over me … people think me horrible … I want to hide when anyone mentions hair. … I feel so guilty."

Typical Features. First, they had been exposed to a similar parental pattern of behaviour. Mothers were organising, unloving, ungiving, and hard working and, unusually for their culture, had administered physical punishment to their daughters. Attempts at attachment to fathers had met with equivocal responses. Secondly, each had a similar sibling pattern of numerous elder brothers and because they felt mother loved the boys best, they responded by becoming tomboys themselves. They emphasised their dislike of playing with dolls. Thirdly, their education was reduced to a minimum because the boys had to have a good start. Fourthly, they had all experienced emotionally damaging deaths of significant figures in early childgood. These events emerged during therapy and were related by them as hateful wishes about their mothers which were then repeated in the transference (Chap. 2) to the therapist with fear of *her* death. June's hate wishes for her baby sister have already been described, Mary's related to a death of a small boyfriend and Jill's to a cousin. Mary's hate wishes intensified at the sudden death of her father just before the onset of her hirsutism, Jill's on her husband's death, and June's on her elder sister's death from cancer. These deaths of parental figures appeared to echo the omnipotence of childhood, and to reawaken dormant fears of the magical power of their wishes. It was following these events that all three developed, in addition to hirsutism, difficulties with menstruation and increases in psychoneurotic symptoms.

The need for power, its danger and the fearful omnipotence of their wishes came up frequently in therapy with remarks such as: "I dare not wish anything … I have to say, 'Please God, I didn't really wish it.'" They equated magic and their power over death with danger to people close to them and in particular to their children. June felt unable to have children because she said "they will be damaged." Mary was constantly dreaming of the death of her son.

Outcome of Psychotherapy or Psychological Management. It was not possible in this study to measure objectively any reduction of hirsutism, but two of the women claimed a diminution in the strength of their facial and body hair. However, the concomitant menstrual dysfunction disappeared and two discovered the joy of orgasm and were able to relinquish psychoneurotic symptoms. A major benefit of therapy was a lessening of the somatopsychic component of their hirsutism. They were now able to accept it and no longer saw it as a shameful symbol of their need to pay for long-repressed feelings of guilt over their omnipotence and magical power "to kill" people close to them.

11.5 Hyperprolactinaemia

At the 14th European Conference on Psychosomatic Research in 1982, Fava et al. [24] reviewed previous reports on somatopsychic effects of hyperprolactinaemia and also those pointing to its possible psychosomatic aetiology. The commonest somatopsychic effects were in women, and were depression and hostility, whereas in six out of nine male patients [25] the presenting symptom was loss of libido. The males were not significantly more depressed than a control group of medical patients and the greater behavioural changes found in women were felt to be due to a interaction of prolactin with oestrogen and progesterone.

Animal studies have shown that stressful stimuli may raise prolactin levels, and what is at present known about a psychosomatic aetiology for hyperprolactinaemia in man has been reviewed by Nunes et al. [26]. The same authors have added an important study of their own on 101 patients with hyperprolactinaemia and/or galactorrhoea. Of these 101 patients, 51 were reared without their fathers and 18 with an alcoholic and violent one, whereas such situations were uncommon in the population from which these women were drawn. There was also a significant temporal relationship of both onset and exacerbations of the condition to external events such as marriage, birth of a child or actual or threatened loss of a significant person either by death or separation, including abortions. It was concluded that the adverse childhood experiences already mentioned appeared to have conditioned these women to develop hyperprolactinaemia and/or galactorrhoea later in life in response to this type of event.

The most recent contribution on this topic was made by Strauss et al. [27] at the 17th European Conference on Psychosomatic Research. They reported on the psychological characteristics of patients and evidence for psychological factors determining the development of hyperandrogenaemia, amenorrhoea and hirsutism as well as hyperprolactinaemic symptoms.

Psychological Management. Although the authors have no experiences of treating hyperprolactinaemia by psychological means, whether alone or in combination with the more usually prescribed bromocryptine, they suggest that some of the concepts and approaches described in the section on idiopathic hirsutism (Sect. 11.4) may also be applicable to patients with hyperprolactinaemia and should be tried.

11.6 Thyroiditis

For psychological management of thyroiditis, see Chap. 10, and the case histories of Mrs. K. G. and Mrs. J. T.

References

1. Reame NE, Sauder SE, Case GD, Kelch RP, Marshall JC (1985) Pulsatile gonadotropin secretion in women with hypothalamic amenorrhea: evidence that reduced frequency of gonadotropin-releasing hormone secretion is the mechanism of persistent anovulation. J Clin Endocrinol Metab 61:851–858
2. Grossman A, Moult PJA, McIntyre H, Evans J, Silverstone T, Rees LH, Besser GM (1982) Opiate mediation of amenorrhea in hyperprolactemia and in weight loss-related amenorrhea. Clin Endocrinol 17:379–388
3. Groen JJ, de Loos WS (1973) Psychosomatische Aspecten van Diabetes Mellitus. De Erven Bohn, Utrecht
4. Groen JJ (1982) Clinical research in psychosomatic medicine. Van Gorcum, Assen, The Netherlands, (Chap 13, pp 224–241)
5. Spencer KM, Tarny A, Dean BM, Lister J, Bottazzo GR (1984) Fluctuating Islet cell autoimmunity in unaffected relations of patients with insulin dependent diabetes. Lancet 1:764–766
6. Plotz, PH (1983) Autoantibodies an anti-idiotype antibodies to antiviral antibodies. Lancet 2:824–826
7. Assal J-Ph, Berger M, Gay N, Canivet J (eds) (1983) Diabetes education: how to improve patient education. Excerpta Medica, Amsterdam
8. Pelser HE, Groen JJ (1989) Diabetes mellitus. In: Lacey JH, Burns T (eds) Psychological management of the physically ill. Churchill Livingstone, London
9. Minuchin S (1974) Families and family therapy. Tavistock, London
10 Minuchin S. Rosman BL, Baker L (1978) Psychosomatic families. Harvard University Press, Cambridge, Mass.
11. Groen JJ, Pelser HE (1982) Newer concepts of teaching learning and education and their application to the patient-doctor cooperation in the treatment of diabetes mellitus. Pediatr Adolescent Endocrino 10:168–177
12. Yalom ID (1975) Theory and practice of group psychotherapy. Basic Books, New York
13. Pelser HE, Groen JJ, Stuyling de Lange MJ, Dix PG (1979) Experiences in group discussions with diabetic patients. Psychother Psychosomatics 32:257–269
14. Bottazzo GF (1986) Death of a beta cell: homicide or suicide? Diabetic Med 3:119–130
15. Spencer KM, Dean BM, Bottazzo GF, et al. (1982) Preliminary evidence for possible therapeutic intervention in early Type 1 (insulin dependent) diabetes. Diabetologia 23:44
16. Bottazzo GF, Florin L, Christensen R, Doniach D (1974) Iselt cell antibodies in diabetes mellitus with autoimmune polyendocrine deficiencies. Lancet 2:1279–1282
17. Bottazzo GF, Dean BM, Gavruch AN, Cudworth AG, Doniach D (1980) Complement fixing islet cell antibodies in Type 1 diabetes: Possible monitors of active beta-cell damage. Lancet 1:668–672
18. Patton RG, Gardner LI (1962) Growth failure in maternal deprivation. Thomas, Springfield, Ill., p 94
19. Powel GF, Brasel JA, Blizzard RM (1967) Emotional deprivation and growth retardation simulating idiopathic hypopituitaryism. New Engl J Med 276:1271–1278, 1279–1283
20. MacCarthy D (1981) The effects of emotional disturbances and deprivation on somatic growth. In: Davis JM, Dobbing JW (eds) Scientific foundations of paediatrics, 2nd ed. Heinemann, London
21. Russell GFM, Szmuker G, Dare C, Eisler I (1987) A controlled trial of family therapy in the management of anorexia nervosa. Arch Gen Psychiatry 44:1047–1056
22. Fava GA, Grandi S, Santarsiero G, et al (1988) Hirsutism and psychopathology. In: 17th European Conference on Psychosomatic Research. Book of Abstracts. Klinikum der Philipps Universität, Marburg, p 70 (ISBN 3-8185 0025-8)

23. Strauss B, Appelt H, Bohnet S, et al (1988) Hyperprolactinaemic and hyperandrogenemic states in women. In: 17th European Conference on Psychosomatic Research, Marburg. Book of Abstracts. Klinikum der Philipps Universität, Marburg
24. Fava M, Fava GA, Kellner R, Buchman T, et al (1983) Psychosomatic aspects of hyperprolactinaemia. Psychother Psychosom 40:257–262
25. Fava M, Fava GA, Kellner R, et al (1982) Psychological correlates of hyperprolactinaemia in males. Psychother Psychosom 37:214–217
26. Nunes MCP, Sobrinho LG, Calhaz-Jorge C, et al (1980) Psychosomatic factors in patients with hyperprolactinaemia and/or galactorrhoea. Obstet Gynecol 55:591–595
27. Strauss B, Appelt B, Bohnet HG, et al (1988) Hyperprolactinaemia and hyperandrogenic states in women: a future task of psychosomatic research. In: Abstract Book, 17th European Conference on Psychosomatic Research 1988, p 208

12 Musculoskeletal System

It has long been recognised that posture may reflect emotions both in man and animals, e.g. the hangdog look. Expressions such as "bowed down with worry" or "they are a stiff-necked lot" are self-explanatory, while "being puffed up" with pride or "thrusting your chest out" suggest overfilling of the chest as seen in some sergeants or hostesses unsure of their position. A great variety of facial expressions, hand movements, scratching, shrugging of the shoulders and crossing of legs are all accepted forms of non-verbal communication. However, maintained positions of the head, neck, shoulders and spine have received less attention although long-standing imbalance or insufficient muscular support may lead to backache, neckache, arm and leg pains. Barlow, a senior member of the British Society of Psychosomatic Research, has done more than most to alert clinicians to the relationship of unconsciously adopted faulty postures to symptoms. He encourages a degree of awareness in the sufferer by use of the Alexander Principle [1, 2], and many of his patients have benefited. Orthopaedic surgeons, physiotherapists and chiropractors are also aware of the importance of posture and employ varying techniques to improve it, but few have been as single minded about it as Barlow.

It is not difficult to recognise psychological reasons for a child seeing itself as an ugly duckling, and then starting to behave like one, perhaps with its head on one side, one shoulder dropped and its spine scoliotic. If the problem is recognised early enough, competent psychotherapy and/or management should be offered to the parents, and physiotherapy or Alexander Principle therapy to the child. All too often postural abnormalities are not perceived until later in life when wear and tear has affected ligaments and bones. At that point re-education and techniques encouraging self-awareness are more likely to be effective than a psychological approach.

Muscles. Unlike smooth muscle activated by the autonomic nervous system, of which the individual is wholly unconscious, striped muscle fibres are innervated by the voluntary nervous system and to that extent are under voluntary control. However, some such functions are so automatic that they can be termed unconscious, for example, breathing and swallowing. Psychosomatic disorders of both are common but are not always recognised by specialists or GPs (see, for example, Chap. 7 for hyperventilation and Chap 6. for aerophagy and pharyngeal spasm).

12.1 The Dropped Shoulder Syndrome – Costoclavicular Compression

Wood Jones, an Australian anatomist, was responsible 50 years ago for a perceptive psychosomatic observation when he said that the typical patient with this disorder was the widow who had to take in washing, thus illustrating the interplay of a musculature unaccustomed to heavy toil, coupled with the effect of depression on posture. Ask any patient to draw a rough sketch of a woman recently widowed and with 3 children under 5, and the result is a bowed figure.

This condition is the most common cause of arm pain, but it is frequently misdiagnosed as carpal tunnel syndrome, cervical spondylosis or PID. Traumatic ulnar neuritis is a less common diagnostic error because it is rarer and also because the distribution of muscle wasting and sensory changes are clear cut, as indeed are those of carpal tunnel syndrome, but its neurology is often poorly taught. As a result one sees many unfortunate people who have had their carpal retinaculum(a) divided but who remain in great distress from costoclavicular compression which they have had all the time. Doctors should be alert for less common causes of neuritic arm pain such as syringomyelia and spinal tumour when there is a history of Lhermitte's sign or when CNS findings are suggestive.

12.1.1 Diagnosis

Appropriate psychological management depends as much on correct diagnosis as in any other from of treatment. Because arm pains are frequently misdiagnosed, and therefore treated badly, we are making an exception in offering diagnostic pointers.

12.1.1.1 History

The history in costoclavicular compression is so characteristic that one can be sure of the diagnosis in 75% of cases.

1. Pain usually affects the whole arm and hand. By contrast, in carpal tunnel syndrome and ulnar neuritis the pain is usually confined to the lower arm and the thumb and the 2nd and 3rd digits in the former, and to the ulnar border and the 4th and 5th digits in the latter. In cervical spondylosis and acute cervical disc prolapse the distribution of pain and sensory impairment is either related to the C5/6 dermatome or to that of C7 depending on which roots are involved, and with reduction of either biceps/supinator jerks or triceps jerk when C7 is affected.

Diagnosis is sometimes made difficult by a dropped shoulder syndrome developing secondarily to one of these other causes of arm pain because they may lead to awkward carriage of the arm and shoulder, fatigue and depression. Patients should be asked if anything makes the pain worse. Heavy shopping baskets, heavy overcoats and ironing almost always do.

2. Paraesthesia and sensory impairment may affect all the fingers, not just those in C7 and C8 distribution, because the cause is ischaemic from the subclavian artery being squeezed between the first rib and the clavicle rather than from direct nerve pressure. This explains why numbness of the hands on waking is quickly relieved by waving the arm about with temporary return of circulation only for the patient to be woken again about an hour later. Because of costoclavicular compression patients experience exacerbation of symptoms if they work long with their arms up, e.g.

putting things on shelves, painting ceilings. A motor mechanic working on his back under a car dropped the spanner on his nose because he lost sensation in his hands.

3. Objective evidence of sensory impairment is usual in carpal tunnel syndrome and limited to the 1st, 2nd and 3rd digits and lateral border of the 4th, while in ulnar neuritis the objective sensory loss is restricted to the ulnar nerve distribution in the lower arm and hand. However, in dropped shoulder syndrome objective signs of sensory loss are rare despite the widespread distribution of sensory symptoms. In severe cases of dropped shoulder syndrome in which the diagnosis remains uncertain, measurement of nerve conduction times can help and certainly should be considered before ressection of the first rib.

4. Ischaemic changes: patients may complain of a cold blue hand on the most affected side. Post-stenotic aneurysms of the subclavian artery may throw off emboli into the digital arteries causing Osler's nodes, but these are rare.

5. The patient may also have signs and symptoms of hyperventilation.

12.1.1.2 Physical Signs

The Subclavian Bruit. If a doctor examining a patient who is standing with the head rotated to the opposite side is unable to elicit a bruit by raising the affected arm through 90°–120°, costoclavicular compression is unlikely. In such cases further elevation of the arm should result in obliteration of the radial pulse leading 2 or 3 min later to the development of the paraesthesia and pain of which the patient was originally complaining.

Posture. The patient may not be stooped when seen, but the shoulder girdle muscles are often poorly developed, and the build is asthenic.

Overfilled Upper Chest. This cause of costoclavicular compression has not to date received the attention it deserves, but it is almost as common a cause as drooping of the shoulder. For example, a woman with symptoms of hyperventilation since her 'teens recalled painting a ceiling with her mother and not being able to hold a brush for more than a minute or two at a time. Her mother thought she was shirking.

12.1.2 Psychological Management

With Wood Jones' dictum in mind, doctors should try to identify any recent change in physical activity at work or domestically. A new house with a large derelict garden may cause unwonted physical effort by a man or woman, and if a man he may have recently retired from a sedentary job.

Widowhood, separation or divorce may affect posture not only through depression but also because the woman takes on physical tasks which her partner did previously. Equally, if she is lonely and sad, she is likely to try and keep these feelings at bay by physical activity, thus becoming exhausted. The same to a lesser degree may affect widowers who have to do the housework and ironing in addition to their normal job.

Psychological management first involves explaining to the patient the mechanisms of the symptoms in relation to unconsciously adopted shoulder posture and/or hyperventilation.

Second, patients with this disorder tend to exploit themselves or allow themselves to be exploited by spouse or children, e.g. Mrs. J. W. who said: "I still do all my three daughters' washing for them." Therefore, insistence by the doctor that the patient should not be allowed to wash up, get the coal in, do the ironing or carry heavy shopping for at least 3 months is often therapeutic, as is making sure that the patient attends the physiotherapy department at least twice a week for shoulder elevating exercises. Unless this is done, the family does not take the sufferer's symptoms seriously! The most responsible member of the family, who is not necessarily the spouse, should be told this.

If acute depression is being kept at bay by work, it is necessary to help patients to express their feelings, e.g. guilt over a daughter in and out of mental hospital following puerperal depression, e.g. case Mrs. J. W. "Where did I go wrong?"

If overfilling of the chest is present, re-education in posture and breathing should be combined with exploration of why (see Chap. 7).

12.1.3 Case Histories

Mrs. L. Q., aged 53, who had lost her father when she was 12, developed costoclavicular compression after she and her husband took over a small business which involved heavy lifting and very long hours. In addition there was decorating and a lot to do in the garden.

That she had a past history of migraine was not surprising. She was the youngest of the family. Her father's death had meant that money was short, and she strove for success at school and later at work. The tragic loss of her only daughter led her to adopt two children and to work harder than ever.

(Therefore in this case costoclavicular compression followed unwonted heavy manual work by a woman who had habitually used work and occupation to keep away unresolved feelings of loss for her father and for her daughter.)

Psychological management involved explanation of the cause of her symptoms (by enabling her to hear her own subclavian bruit through a stethoscope) and encouraging self-awareness by asking her to draw someone overburdened with work and grief, and helping her to talk and weep over her unresolved losses.

Physiotherapy was simultaneously directed to reducing habitual overfilling of her chest which was pushing her 1st rib upwards, and to making her aware of her slumped posture when tired and/ or depressed. Her family were asked to take over the heaviest physical work for 3 months. Psychological management enabled her to accept this help, something which she would previously have rejected.

Mrs. Y. T. suffered syndrome shifts from dropped shoulder syndrome to IBS with cancer phobia and then to depression and finally a return of dropped shoulder syndrome. This married woman first consulted a specialist in physical medicine with arm pain when she was 43, which was diagnosed as left brachial neuritis and treated with exercises. Five years later an orthopaedic surgeon said the pain was due to cervical spondylosis, and she received traction and short wave diathermy. Four years later, in 1978 she was seen by one of us with pain in both arms, worse at night and when carrying her shopping. Digits 2, 3 and 4 were paraesthetic, and subclavian bruits were present on raising her arms just above 90°, followed by obliteration of the radial pulse. Her husband, who had asthma and heart disease, was a long-standing source of worry and work. For the past year she had been worried about her daughter who was sterile and had been negotiating an adoption. This fell through, and she wept as she spoke of her distress for her daughter and herself and the probability of her daughter's marriage breaking up. Her symptoms improved after three sessions in which she was able to talk and weep, and a course of shoulder elevating exercises.

Follow-up of her case notes in 1986 revealed that syndrome shift to IBS had occurred in 1977 when she became phobic for cancer of the bowel and was referred to a surgeon. She told him that she was "sitting on a lump". Investigations were negative. She had unresolved double feelings for her father who had died of cancer of the bowel shortly before. Three years later there was a further syndrome shift to depression and she was admitted to a mental hospital. The last entry in her notes revealed that she had reverted to her earlier psychosomatic presentation of costoclavicular compression.

Summary. This history illustrates (a) the tendency of psychosomatic patients to split their caregivers through syndrome shifts; (b) the dangers of multiple referrals as a result; and (c) the difficulty in "holding" psychosomatic patients long enough in psychological management once their presenting somatic symptom has remitted. As a result Mrs. Y. T. failed to receive sufficient psychological help to resolve the psychopathology basic to all her presentations, pathological guilt over loss and fear of retribution.

Mrs. J. W., a married woman whose asthma remitted with psychological management and re-education in breathing and posture (details in Chap. 7) experienced syndrome shift to migraine 2 years later when driving herself hard at work and at home because her teenage daughters still expected her to do their laundry. The migraine lessened with the type of management described in Chap. 9 only for a shift to occur to her musculoskeletal system, first a dropped shoulder syndrome, then 3 years later backache and intervertebral disc degenerative changes. She had had an earlier attack of back pain and sciatica when she was 21.

The provocative life situation at the time of her dropped shoulder syndrome was her daughter's puerperal depression. For 2 years the patient cared for the baby and visited her daughter in a mental hospital nearly every day. She blamed herself for her daughter's illness, felt depressed and also physically exhausted with worry and toil. She was helped to accept her feelings of guilt in therapeutic sessions, and her husband's understanding was sought in easing her physical burdens.

The provocative life situation leading to the development of back pain was her son's return home after the breakdown of his marriage, which she considered his fault as he had become a gambler; at the same time she had to work harder and faster as a cook because of a time and motion study. Significantly, the back trouble occurred just before Christmas when "struggling" to keep things going at work and also (resentfully) having "three men to look after at home".

Summary. Syndrome shifts: asthma → migraine →dropped shoulder syndrome →backache, PID

12.2 Intervertebral Disc Disorders

12.2.1 Acute Disc Prolapse

The onset of severe back pain and/or sciatica commonly occurs when a person is not lifting heavy weights. Characteristically, it strikes first thing in the morning when turning over or getting out of bed. The patient may have felt something "go" in the back while lifting a day or two before but symptoms rarely develop then.

During the Second World War Scott [3], an orthopaedic surgeon in the RAF, later to be Director of the Nuffield Orthopaedic Centre in Oxford, was struck first by the number of young men consulting him for backache, many of them aircrew, and second by the distance between the vertebrae on X-ray and the scalloping required to accommodate the rounded shape of the intervertebral discs. In 1951 Charnley [4] showed that the intervertebral discs of a cadaver behaved like sponges, readily absorbing water or normal saline with very high pressures developing within the disc. Hirsch [5] reproduced typical back pain by increasing the pressure in the disc by injecting it and found evidence of changes in the nucleus preceding those in the annulus, "which habitually ruptures from within upwards".

Scott's experience in the war was in accord with that of Barr [6] who stated: "Low back and sciatic pain signify a state of stimulation of the cerebral cortex." Scott went on to point out that attacks of acute pain had been known to come on after exposure, strenuous exercise without back injury, *and prolonged emotional strain* [our italics], and that emotional strain was potentially a factor in periodic increases in pressure in the nucleus pulposus. In an address to the Psychosomatic Research Society in 1964 he recalled that recruits to the London police before the Second World War had to be 6'0" (183 cm). Those found to be only 5'11 $^1/_2$" were advised by the recruiting sergeant to go to bed for 2 days and come back shortly after getting up, when their height was usually 6'0" due to swelling of their intervertebral discs; an observation which fits with the frequent onset of PID symptoms first thing in the morning and sodium and water retention at night. On a visit to the Scilly Isles Scott learned from the GP there that none of his patients who spent much of the year bent double picking or planting daffodils attended with backache. The only two people on the island of St. Mary's who had had PIDs were the postmistress and the schoolteacher. (See Chap. 9 for frequency of migraine among school teachers.)

After the war Scott and co-workers tested his hypothesis of stress-induced swelling of the nucleus pulposus using Orkney voles [7]. It had been previously noted [8] that these animals, when involved in daily periods of fighting, showed an increase of weight in the adrenals and a decrease in the thymus. The stress of fighting was induced by putting a young male into the cage of a pair of old voles. The animals and controls were killed, and the volume of the nucleus pulposus in relation to the total disc area was measured.

In this manner 79 discs were measured, and the stressed voles were found to have a greater enlargement of their nuclei compared with controls at a level of significance of 1:100–1:1000. Subsequent work was done on litter mates and on the polysaccharide composition of the nucleus pulposus.

12.2.2 Psychological Management

In the sections on aphthous ulcer, IBS and migraine, it has been pointed out that syndrome shift is common not only between these disorders but between intervertebral disc disorders, dysmenorrhoea, PMT and pseudocystitis as well. Migraine patients usually ask at the end of their group therapy whether they are likely to get anything in place of their migraine. We reply: "Not necessarily", but if they did, it might be one of the conditions mentioned. At this point about half the group's heads will be nodding and then they say they have had one or more of these already!

What then determines these syndrome shifts? As far as migraine and IBS are concerned, it appears to be the differing life situations which have already been described. Patients with aphthoses have often experienced loss or alienation in addition to overwork and hyperactivity, and this accords with recent research on altered immunity in the aetiology of aphthous ulcers and Behçet's syndrome. A *typically* provocative life situation appears to be present in disc disorders, which is distinct from those provocative in migraine or IBS and may be termed "struggle" (see transcripts Mrs. J. W., Mrs. B. R., Mrs. F. R.).

Typical Life Situation. The *struggle* in which the individual is involved may be domestic, social or at work. Release by victory or defeat does not occur because neither a verbal nor a physical confrontation takes place, or if it does, only after many weeks or months. To distinguish the difference from *fight*, we quote an OED definition of struggle as implying *continued effort*. For example, it may occur when the patient becomes very tense in long *anticipation* of a possible quarrel or showdown which he knows he cannot avoid at a coming meeting. Once the confrontation is over, tension may subside unless the outcome is deferred to some future meeting. Enquiry shows that stresses of this kind commonly precede sciatica, neck pain or brachialgia. In this respect the fighting Orkney vole experiment may have significance.

Faced with a patient with these symptoms and signs, the following question may be put: "I wonder whether you think you are, or have recently been, involved in a sustained *struggle* in any area of your life?"

As the appended case histories illustrate, the struggle commonly involves their own rigidity in dealing with spouses or children, a re-enactment of rigidity and hostility from their own childhood. However, the struggle may be secret and internal; as for example, over a forbidden, undeclared, adulterous wish in a very upright person.

12.2.3 Case Histories

Mrs. B. R. complained of backache, neckache and sciatica with previous syndrome shifts from travel sickness, migraine, urethral syndrome, IBS, hyperventilation and heart phobia. Multiple degenerate intervertebral discs were visible on X-ray examination. This uptight (tense), obsessional woman typifies multiple syndrome shifts between the lesser afflictions. Her mother, a perfectionistic school teacher, had had migraine, and her father was strict and meticulous. Despite academic success she felt she had never pleased him, and when at 18 she would not marry the older man of his choice, he threw her out of the house, and she developed back pain and sciatica. "I could never win and I am still trying – I never have time to do what I want to do and work to a schedule." As so often happens, she married a man almost as meticulous as her father. She has always disliked herself, and she feels guilty over everything, especially her double feelings for both parents.

Prior to referral she had suffered from the following: (a) travel sickness as a child when her parents were always quarreling; (b) migraine and migrainous headaches from puberty onwards while striving for success at school; (c) severe low back pain and sciatica at age 18 when turned out of the house; and (d) attacks of pseudocystitis between age 20–30.

She was first seen when aged 32 with IBS and a cancer phobia. Four years later she returned with hyperventilation and fear that the chest pain was breast cancer. Her phobia was due to guilt over unresolved mourning for a great aunt who had given her the demonstrative love her parents had failed to do. She blamed herself for not taking her to the GP when she first had dyspepsia 3 years previously. In her recurrent dreams her great aunt was always bald, her hair having fallen out in the last month of her life when her impending death was kept from the patient. She saw the loss of the person she loved most as punishment for her bad feelings for her parents. After four sessions of psychological management, although dreams of her aunt continued, they were less distressing because in them her aunt had her hair back. Improvement followed psychological management coupled with re-education in breathing. Hyperventilation recurred 2 years later after her father's cardiac infarction a month after his retirement. She feared she had heart disease, too.

A relapse of IBS occurred when a man living opposite died of cancer aged 39 – the same age as herself. "I'll never get over losing my great aunt – I feel guilty when my mother comes every Friday to get her hair done – it screws me up inside."

Two years later she returned with severe neck pain and back pain over 4 months. To the question: "I wonder if you are involved in any kind of a struggle?" she replied: "Yes, with my eldest daughter, I feel like hitting her – I am so angry with her I could cut her off – she has a woman friend the same age as I am and she comes in and refuses to talk to me and then goes out with this woman." She then made an effort to find out why her daughter had withdrawn from her. After talking they went out together for the first time for a year, and her back and neckache improved dramatically. A family meeting with her and her husband and both daughters followed.

Summary. Mrs. B. R. like Mrs. Y. T. illustrates the problems arising from multiple referrals (scattering/splitting [9]) and also the difficulty of holding such patients in therapy once one or other somatic manifestation has subsided.

Albert and Frank, two young men with intractable severe back pain who had radiological appearances of scalloping of vertebral bodies (see Sect. 12.2.1). One had been invalided from the Army because of intervertebral disc prolapse, the other had been admitted to an orthopaedic ward with an incorrect diagnosis of transverse myelitis. Despite normal CNS signs a myelogram had already been done when first seen! The first said that his disability had prevented him from finding a satisfactory job and was angry with his wife for her denigrating attitude and lack of understanding that his chosen career had been ruined (*struggle*). The second man was in conflict with his future mother-in-law over his girlfriend. The exacerbation occurred after a weekend of intensified conflict which also involved his girlfriend walking out on him.

Both patients' back symptoms remitted when they were able to express their emotions verbally rather than somatically. Instead of being rewarded for their somatic presentation by frequent examination and investigations by doctors and questions by nurses about their backs, a team policy of not "feeding" the somatic aspect was adopted. Listening was substituted, and they were encouraged to talk about their lives, feelings and families. They were also given a relaxation technique and recovered. It is patients like these who become orthopaedic cripples following multiple investigations and injudicious operations.

Mrs. F. R. presented with intervertebral disc degeneration as a syndrome shift from RA. This woman (see also Chap. 10) had been in remission for several years and then returned with severe lower back pain for 12 months, made worse by lifting, ironing, etc. Her only remission had been for 2 weeks while on holiday in Italy, away from her *typically* provocative stress. X-ray examination showed several arthritic and degenerative intervertebral discs.

At a suitable point in interview she was asked if she was in any kind of emotional struggle or battle. "Yes, my son-in-law returned to his first wife a year ago, leaving my daughter with their two children aged three and five." She expressed feelings of hatred for her son-in-law and said that he was seldom out of her thoughts because when at home, she was reminded of it by her daughter and grandchildren's distress. She added that she would not trust herself not to kill him and that "if they got together again, I couldn't have him in the house." Her husband had been suicidal over it. The patient's symptoms lessened following two interviews during which she expressed her feelings freely, coupled with relaxation exercises.

Summary. In contrast to Mrs. Y. T., Mrs. B. R. and Mrs. J. W., this patient had only one syndrome shift, if the mild depression a year before her RA is omitted. The stressful provocative life situations for both presentations were *typical*, as were her attitudes to each. Because her RA was protracted and did not remit quickly, it was possible to hold her in psychological management over a longer period than the two previous cases. In resolving her pathological mourning she learned new ways of coping with loss and guilt, but her anger with her son-in-law, for which she had no outlet until she sought consultation, was a new situation for which initially she had no adequate response.

References

1. Barlow W (1955) Psychosomatic problems in postural re-education. Lancet 2:659–664
2. Barlow W (1981) The Alexander Principle. Arrow, London
3. Scott JC (1955) Stress factor in the disc syndrome. Br Jt Bone Surg 37B:107–111
4. Charnley J (1952) The inhibition of fluid as a cause of herniation of the nucleus pulposus. Lancet 1:124–126
5. Hirsch C (1951) Morbid anatomy of lumbar discs. J Bone Jt Surg 33B:472
6. Barr JS (1951) Low back pain and sciatica. J Bone Jt Surg 33B:469–470
7. Chitty D, Chitty H, Leslie PH, Scott JC (1956) Changes in the relative size of the nucleus in the intervertebral discs of stressed Orkney voles. J Pathol Bacteriol 72 [2]:459–470
8. Clarke JR (1953) The effect of fighting on the adrenals, thymus and spleen of the vole. J Endocrind 9:114–126
9. Winnicott DW (1966) Psychosomatic illness in its positive and negative aspects. Int J Psychoanl 47:510–516

13 Urological Disorders

Emotionally induced bladder dysfunction was described by Janet [1] in a classical monograph, and he quoted Guyon on how to differentiate psychic cystitis from true cystitis. Psychophysiological research on the bladders of 26 patients was carried out by Straub, Ripley and Wolf [2] in 1949 with the same scientific rigour as members of their group had previously applied to the stomach, nose and colon. Hyperfunction was found to be associated with anxiety (tension), while hypofunction and retention, more usually with feelings of depression or being overwhelmed.

For studies on the effect of emotional stress on renal circulation and output, the reader is referred to the animal work of Blomstrand and Lofgren [3], and on the role of the hypothalamus in this to Verney [4]. Rates of excretion of sodium, potassium and creatinine were measured by Schottstaedt, Grace and Wolf [5] in both stressful and tranquil situations. Oliguria and fluid retention were associated with anxiety (tension) and diuresis with return of tranquillity.

The reports quoted provide a sufficient rationale for accepting a psychosomatic determinant in most cases of enuresis in childhood and some cases of idiopathic oedema. An emotionally based disposition to renal calculi is also possible but less certain. However, the studies have their greatest clinical application in the psychological management of the urethral syndrome (psychosomatic "cystitis") and to the rarer interstitial cystitis (Hunner's ulcer) which we will describe.

In other urological disorders such as acute nephritis, nephrotic syndrome and retroperitoneal fibrosis, abnormal immunological responses are involved. It is our experience that loss and/or alienation has provoked severe emotional stress in sufferers from these disorders a few weeks or months prior to onset. Psychological management of unresolved loss as described in Chap 10 is therefore appropriate in this section if the response to orthodox treatment is refractory or in the event of frequent relapses.

13.1 Case Histories

A girl of 14, the youngest of six, developed acute nephritis in January. Her mother had abandoned the family the previous August, only leaving a note. The father, when interviewed, said that he and five of the elder children were weeping for a week but that the patient had not broken down, had remained strong and had done all the housework and cooking. At Christmas a friend had heard from the mother that she might return for a few days, and the patient spent several evenings in a telephone box waiting for news from the friend about her mother. Her hopes that her mother would return were finally dashed.

An only girl of 18 who had had Hodgkin's disease 4 years previously developed nephrotic syndrome 3 weeks after her father's sudden death from MI. He had always had great expectations of his daughter and had urged her to take the necessary exams to get a good job in a bank or public enterprise. He felt everything was lost when she was repeatedly rejected on the grounds of her previous medical history and was forced to take a job her father felt was below her (him?), and MI ensued.

An emotionally dependent man of 40 developed retroperitoneal fibrosis shortly after his wife discovered that he was having an affair with another woman. She demanded divorce, and despite his pleading she refused to have him back.

All three cases received psychological help in addition to standard treatment. The first two remitted, while the last one required ureterolysis.

13.2 Urethral Syndrome, Detrusor Irritability or Pseudocystitis

This common condition causes much distress to sufferers, mainly women. It results in repeated, costly, negative investigations by GPs, gynaecologists, urologists and sometimes neurologists. Zuffall [6] described it as "A syndrome ... which affects women and consists of urinary frequency, dysuria, "pressure", pain in the low back, flank and suprapubic area." He added: "Although these symptoms are those of inflammation of the lower urinary tract, corroborative physical and laboratory findings are minimal if not absent altogether."

Sufferers from the condition in the UK unable to obtain relief have formed a self-help association (The Cystitis Association).

Substantial clinical and research studies have been carried out by Cardoso et al. [7, 8 and 9], who after confirming detrusor irritability by cystometry, reported that after bladder retraining given for 3 months, 82.5% of 40 patients were in remission. In a recent study Macaulay, Holmes et al. 1987 [10] evaluated psychotherapy and bladder drill against controls. Previous reports [8, 9] had shown that biofeedback was less satisfactory because of patients dropping out and the high cost in therapists' time. Zuffall [6] studied 190 patients over 8 years and reported that of the many treatments tried, none appeared superior and concluded that "The urethral syndrome is to a large extent based on factors in the psyche ... These patients were not referred to psychiatrists because none appeared able to accept the idea that her symptoms had a psychic basis."

Readers will note that this aversion to psychiatry is also a feature in migraine, IBS and in other common afflictions such as backache and aphtous ulcers. This is because sufferers do not see themselves as neurotic or different from the rest of the population, of which they make up 10%–20%.

Zuffall added: "Treatment caused temporary improvement, but *the type* of treatment seemed to be immaterial" (providing it was not harmful). By that he meant repeated cystoscopy or catheterisation and which nowadays includes repeated courses of broad spectrum antibiotics for non-existent infection and which predisposes to thrush (candidiasis).

13.2.1 Psychological Management

This is similar to that for migraine. In that section we detailed the approach such patients require before being able to accept that being uptight (tense) in the face of a particular life situation (a) does not imply that they are any more neurotic than any other section of the population, or (b) that it is being suggested that they are imagining or overstating their symptoms. It is helpful to explain that being unrelaxed or tense for long periods may increase the irritability and contractility of smooth muscle in the bladder, as in the colon in IBS [2]. Patients should also be reminded that lay people, including children, know that anticipatory tension before examinations or interviews provokes frequency of micturition or defaecation in about half the population. Animals react in this way as part of the normal fight or flight response. However, it may be pointed out that some life situations which provoke "uptight-ness" (tension) are not as easily resolved as sitting an exam, or having the interview but may persist for days, weeks or years, e.g. in people fighting the clock against a heavy workload and/or an inability to lower their high standards (migraine), or who have difficulty in making decisions (IBS) or in resolving the *struggle* (backache and intervertebral disc disease). This kind of introduction and clarification helps women, initially resistant to any emotional basis for their symptoms, to be able to accept a combination of a relaxation technique and/or bladder drill training together with psychological management of the type suggested for migraine in Chap. 9. Frewen [9] put it this way:

> As patients are always unaware of the cause of their symptoms, it is essential that they have a clear understanding not only of the aetiology, but also of the physical and psychological components of their urinary symptoms .... Those who live in conflict with their environment or who are unable to adapt themselves to their social circumstances will not respond favourably.

In another study Rees and Farhoumand [11] found 60% of such patients had had psychiatric symptoms compared with 6% of the general population and their obsessionality/anxiety scores were high. However, other psychological studies have been less clear cut. The *somatopsychic* effects of this distressing complaint are considerable after weeks, months or years of suffering. However, careful history taking will reveal that uptightness (tension) long antedating their symptoms has been associated with certain provocative *typical* life situations in this group of the population (10%–20%).

We suggest that when inventories and psychological tests refer to anxiety, this includes what we prefer to call "uptightness" (tension). Our reasons for avoiding the term *anxiety* or even *tension* in dealing with these patients has been explained in the section on migraine (see Chap. 9). Although some people with these disorders have anxiety states, most do not, and it is unhelpful if doctors label them as such or give them psychotropic drugs. Free-flowing anxiety is probably no more common in this large subgroup than in the rest of the population.

13.2.1.1 Causes of Uptightness

Having listened and examined empathetically, the next priority is to encourage patients to describe situations or other people's behaviour which makes them feel uptight. This may require facilitation as in migraine.

Causes vary from hostility to authoritarian figures dating from childhood who may still be alive, to incorporation of high standards of behaviour from which they cannot escape, or to relatively minor sources of tension involving surrogates whose attitudes or behaviour provoke it, e.g. sniffing, smoking, scratching, etc. These may emanate from a spouse, in-law, child, neighbour, employer, colleague at work, or some individual on a committee. In migraine, some early workers considered the essential psychodynamic to be a hostile-dependent relationship with a parent. That is also usually so in urethral syndrome, but it requires careful translation before it is acceptable to the patient and his or her doctor. Sexual frustration and guilt were originally thought to be important in psychosomatic cystitis [2, 11], and as symptoms are perineally situated, it is not surprising that some patients and doctors jump to that conclusion; Mrs. T. L. might at first sight be thought to support this. Pursuit of this particular quarry is not wrong but in practice it rarely relieves the symptoms which are always based (as in Mrs. T. L.) on tension (uptightness), just as in migraine or proctalgia fugax, arising from hostility to authoritarian figures in childhood. Relief depends on bringing those ingrained coping responses to awareness and then helping the patient modify them.

Most patients with relatively minor provocative tension can be relieved quickly once they become aware that their responses are related to their symptoms, but patients with more intractable problems such as an illness or alcoholism in a spouse require longer psychological management/psychotherapy. In the first group attainment of awareness as described, together with relaxation exercises as for migraine, is usually enough to bring about remission or reduction in symptoms; others may also require bladder drill retraining [8, 9]. A nurse attached to a GP (or group) can learn the technique; otherwise, referral to a urologist or gynaecologist able to offer the service will be necessary.

People with the urethral syndrome, as with migraine or IBS, like to have their t's crossed and i's dotted. They are understandably intolerant of doctors who are dismissive. Only when the mechanism of their symptoms in the absence of infection has been explained will they allow themselves to accept the combination of psychological management and training in awareness we have described.

13.2.2 Case History

Mrs. T. L., a married woman of 38, had had repeated attacks of so-called cystitis and pain in the vagina from the age of 14, with nothing found after repeated and intensive investigations. She had also had dysmenorrhoea, colon spasm, migraine, travel sickness, and occasional hyperventilation with claustrophobia.

Her resentment of males appeared to date from her birth, which she was told was an accident; as her father had wanted a boy, he refused to visit her mother in hospital or to see his daughter for 6 weeks.

She became a tomboy and became very close to her father until her 'teens when he became increasingly strict and later resented her marriage. Her ambivalence for males was subsequently transferred to her husband, her son and her doctors. At the second interview she revealed a hidden secret about a teenage girlfriend who had left home. The patient was approached by the police in a cinema and told that this girl had had a baby and put it in a dustbin. "I was terrified and panicked ... my mother had caught my sister playing with her boyfriend and there had been a rumpus." Guilt over her own first sexual experience at 14 led to the belief that her bladder and vaginal symptoms were due to venereal infection contracted then.

The patient said she could never relax and had to be busy, e.g. dressmaking, ballroom dancing and swimming, and was obsessive about cleanliness.

After her first interview for the above, she developed such terrible backache that "I could not even put a plug in to play my cassette player ... I am in a very *infuriating* battle with my husband. He thinks the house is too tidy, and my 8-year-old son *infuriates* me – I feel inadequate because my husband can control him." She said she preferred men with a sense of humour, and her husband had not got one and that also annoyed her intensely.

She was taught relaxation and her vaginal pains and urinary symptoms lessened after a joint interview with her husband and sharing with him both her hidden secret and acceptance of her long-standing resentment of males and awareness that uptightness arising from it provoked her symptoms.

Despite her long history and 7 years of being treated by antidepressants and ECT, she had never been offered psychotherapy or psychological management, and throughout that time she had not dared to tell anyone of her hidden secret and guilt, including her husband.

Duration of management: 9 h over 6 months. Greatly improved. (See also Mrs. B. R., Chap. 12.)

Summary. It was felt at one time that pseudocystitis, like many other psychosomatic disorders, was predominantly due to sexual hang-ups [19]. At first sight Mrs. T. L.'s history might be thought to support this view. However, in practice pursuit of a purely sexually based psychopathology is unhelpful in the majority of these patients, and those who sense that it is largely irrelevant become impatient and drop out of treatment. Certainly, many sufferers admit to, or complain of, sexual difficulties such as vaginismus, dyspareunia or lack of orgasm, but that is to be expected in a group of tense, rather obsessional people who may suffer at other times from migraine, dysmenorrhoea, IBS, intervertebral disc problems, etc. Their hostility to authority, female as well as male, which originated in childhood, comes through in their response to doctors who may resent it and reject them. The perineal locus of their symptoms inevitably leads them to dredge up from the past feelings of sexual guilt, however apparently minor, from masturbation to possible venereal infection from lavatory seats, or to become suspicious of an innocent partner. Doctors should certainly not be dismissive of such fears and hidden secrets but encourage their ventilation. Unless the deep seated causes of these patients' hostility and uptightness are recognised and treated by bladder drill and relaxation techniques, combined with psychodynamically orientated psychological management, most will remain angry, continue to suffer and think doctors are stupid.

Mrs. B. R. (Chap. 12) with multiple syndrome shifts is more characteristic of the majority than Mrs. T. L. In short, psychosexual frustrations are usually concomitant, rather than primary.

13.3 Hunner's Ulcer – Interstitial Cystitis

In 1914 Hunner [12] described eight instances of chronic recurrent oedematous ulceration of the bladder. Common presentations are lower abdominal pain, frequency, dysuria and haematuria. Hand [13] believed that interstitial cystitis (IC) was initiated by a neurogenic factor. Several authors [14, 15] have found a relationship between emotional problems, hyperfunction of the bladder and IC, while the consistent finding of increased numbers of mast cells suggests that histamine release may cause a bleb which may then ulcerate. A similar pathogenesis has been suggested for oral aphthous ulcers (described in Chap. 6) together with suggested psychological management.

Henriques (personal communication) referred to J.W.P. four such patients 15 years ago because he had been impressed by these patients uptight (tense) personality and the close temporal relationship to interpersonal emotional stress. His suspicions were supported by the detailed history in each case. Gil Vernet et al. [14] found a state of tension in patients with IC, and Weaver et al. [16] observed that the original diagnosis in a relatively large number had been some form of neurosis.

13.3.1 Psychological Management

Cohen [17] suggested that IC should be regarded as a migraine equivalent and treated as such. This accords with our experience and parallels our recommendation for the management of the much more common oral aphthous ulcers and the urethral syndrome.

13.4 Factitious Haematuria

A condition consciously self-induced by adding blood from a pricked finger or excoriating the urethra is not by our definition psychosomatic and should really have no place here. However, as it is not as well recognised as dermatitis artefacta or other forms of malingering, it should be remembered in the differential diagnosis of haematuria and low pain when investigations are negative [18].

References

1. Janet J (1890) Les troubles psychopathiques de miction de psychophysiologie normale et pathologique. Librairie le François, Paris
2. Straub LR, Ripley HS, Wolf S (1949) Disturbances of bladder function associated with emotional states. JAMA 141:1139–1143
3. Blomstrand R, Lofgren F (1956) Influence of emotional stress on the renal circulation. Psychosom Med 18:420–426
4. Verney EB (1958) Some aspects of water and electrolyte secretion. Surg Gynecol Obstet 106:441–452
5. Schottstaedt WW, Grace WJ, Wolf HG (1955) Life situation, behaviour patterns and renal excretion of fluid and electrolytes. JAMA 157:1485–1488

6. Zuffall R (1963) Treatment of the urethral syndrome in women. JAMA 184:894–895

7. Cardozo L, Stanton LS, Hafner J et al (1978) Biofeedback in the treatment of detrusor instability. Br J Urol 50:250–254

8. Cardozo LD, Abraus PD, Stanton LS et al (1978) Idiopathic bladder instability treated by biofeedback. Br J Urol 50:521–523

9. Frewen WK (1978) An objective assessment of the unstable bladder of psychosomatic origin. Br J Urol 50:246–249

10. Macaulay AJ, Stearn RS, Holmes DM, Stanton SL (1987) Micturition and the mind. Br Med J 294:540–543

11. Rees DLP, Farhoumand N (1977) Psychiatric aspects of recurrent cystitis in women. Br J Urol 49:651–658

12. Hunner GL (1914) A rare type of bladder ulcer in women. Trans Soc Surg Gyn Assoc 27:247–272

13. Hand JR (1949) Interstitial cystitis: a report of 223 cases. J Urol 61:291–310

14. Gil Vernet JM, Gonzalez V, Fernandez E (1960) Etiopathogenesis, etiology, pathology and treatment of interstitial cystitis. Acta Urol Belg 28:425–440

15. Bowers JE, Schwarz BE, Leon MJ (1958) Masochism and interstitial cystitis. Psychosom Med 20:296–302

16. Weaver RG, Dougherty TF, Natoli A (1963) Recent concepts of interstitial cystitis. J Urol 89:377–383

17. Cohen RL (1963) The treatment of "interstitial cystitis" also a migraine equivalent. Compr Psychiatry 4:58–61

18. Kerr DD, Wilkinson R, Horler AR et al (1980) Factitions haematuria and urinary tract infection. Arch Intern Med 140:631–633

14 Disorders of Blood

Emotional stress has been observed by us and others to have preceded the onset of several disorders of blood and the reticuloendothelial system. A close time relationship combined with the frequency of such an occurrence suggests that chance is an unlikely explanation.

Some of these conditions are now generally recognised as disorders of immunological competence, while others involve autoimmunity. A form of psychological management which has been found appropriate for this group has been described in Chap. 10. However, in a disorder such as pernicious anaemia, which may follow pathological loss or threatened loss of a surrogate, the parietal cell damage is irreversible by the time of diagnosis, and no amount of psychological help will change it. The only conceivable place for psychological management would be to try to avert other AI disorders such as thyroiditis, Addison's disease or diabetes which in our experience not infrequently follow further losses of key figures or surrogates. Examples of multiple AI disorders affecting one patient are quoted in Chap. 10.

14.1 Pernicious Anaemia

Psychological symptoms of pernicious anaemia include apathy, dizziness, and feelings of unreality; these are frequently misdiagnosed as depression and inappropriately treated with psychotropic drugs until someone suggests a blood count. These symptoms of anaemia and the postural hypotension from the associated neuropathy are truly somatopsychic as revealed by their dramatic remission *within a few hours* or days of vitamin B12 treatment.

However, in PA, as in some other disorders such as Hashimoto's thyroiditis, thyrotoxicosis, Addison's disease and SLE, the original psychosomatic determinant of unresolved loss is commonly obscured by the prominence of the somatopsychic symptomatology. The same point was made in Chap. 1, and the symptomatology is typified by the occasional suicidal attempt by characteristically intrepid and *superstable* elderly patients with giant cell (temporal) arteritis or polymyalgia when their compensatory coping mechanism of activity is prevented by overwhelming pain or disability.

14.2 Infectious Mononucleosis

Although the EB virus has an aetiological role, it has long been accepted that an abnormal immunological response is also involved. That is reflected in false-positive serological results and formation of antibodies to red cells, platelets, etc. Here as in other disorders in which viruses are involved, the frequency of infection with EB virus is much higher than the frequency of clinical manifestations. Similarly, only a small percentage of those innoculated with swine 'flu vaccine developed clinical Guillain-Barré syndrome [1].

In Chap. 10 we have described the kind of psychological management which is appropriate in the relapsing or refractory case which can be so damaging to young people career prospects, if not tackled. Reference is also made to an earlier article [2].

14.3 Acquired Haemolytic Anaemia and Essential Thrombocytopenia

Both these conditions, in which antibody formation is involved, and of which infectious mononucleosis is an occasional cause, might be expected to benefit from psychological management of the precipitating condition of unresolved stress of alienation/loss/mourning. However, to date we have been unable to provide conclusive evidence that it does so. That may possibly be because the number of cases in which the opportunity has presented is too small.

14.3.1 Case History

Ms. K. G., a girl of 20, was beset by unresolved feelings of guilt and loss over several key figures. The oldest of three and her father's favourite, she felt responsible for her parents' quarrels and that she had taken love belonging to her mother. She was only 11 when her mother nearly died from a hysterectomy, and she saw her badness as the reason. Her maternal grandmother died when the patient was 14, after a leg amputation, and she felt guilt at not visiting her during the last 10 days of her life because she feared seeing her so ill. "I couldn't believe Nanna was dead until 3 years later."

Two years before onset of the thrombocytopenia her father, aged 38, had a severe MI, and remained too ill to work, with hypertension and renal failure. She was anticipating his death and felt guilty if she went out and left him.

The boyfriend whom she had known since she was 15 left her a year before onset. "I didn't want to live and I slashed my left wrist." Not long afterwards she became engaged to a steady young man but felt guilty that she had refused to see the first boyfriend when he wanted to try to resolve mutually hurt feelings. When her purpura began, she was also having nightmares about the girl who had taken him away and feared she would have to "pay" by losing her fiancé in an accident on the icy roads. Finally, she added that all such fears took her mind back to the time a man threatened to shoot her paternal grandfather when she was a child.

She was helped to work through these feelings of loss and anticipated loss, and it enabled her to decide to meet her first boyfriend and resolve most of her bitter feelings towards him. Emotional improvement and increase in platelet count followed, but the improvement did not last long enough to save her from splenectomy. Since her marriage her purpura has remitted.

A past history of glandular fever at age 9 and a sensitivity rash to trimethoprimphis-sulphamethoxazole at age 15 suggest previous immunological vulnerability.

14.4 Hypereosinophilic Syndrome

Although comparatively rare, this often fatal condition has in our experience always been closely related to actual or anticipated unresolved loss and mourning [3]. Like polyarteritis nodosa the syndrome may also follow long-standing asthma.

14.4.1 Case Histories

Miss E. J., aged 19, the second of three girls, presented with severe asthma in December 1977 which alternated with hyperventilation and migraine. She said her mother wanted to come in with her, "She always does." In the waiting room there was not only mother but the patient's boyfriend who also said he wanted to come in, to which mother very reluctantly agreed. From then on these two talked as if the patient was a child who could be ignored. Mother's attitude was oppressive and overconcerned. Her voice was strident. The boyfriend's attitude was proprietary, and neither he nor her mother asked the patient what she thought.

Outpatient psychological management followed on the lines described for asthma in Chap. 7, and during the first 12 months her doctor admitted her on three occasions in status asthmaticus. As an inpatient she courted rejection and nearly succeeded in achieving it, despite the tolerance of nurses with long experience and understanding of asthmatic patients' manipulative behaviour.

The patient said that her asthma had started when she was 18, when she began to feel rebellious against her mother's dominance and oppressiveness which she had accepted as a child. She also had feelings of inferiority to her clever and bossy younger sister. Gradually, she was helped to express her feelings of anger and rejection and to feel she was well enough to resume her training as a teacher.

Because of family pressure she was referred elsewhere by her GP, and in 1980 to a clinic in London where her eosinophil count was normal. She returned in July 1981 with additional symptoms of fatigue, muscle pains and paraesthesia.

Her WBC count was 14.8, with eosinophils 43%. There was a low grade fever, dense shadowing on X-ray on both lungs reported as typical of eosinophilic infiltration. The diagnosis lay between polyarteritis nodosa, sensitisation angiitis superimposed on long-standing asthma or hypereosinophilic syndrome. Three months later, after initial improvement on oral corticosteroids and gradual reduction of the latter, she developed a purpuric rash, peripheral neuropathy, polyarthritis, myocarditis and pericarditis. Despite negative biopsies PAN now seemed the likely diagnosis, but there was no evidence of renal involvement. Corticotropin was substituted for oral steroids, and psychological management was resumed.

From then on her symptoms remitted, her lungs cleared, and her eosinophil count never again exceeded 10%. Interviews over the next year showed that she was maturing emotionally. She recognised that her inadequate way of "coping" with her younger sister had always been not to compete with her. This feeling of inferiority began to trouble her less, and she began applying for good jobs. She then decided to become engaged to her boyfriend and announced the date of the wedding in 1983. In all follow-ups since, she has remained well. In January 1987 her eosinophil count was 9% and WBC 7.2 and she was pregnant. A maintenance dose of ACTH had been continued for 5 years.

Summary. Childhood background and life situation at onset are typical for asthma. At onset of hypereosinophilic syndrome, feelings of alienation for her mother intensified as the latter opposed her love affair. She then mentioned dreams and fears about death and loss of her mother, father and her clever sister 4 years younger to whom she had always seen herself as second mother. This was the coping mechanism she had adopted to compensate for feelings of intellectual inferiority.

Mrs. D. M. Hypereosinophilic syndrome occurred in this woman when aged 35, 2 months after her father's sudden death. She was the youngest of four children and the devoted younger sister of the patient with Crohn's disease who died of cancer of the jejunum mentioned in Chap. 6. That sister's prolonged illness began when the patient was only 4 years old. Her parents' anxiety and concern resulted in relative neglect of the patient. She idolised her sick sister but not until she was in psychological management for her hypereosionophilia was she able to acknowledge her double feelings, i.e. hate as well as love. During her sister's terminal illness she had been busy with three young children of her own and felt that she had not been as supportive as she should have been. She had been unable to weep after the death, and 15 years later the fact that mention of her sister brought tears to her eyes covered by a smile indicated that her mourning was still unresolved. Her next loss was her mother, but because her ambivalence for the latter was minimal she had got through her grief in a few months. However, her father continued to grieve but later remarried. She experienced a mixture of happiness for him but also a feeling of anger that he was betraying her mother. Such were her feelings when her father died of a heart attack only a month after his wedding. She took ill 2 months later with high fever, breathlessness, dense shadowing in both lungs and an eosinophil count of 50% with WBC 18000. Investigations revealed no evidence of polyarteritis. Treated with corticotrophin in declining dosage for 9 months together with psychological management of her unresolved mourning, she remitted. Four years later her doctor confirmed that she had remained well.

14.5 Psychogenic Purpura: Autoerythrocyte Sensitisation

We have no personal experience of this syndrome. It may follow trivial injuries [4] contracted in everyday life but it has also followed severe bruising from beating [5]. Agle and Ratnoff [6] were the first to note that these patients had severe emotional disturbances antedating their purpura. They were also considered to have hysterical and masochistic personality traits. It is reported that these patients *profit* from a supportive relationship with a primary physician rather than by traditional psychotherapy [6].

14.6 Thrombosis

Clotting of blood, while an essential part of the flight or fight response [7] against wounding in combat, or placental bed following childbirth, can, if excessive or inappropriate, be a hazard to life. Judine [8] and MacFarlane [9] found increases in fibrinolytic activity to compensate for thrombotic tendencies following the physical stress of surgical operations and trauma. Biggs et al. [10] extended these studies and found that adrenalin was a mediator, quite apart from shock. They also found that levels of fibrinolysis could be as high after a minor operation, such as circumcision, as after major surgery. Most importantly they showed that increased fibrinolysis not only followed surgical operations but preceded them. Thus, fear of impending operation appeared to be the cause of a proportion of the positive results.

Britton et al. [11] in an article entitled "Stress – a significant factor in venous thrombosis?" showed that the coagulation response could be modified by β-adrenergic blockade, but that fibrinolysis was not affected. As a result they suggested that this hazard of stress associated with surgical operations, whether physical or emotional, might be controlled in this way.

14.7 The Haematological Stress Syndrome

Reizenstein [12] reviewed a range of haematological abnormalities under this title but made no reference to the nature of the stress.

Gaisbock's polycythaemia has long been recognised to occur in anxious and unstable people, some but not all of whom have been addicted to alcohol and tobacco [13].

Similarly, shifts to the left in WBC counts have been observed in people emotionally stressed. Such a combination is one of the less known manifestations of giant cell (temporal) arteritis [4, 15]. In these cases anaemia persists until diagnosis and treatment with corticosteroids [16]. As giant cell (temporal) arteritis is precipitated by pathological grief and loss [17], it is not surprising that recent widowhood is a common finding in this groups of patients and that many also suffer from depression. It is likely that Reizenstein's patients with anaemia and raised ESR come into this diagnostic bracket.

References

1. Grouse LD (1980) Swine flu sequelae. JAMA 243:2489
2. Hughes JP, Paulley JW (1960) Steroid therapy in glandular fever. Postgrad Med J 36:553–556
3. Parillo JE, Fonci AS, Wolff SM (1978) Therapy of the hypereosinophilic syndrome. Ann Intern Med 89:167–172
4. Gardner FH, Diamond LK (1955) Autoerythrocyte sensitization. Blood 10:675–690
5. Ratnoff OD, Agle DP (1968) Psychogenic purpura: syndrome of autoerythrocyte sensitization. Medicine 47:475–500
6. Agle DP, Ratnoff OD (1962) Purpura as a psychosomatic entity. A psychiatric study of autoerythrocyte sensitization. Arch Intern Med 109:685–694
7. Cannon WB, Gray H (1914) Factors affecting the coagulation time of blood. Am J Physiol 34:232–242
8. Judine SS (1936) La transfusion du sang de cadavre aux êtres humains. Press Med 4:68–71
9. MacFarlane RG, Biggs R (1946) Observations on fibrinolysis. Lancet 2:862–864
10. Biggs R, MacFarlane RG, Pilling J (1947) Observations on fibrinolysis. Lancet 1: 402–405
11. Britton BJ, Hawkey C, Wood WG, Peck M (1974) Stress – a significant factor in nervous thrombosis. Br J Surg 61:814–820
12. Reizenstein P (1979) The haematological stress syndrome. Br J Haematol 43:329–334
13. Gaisbock F (1922) Die Polyzythämie. Ergeb Inn Med Kinderheilkd 21:204–250
14. Paulley JW, Hughes JP (1960) Giant cell arteritis, or arteritis of the aged. Br Med J 11:1562–1567
15. Hamilton CR, Shelley WM, Tumulty PA (1971) Giant cell arteritis including temporal arteritis and polymyalgia rheumatica. Medicine (Baltimore) 50:1
16. Allison MC, Gough KR (1985) Steroid sensitive systemic disease with anaemia in the elderly: a manifestation of giant cell arteritis. Postgrad Med J 61:501–503
17. Paulley JW (1983) Pathological mourning: a key factor in the psychopathogenesis of autoimmune disorders. Psychother Psychosom 40:181–190

15 Disorders of the Skin

15.1 Psoriasis

R. B. Coles and R. H. Seville

It seems to be agreed generally that there is a genetic element which determines psoriasis, but usually of more importance are the factors that precipitate or trigger the condition. Treatment and even prevention of these may considerably improve the prognosis; they include infection, trauma or endocrine factors and have been described elsewhere [1]. Major psychological stress precipitates psoriasis in over 40% of first attacks [2], and worry or stress can exacerbate pre-existing lesions in 70% of patients [1]. The treatment of this stress by psychotherapy will be detailed in this chapter [3–5]. Physical treatment is usually needed in addition, often with dithranol, and continued until no trace of the rash remains [6]. Early and complete therapy is followed by a significantly better prognosis [7].

15.1.1 Consultation

This is fundamental to patient management and is part of therapy. Consultation need not be exhaustive if carried out early in the illness when the upset is much more recent and usually before it is overlaid by rationalisation or psychological forgetting; a short time, therefore, spent at the onset may save years of illness. It must first be ascertained when the skin was first affected and the times of any exacerbations. As the incubation time from stress to the onset of psoriasis is within 1 month, attention should be paid to this period, particularly with regard to interpersonal relationships and conflict. Knowledge of the patients and their background, as occurs in general practice, makes this much easier as the conversation can be guided into those areas patients may not wish to remember. This may be indicated by blankness, hesitancy, hostility, altered voice tone or attacks of scratching. When patients cannot remember, it is then a great time saver to encourage them to ask their partner, parents or trusted friend whether they recollected any prior events which were upsetting, checking diaries or other records as required. The aim is to help the patients gain insight into the nature of the emotional trauma they have suppressed or brooded over and the part they have played in it; there is then a significant improvement in the prognosis [5] as can be seen in Fig. 3.

Insight is here defined as self-knowledge: that is, observation and appreciation by the patients of the significance of what has happened that upset, i.e. distressed them, resulting in an understanding in depth with acceptance of reality – the veneer of superficial recognition only evades real awareness. In other words there has to be

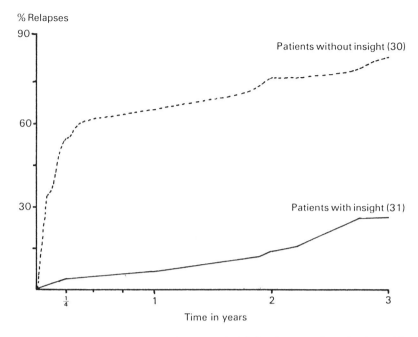

Fig. 3. The rate of relapse after discharge from hospital following complete clearing with dithranol is significantly slower in patients with insight compared to those judged to have none. (From [17])

complete understanding, acceptance, and willingness to relearn and adjust. No longer is the patient being ruled by the effects of retained upsets or habit programmes from the past. It is only then that these upsets truly become past history, no longer an upsetting event when remembered, and no longer a conditioned reflex (the layman's scar on the mind) that perpetuates the illness or psoriasis.

Insight at consultation is dependent on a gentle and sympathetic approach. It does not come with persistent introspection by the patient; it certainly does not follow an unsympathetic inquisition. There must be real caring so that the patient feels free to recollect what has happened; this only comes if there is the right atmosphere in which the patient feels secure, the doctor acting mainly as a mirror. To gain insight is always of the patient's own doing and cannot be enforced or imposed by another.

It follows that to establish rapport and share such personal information, consultation should be in private and without interruption. Patients will not talk easily about their problems if they are unclothed. It is better for them to sit facing across the corner of a desk rather than be separated by its imposing expanse.

A handshake at the beginning reassures the patients, helps to convince them that they are not infectious and gives some indication of their character. The doctor should be able to interpret body language and the subtleties of voice tone. Communication should be at the patients' level, in a language they can understand and to which they can respond.

Failure to find a precipitating factor for the psoriasis, whether physical or psychological, should be followed by retaking the history on the lines already

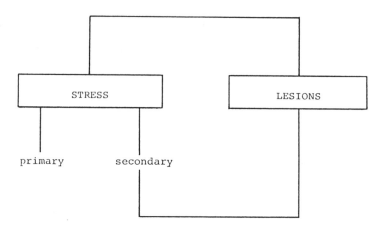

Fig. 4. The vicious circle of events that may follow precipitating factors for psoriasis. (From [7])

suggested in Chap. 4. Details of the patient's individual development should be recorded in case some lead is discovered. Koblenzer has suggested that the physician keeps a number of questions in mind [8]:

> To what degree do the symptoms interfere with the quality of life for the patient? What purpose do they seem to serve in the psychic economy? Does the patient seem to be seriously anxious or depressed? Is the concern he expresses consistent with the severity of the symptoms? Does he seem to have sufficient ego strength [i.e. ability and maturity to face reality] to tolerate the physician's belief that he is causing, or contributing to the perpetuation of his illness, or will he flee if faced with this information? Is he capable of forming a therapeutic alliance? Is he psychotic, with disordered thought patterns, hallucinations, or delusions?

It should not be forgotten that the presence of psoriasis may be so distressing to the patient that the condition then continues as a stress response, as can be seen in Fig. 4 [7]. It should be clear from the patient's history as to whether stress has precipitated or is secondary to the development of the condition. Secondary stress, if found, should be reduced by explaining how the rash may be cleared, and if applicable colour photos shown of before, during and after dithranol therapy [6]. A confident therapeutic approach, when justified, is beneficial [9].

Clinical evaluation is sometimes complicated by the fact that the same rash can be provoked in the same patient on different occasions by any of the physical or psychological precipitating factors; also, like most constitutional reaction patterns, psoriasis may persist or extend for a while after the provoking stimulus is removed.

Initial failure to clear the rash completely should be followed by specialist referral, usually to the dermatologist. There may be physical reasons for the persistence of the rash, specialised treatments may be necessary, or continued in-depth consultation required. Communication in any of these events then becomes even more vital and will now be dealt with in detail [10, 11].

15.1.2 Communication

Patient and doctor must always be free to communicate with each other, and when a hospital doctor is involved there is an increase in the need for free and useful communication and education. However, all of us show bias in some aspect of our thinking. Patients may communicate at a purely physical level, not wishing to discuss their background or they may well not realise that it is important. Similarly, doctors may regard the psoriasis as a physical entity to be treated with ointment or other agents. On the other hand, they may be interested in the psychodynamic, social and personal background of the patients, and they may wish to take a detailed history, enabling the patients to talk about their difficulties freely along the lines already described. Ideally, the family doctor has to take a social receptive attitude on one side, and a physical attitude on the other. All this needs to be varied according to the requirements of the patient. However, bias will obviously be present in many cases, and when a hospital doctor is involved further difficulties may ensue [10].

Some of these patients are shown diagrammatically in Figs. 5–12. (In these drawings bias on the physical side is indicated by a *continuous* line or circle, and bias on a social/psychosomatic/psychodynamic side is indicated by *broken* lines. The patient is abbreviated to *P*, the general practitioner to *GP* and the consultant to *C*.)

There are all sorts of variations of these patterns, and drawings of this may be produced ad lib as a sort of intellectual exercise. Their only value is in pointing out that communication in this triad of people is biased in all sorts of ways, and every effort must be made by the family doctor and the consultant to improve the communication situation. How can this be done?

As has been mentioned, the consultation setting is all important. The patient needs a peaceful, quiet environment to communicate with the doctors concerned. There must be no element of hurry, and in both the family doctor situation and the hospital situation this is difficult. The family doctor may have a big queue of patients

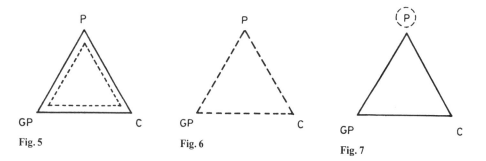

Fig. 5   Fig. 6   Fig. 7

Fig. 5. The hospital doctor(s), patient (*P*) and family doctor (*GP*) all communicate freely, both on the social/psychosomatic level (*broken line*) and on the physical level (*solid line*); unfortunately, this ideal state is rarely attained

Fig. 6. The three members of the triangle communicate only on psychosocial lines (*broken line*)

Fig. 7. The patient's (*P*) psychosocial problems are not discussed, and the consultant (*C*) and the family doctor (*GP*) communicate with the patient only in physical terms (*solid line*)

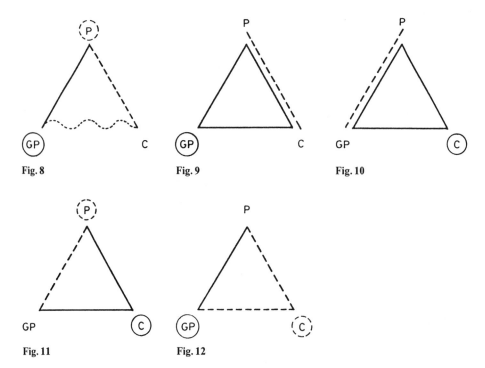

Fig. 8. The patient (*P*) has psychological problems (*broken line*) but the GP only accepts mechanical communication (*solid line*). The patient and the consultant (*C*) communicate on a psychosomatic basis, and then the consultant has the difficulty of communicating with the GP, hence the *wavy line*! The difficulty will lie in the fact that if he or she communicates exactly what he or she feels, he or she is likely to be rejected by the GP, who may well have strong negative feelings towards this mode of thought

Fig. 9. Again the GP accepts only mechanistic problems (*solid line*) and the patient (*P*) and consultant (*C*) communicate along both paths. The consultant, knowing the GP's feelings, will only communicate mechanically to the GP, hence a collusion occurs between the patient and the consultant, the latter being aware that the GP will not tolerate psychosomatic statements (*broken line*) and may block this side of the communication because of his or her own unconscious difficulty

Fig. 10 This is parallel to Fig. 7 in which the patient (*P*) and (*GP*) collude on the emotional side (*broken line*)

Fig. 11. A patient (*P*) with an emotional problem (*broken line*). The family doctor (*GP*) realises this, but he or she wants the physical problems (*solid line*) checked because there is always the nightmare of failing to detect something organic. He or she therefore sends the patient to a physically orientated consultant who communicates back to the GP a physically biased report. This may add to the problem of treatment

Fig. 12. The reverse situation to Fig. 9. The GP is convinced that there is an organic physical problem (*solid line*) and the unconsciously biased consultant (*C*) tends to regard the patient's (*P*) symptoms as caused by emotional problems (*broken line*)

and may have allowed a certain number of minutes for each interview in the appointment system. After the diagnosis has been made, it might be possible for him or her to make a special arrangement to spend time with the psoriasis sufferer so that the patient's story can be told in full. It is very common for patients to talk only about their skin, and only time will allow them to go behind the defence so to speak, to give tongue to the many difficulties which they may have been experiencing. The hospital situation is even more difficult in that the consultants often see patients with other people present, and students, nurses and secretaries do not improve the chance of communication. The consultant concerned may wish to teach on the patient's problems. In most cases, this teaching constitutes discussion about the visual changes that the patient shows. In other words, the patient's external boundary is discussed without any free discussion with the patient. Questions are asked, and as Balint pointed out years ago: "People who ask questions get answers, but very little else" [12].

Some dermatologists are committed to organising a certain set of physical treatments for patients with psoriasis; although these may be excellent, education and teaching are required for the patient to learn to use them properly. Lack of this organisation may be responsible for treatment failure [13]. Patients should have some say with regard to the nature of their treatment, for example whether to have intensive dithranol therapy with its associated mahogany staining of the skin or to use weaker strengths with consequent less staining but a longer time for complete clearance. The personal economics of the interaction of each patient and the treatment must be explained in advance so that there are no surprises and no disappointments, so the patient understands what the proposed treatments can do and what commitment is involved in time, discomfort and money. This co-operative approach leads to the patient's responsible involvement in the treatment.

Above all, patients need time, and because of this, one way is to work with them in groups. This improves their education, and with increased understanding both at a physical and psychological level there is a better response to therapy [3]. This type of educative, open group approach does not substitute for regular attendance at a clinic and for physical treatment, but it does give a chance for patients to learn about their psoriasis in detail, not only from the doctor but also from other patients. Insight may be gained on these occasions with improvement to the prognosis, as has been mentioned earlier.

15.1.3 Psoriasis Associations

Self help and mutual aid groups are a feature of this part of the century. Killilea [14] identified six basic characteristics of self help groups, namely, common experience of members; regular contact between members; beneficial experience helping others; confirmation of feelings and expectations; sharing of factual information; and general education about the condition. Groups of this kind are active, the members setting out to achieve and do something about their condition and the circumstances related to it. Individually and collectively, this activity seems to be beneficial, and insight may be gained.

Time spent at group therapy, the Psoriasis Association or at consultations helps the patient gain a balanced perspective and to face reality. The confidence inspired by others that one's assessment and solution to a problem is correct takes much of the stress from a patient weighed down by negative emotions.

15.1.4 Learning to Live with Psoriasis

So far in this chapter an optimistic approach has been described, and this should be pursued provided the patient is fundamentally willing to be cleared completely. Any failure should not be taken personally, and the patient's need for an illness, personal inflexibility or genetic susceptibility should not be attacked with therapeutic arrogance; the aim should then be to alleviate symptoms rather than effect clearance. These patients may have found that the only way of expressing some emotions has been via their skin, and they are unconsciously threatened by the clinician's aggressive claims to have a cure; if so, they will always defeat him or her. If the clinician is more humble, they will often feel safe to part with some of their psychosomatic disorder especially if he or she helps them to feel emotions possibly for the first time and express them verbally.

Jobling and Coles [15] pointed out that the standard pattern of medical consultation takes the form of the patient presenting symptoms, that is those most evident to him or her, while the doctor may amplify the problems by questions directed towards an original diagnosis. Patients' questions are often badly articulated. What's wrong with me? What causes it? What can be done about it? How soon will it go? How can it be prevented? Will it come back? There is great anxiety present, no doubt, and it must be borne in mind that skin disease provides the classic example of stigmatised illness. It's a major exception to the rule that the sick are not held responsible for their misfortune. The daunting fear of what may seem like a lifelong career by a psoriasis sufferer needs recognition [16]. The vicious circle of events that the last mentioned can cause has already been shown diagrammatically in Fig. 4.

The patient may feel that psoriasis is an incurable condition, and the fear of the future handicapped by psoriasis is an increasing black cloud on the horizon. Some patients have met other people who have been cleared, only to relapse later – perhaps even to worsen – after a period of treatment which was initially an apparent success. These factors will influence the patient, enhance anxiety and increase the need for steady communication to put the situation into perspective. Firstly, therefore, patients must be given every opportunity to express their fears, either on a one-to-one basis, in the group situation or in a combination of both. With that the gentle training about the actual prognosis, what can be done, how it can be done, and various problems in relationship to treatments can be explained to the patient. Treatments are expensive in time from the patient's point of view. Time may be lost from work and also some treatments are messy; however he or she may feel that it is a good price to pay for a period of clearance.

Comforting your patient through all the vicissitudes of the illness is part of the doctor-patient relationship; the approach comes from knowing your patient and his or her illness and background, and knowing the most efficacious therapies to suit his or her individual needs – it is then that there is true caring.

15.1.5 Summary

Early and complete treatment is followed by a significantly better prognosis. This envisages psychotherapy, which need not be exhaustive, and some physical treatment, both of which are best initiated early in general practice. Good communication is fundamental to consultation, and when consultants are involved this becomes more vital. Details are given of a consultation setting in which the patient feels secure enough to gain insight into personal emotional problems with significant improvement to the prognosis.

References

1. Farber EM, Nall L (1984) An appraisal of measures to prevent and control psoriasis. J Am Acad Dermatol 10:511–517
2. Seville RH (1977) Psoriasis and stress. Br J Dermatol 97:297–302
3. Coles RB (1965) The treatment of psoriasis in groups. Med World 2:1–8
4. Coles RB (1967) Group treatment in the skin department. Trans St John's Hosp Dermatol Soc 53:82–85
5. Seville RH (1978) Psoriasis and stress II. Br J Dermatol 98:151–153
6. Seville RH, Martin E (1981) Dermatological nursing and therapy. Blackwell, Oxford, pp 1–38
7. Seville RH (1987) Dithranol based therapies (pp 185–186) and Doctor–patient relationship (pp 276–284). In: Mier PD, van der Kerkhof PCM (eds) Textbook of psoriasis. Churchill Livingstone, Edinburgh
8. Koblenzer CS (1983) Psychosomatic concepts in dermatology. Arch Dermatol 119:501–512
9. Thomas KB (1987) General practice consultations: is there any point in being positive? Br Med J 294:1200–1202
10. Coles RB, Bridger H (1969) The consultant and his roles. Br J Med Psychol 42:231–241
11. Freeling P (1985) My doctor. J R Soc Med 78:8–17
12. Balint M (1964) The doctor, his patient and the illness. Pitman, London
13. Coles RB, Ryan TJ (1975) The psoriasis sufferer in the community. Br J Dermatol 93:111–112
14. Killilea M (1976) Mutual help organizations. In: Caplan G, Killilea M (eds) Support systems and mutual help. Grune and Stratton, New York, pp 37–93
15. Jobling RG, Coles RB (1985) Dermatol Pract 3:6–7
16. Jobling RG (1977) Medical encounters. Davis A, Horobin G (eds) Croom Helm, London, pp 72–86
17. Practitioner (1977) 834

Addresses of the Psoriasis Associations

Canadian Psoriasis Foundation,
P.O. Box 5036,
Armdale,
Halifax,
Nova Scotia B3L 4M6,
Canada

Anne Cullen, R. N.,
Psoriasis Centre,
c/o Elisabeth Bruyers Health Centre,
43 Bruyers Street,
Ottawa,
Ontario K1N 5C8,
Canada

Mrs. Judy Misner, President,
Canadian Psoriasis Society,
168 Harlington Crescent,
Halifax,
Nova Scotia B3M 3N1,
Canada

Mrs. M. Oaks, President,
Vancouver Island Psoriasis Society,
841 Fairfield Road,
Victoria,
British Columbia V8V 3B6,
Canada

R. Schachter,
Canadian Psoriasis Association,
The Women's College Hospital,
Toronto
Ontario,
Canada

Mrs. D. Mullins,
Psoriasis Research Association,
107 Vista del Grande,
San Carlos,
California 94070,
USA

Gail Zimmerman,
National Psoriasis Foundation,
6443 S. W. Beaverton Highway,
Suite 210,
Portland,
Oregon 97221,
USA

Deutscher Psoriasis Bund,
Chilehaus A OE,
Fischertwiete 2,
2000 Hamburg 1,
FRG

Dutch Psoriasis Association,
Bouriciusstraat 4,
6814 CW Arnhem,
The Netherlands

The Psoriasis Association,
7 Milton Street,
Northampton NN2 7JG,
UK

Mrs. Elaine Upton,
Psoriasis Self-Help Group,
24 Monash Drive,
Mulgrave 3170,
Victoria,
Australia

15.2 Atopic Dermatitis

U. Gieler

Atopic dermatitis is a chronic or recurrent skin disease which can be classified according to morphological aspects and course. Inflammatory reactions and strong itching represent the main symptoms. It has an hereditary component: patients and other members of the family often suffer from other atopic diseases, especially allergic rhinitis and bronchial asthma [1].

Very early in the history of dermatology, psychosomatic components were considered to be important in this disease. Brocq and Jaquet [2] introduced the term "neurodermatitis" and underlined the close relationship of this disorder with the activity of the central nervous system.

According to Hanifin and Rajka [3] the diagnosis of atopic dermatitis is made if at least three main symptoms and three optional symptoms are present. Main symptoms are pruritus, typical morphological features, distribution of lesions, chronic or recurrent dermatitis and atopic diseases in the family history. Accessory symptoms include more than 23 very different criteria.

The great variety of clinical and morphological aspects corresponds to the heterogenity of psychological characteristics which the patients present in practice as well. About one-third of the population have an atopic disposition: atopic dermatitis is globally spread and affects 0.7% of the population [4]. At least 5% of all children present symptoms at some time. It should be noted that an early beginning can have important implications for the emotional development.

However, according to a longitudinal study of 2000 children, in 84% the symptoms clear up within a period of 20 years [5]. A late onset, reverse patterns of affected skin areas and social factors were found to contribute to a worse prognosis [6].

Although atopic dermatitis is one of the most frequent diseases seen in general practice and dermatology, its etiology is not yet well understood. Besides the genetic disposition, physiological abnormalities of the skin, dysfunctions of the cellular and humoral immune system, a defect of leucocyte chemotaxis and effector cells and pharmacological defects have been suggested to be important (Fig. 13). However, it is not quite clear which of these factors represent secondary abnormalities or primary defects [7].

It is widely accepted that climate, profession and emotional stress are important triggering factors [8], whereas nutrition plays a minor role in adults. Although the present article focuses on psychological aspects, it should be kept in mind that multiple factors may contribute to the disease and that a distinction between somatogenesis and psychogenesis is artifical. For practical reasons, it is useful to recognise that emotional stress and personality may represent crucial factors which increase the risk of developing atopic dermatitis.

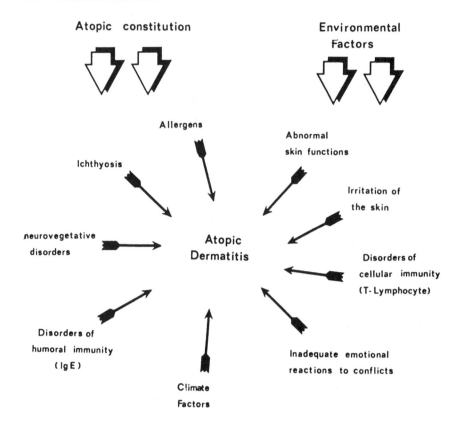

Fig. 13. Pathogenesis of atopic dermatitis [7]

15.2.1 Psychophysiological and Psychoimmunological Mechanisms

A large number of deviations in physiological skin responses have been identified which underline the close relationship between atopic dermatitis and the autonomic nervous system. A basic defect of atopic dermatitis is a vagotonia associated with an overirritability of the sympathetically innervated cutaneous functions. This defect is responsible for a number of typical clinical features of atopic dermatitis which can be observed also during symptom-free intervals: white dermographism (a white line following upon the stroking of the skin), marked perinasal and perioral pallor, loss of lateral hairs of the eyebrows, altered reactions of hair follicle muscles and markedly reduced sweat and sebum production. The last alterations mentioned cause an extreme transepidermal water loss, resulting in the typical dry and itchy skin [9].

The main symptom in atopic dermatitis is itching, which can easily be provoked by different external or internal stimuli such as warmth, dryness of the skin, inflammatory reactions and even the mere imagination of the sensation [10]. The itch threshold can also be lowered by stress [11, 12].

An abnormally elevated release of histamine from mast cells is responsible for the strong itch sensation. This alteration seems to be a part of a general "immuno-

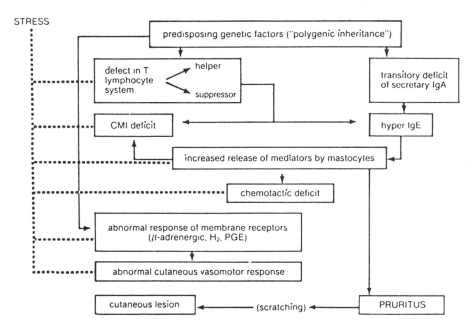

Fig. 14. Psychoimmunological pathways of the influence of stress to pruritus [17]

vegetative" dysregulation [13]. Besides an elevated release of histamine, the production of IgE is increased, possibly due to a defect of the cellular control of the immune system by suppressor lymphocytes. The psychophysiological pathway by which stress stimulates mast-cell degranulation and itching is not quite clear. However, several pathogenetic mechanisms could be taken into account. First, stress hormones such as adrenaline may stimulate the mast cells directly. Since the adrenergic receptors of the mast cells are suggested to be altered in their function, mast cells of patients with atopic dermatitis may be extremely susceptible to endocrine stimuli, associated with autonomic arousal.

Second, the control of IgE production by T-cell subsets may be disturbed. Experimental data indicate that cortisol, which is released under stressful conditions, is capable of suppressing the circulation of specific T-lymphocytes [14]. Therefore, the somatic susceptibility to emotional stress may be increased in patients with atopic dermatitis. Indeed, experimental data suggest that they show stronger autonomic stress reactions than healthy controls [15]. Furthermore, their subjective ability to relax is reduced as compared with patients with other diseases and healthy controls [16].

Panconesi gives a hypothetical model of the interacting triggering factors (Fig. 14) [17].

Since the symptoms themselves represent severe stress, a vicious circle can developed: emotional stress provokes itching and scratching, which are experienced as uncontrollable stress, thus reinforcing the symptoms and resulting in a constant restlessness of the patient.

15.2.2 Personality and Other Psychological Triggering Factors

To cite the host of literature references about personality and psychodynamics would be beyond the scope of this survey. Although empirical research could only yield conflicting results concerning the influence of specific psychological factors, in general psychological factors can cause or influence atopic dermatitis. Patients with atopic dermatitis are suggested to show stronger physiological stress reactions than healthy persons [17–19].

Furthermore, emotional stress has been found to precede the onset of atopic dermatitis in a large majority of the samples of patients investigated [20, 21].

Patients with atopic dermatitis are often characterised by a reduced awareness and/or expression of emotions [19, 22]. This characteristic, generally termed *alexithymia,* is supposed to be a common feature in psychosomatic patients. According to some authors, patients tend to suppress above all emotions associated with the experience of separation, such as aggression, which they would express by scratching their skin. Schur [24] and Marty [25] felt that experiences of loss and bereavement often precede the onset of atopic dermatitis. Furthermore, depression is suggested to be frequent in atopic dermatitis [26]. However, the attempt to find a specific personality pattern failed because individual personality characteristics seemed to represent the consequence, i.e. the attempt to cope with the disease rather than the cause of the disease.

This view is confirmed by Rechardt [27] who analysed patients during acute eruptions and found intense feelings of dependence and hopelessness, overaggression and self-pity. In a follow-up 9 years later, these feelings could no longer be observed. He concluded that emotional disturbances can be attributed above all to the consequences of the disease. Most authors agree that atopic patients frequently are

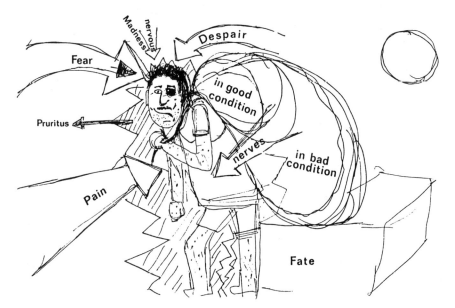

Fig. 15. The burden of the disease: drawing of a patient with atopic dermatitis

not capable of dealing with their emotions, especially anger, hostility and aggression [19, 20, 28]. Therefore, it seems important to support the patients who are coping with the disease to prevent neurotic tendencies.

Itching and scratching, however, can be provoked by emotional stimuli [15]. Possible triggering factors are suggested to be: stress [20, 28–30], emotional tension [30], exhaustion of emotional tolerance [32], even the mentioning of stressful topics [28, 33] and bereavement [26, 27].

The somatopsychic effects, i.e. the belief in being disfigured and the enormous distress caused by itching, are often underestimated by other people. Daily life is often affected by constant itching, since the patient rests only for a few hours during the night. Thus efficiency and concentration frequently decrease during acute eruptions. Furthermore, patients view visible lesions as a restriction of interpersonal attractiveness. Any patient will be able to report how difficult outdoor activities become, due to the reactions of other people to their skin lesions.

The drawing by a patient may illustrate the different stressful aspects of living with such an itchy, painful, disfiguring skin (Fig. 15).

15.2.3 Case History

The following typical example of a consultation illustrates the psychodynamic aspects of patients with atopic dermatitis.

A 21-year-old student consulted the dermatologic outpatient clinic, obviously depressed and somewhat hopeless. He presented the inner sides of his arms to the dermatologist. They were dotted with erythema, lichenification and stroke-like excoriations, especially at the flexures. Being asked how long these lesions had persisted, he spontaneously answered, "For ever!" and then added that it had worsened in the past 6 months. Recently, he could only sleep at night for a few hours. Therefore, he would no longer be able to concentrate on his studies. His apparently indifferent account given in an insistently nonchalant way contrasted with the sad expression of his face. After the application of low-strength topical corticosteroids and sedative antihistamines, the symptoms improved slightly. Since his knowledge about atopic dermatitis was incomplete, an appointment was made to give him more information.

During the 30-min conversation he reported that according to his mother he had had infantile eczema affecting his face and later the flexural areas. Also, a chronic allergic rhinitis had persisted for years during childhood, and an allergy to housedust mites had been diagnosed. His younger brother also suffered from rhinitis but without skin symptoms. During puberty, the skin lesions disappeared, and the rhinitis improved after hyposensitisation. At the beginning of his university studies, in a city far away from home, the skin disease broke out and persisted until the consultation $1^1/_2$ years later.

The patient grew up in a middle-class home. His father, director of a large post office, usually returned home late in the evening and was characterised as an austere and pedantic man. For instances of bad behaviour his father often beat him, whereas the relationship to his mother was intimate and affectionate. In school his classmates teased him because of his eczema and beat him, too. Therefore, he had to take a roundabout way to school to avoid those humiliating confrontations. When he changed to another school, the condition of his skin improved abruptly. He became a member of youth groups and engaged in political activities. He remembered that he had been not only a leader but had suppressed others as he had been suppressed in the earlier school. His skin lesions cleared up almost completely until the beginning of his studies, when he was separated from his parents and his girlfriend. The eczema flared up again, and he retired from social contacts, feeling anxious about presenting his skin to other people. He consulted several dermatologists, non-medical practioners and neurologists without any appreciable success. Since the anamnesis indicated some clearcut psychosomatic correlations, psychotherapy was proposed to him. At first he accepted this proposal gratefully, then, however, stopped the psychotherapy after the third session since the therapist would "not understand anything about his skin disease" (see Chap. 4: "Splitting of care givers"). It was $1^1/_2$ years before he started psychotherapy again. Since that time no further inpatient treatment has been necessary, although some slight eruptions recurred, especially during intervals without treatment sessions.

15.2.4 Psychological Management

This example above illustrates several essential aspects concerning the psychological management of patients with atopic dermatitis:

1. The patients appear in most cases depressive, and they show submissive behaviour. Furthermore, they expose the physician's inability to make the atopic dermatitis better, thereby often provoking initial compassion and then rejection. It is precisely this reaction which the key figure in their emotional development, usually the mother, showed to him, and which the physician can feel as countertransference.

2. Even the death of an intimate person or other emotionally touching events are reported in a strangely neutral way. In the first interviews, affections such as weeping are rarely shown.

3. The initial attempt to introduce a psychosomatic perspective – for instance through the comment: "This is an emotional problem" – will not be successful, since the patient is not aware of this relationsship. A short, additional example may illustrate this: A patient reports in the first consultation: "Decisive in my disease was the divorce from my wife." By this formulation, he obviously offers a psychosomatic explanation. However, if one refers to this remark directly, the patient will make assurances that he could handle it and that he could not imagine that it would have anything to do with his disease (see Chap. 4: "Denial").

   Thus, we cannot assume that the patient is conscious of his problem. Furthermore, he considers his skin as an autonomous organ which has nothing to do with himself: "My skin is not as well as I am!"

4. The somatic anamnesis also give the opportunity to assess the social background, the family structure and actual problems. Therefore, it is better to refer more directly to emotional problems after some consultation.

5. A more extended conversation will often reveal the *typical* psychosomatic personality structure in the sense of Balint [34]. In atopic dermatitis, this characteristic can be explained by an experience the infant gains before his personality structure is stable: the simultaneous perception of tender stimulation through the application of ointment, and of itch and pain through tight rubbing of the wounded skin. The infant is not able to discriminate between those two stimuli. The mother often represses her own rejection of the "abnormal" child and compensates by excessive affection and love. This theory was advanced by Pines [35]

and Spitz [36] and confirmed by numerous well-documented case studies. Schur [26] and Marty [27] underlined the importance of an early disturbance in the emotional development of atopic dermatitis patients, introducing the term *allergic object relation.*

6. Usually, it often takes several years until an atopic dermatitis patient gains some insight into the emotional aspects and decides to start psychotherapy. It is important to give them this time, because otherwise we are repeating the action of their parents, who always gave them advice on how to deal with the itch in a better way.

7. Sometimes when experiences of separation are worked through in therapy, a relapse may occur, leading the physician to question the therapy. However, this experience of separation without complete disappearance is important for the patient, since he may better recognise and feel those relationships.

The course of a consultation with atopic children is different, and the following examples, in accordance with Bosse and Hünecke [40] and Schröpl [27], may illustrate typical aspects.

A vigorous, very active mother (sometimes they are also resigned and depressed) enters the consulting room, pushing a 4-years-old girl in front of her. The child appears helpless but obstinate, often beginning to weep or scratch. An old face with a desperate expression is a striking feature of those children. She is nervous, not knowing where to go, her hands and body and especially her eyes moving around anxiously and restlessly. Most often the cheeks are sore from scratching. As soon as the child scratches again, her mother gives her an order such as, "Sit down there! Don't scratch! Keep your seat like a good girl! Don't make such a fuss!" When asked about her child's complaints the mother takes her child in an unusually hard grasp. She takes off her clothes in an aggressive manner, to which the child submits indifferently, sometimes cringing. Then her mother starts to complain aloud about how her daughter is unable to get rid of that "terrible allergy". She adds that she had consulted many physicians and that she would do anything for her daughter's sake.

A similar constellation can be observed with patients in puberty.

A 14-year-old girl, somewhat morose, is urged inside by her mother. Her father keeps in the background, shy and passive, asking whether he is allowed to enter the consulting room, too. The mother at once takes lead of the conversation, whereas the girl sits down with an indifferent expression on her face, immediately starting to scratch. If only two seats are available, the father usually remains standing, saying that it does not matter.

When questioned about the reason for the consultation, the mother immediately begins to complain verbosely. Thus, enough time remains for a closer look at the whole family. The mother reports a host of highly unimportant details. It is important to address oneself soon directly to the child by looking at her firmly. However, before the girl can react, her mother answers like a shot. Children often look to their mother and then think about the possibility that they might answer on their own.

Then the girl is asked again about the itching, and again her mother answers. She rudely grasps her daughter's arm and presents it like a dead object to the physician. The girl submits to this handling indifferently; however, her face expresses intentional disgust. Frequently I ask the mother directly whether she has noticed that I am not talking to her. At this, the mother may be shocked, and from her reaction one can decide in favour of familytherapy or not.

These examples demonstrate the typical course of consultations and the interplay of patients and their relatives. If the physician has succesfully motivated the family towards therapy, it is important to find an adequate psychotherapeutic approach.

15.2.5 Therapeutic Approach to Atopic Dermatitis Patients

Actually, it is impossible to acquire a therapeutic approach to patients by reading theoretical dissertations. Instead, the reader should notice his or her own feelings about the patient and participate in a Balint group [34] for exchange of experiences or, better, in a special practical training course in psychotherapy. Nevertheless, some basic procedures to facilitate a psychotherapeutic approach should be outlined. The advantage of a physician is that a normal clinical anamnesis focusing on somatic aspects already provides a lot of information about the patient. Furthermore, personal perception reveals many essential aspects which must be taken into account in the treatment.

For instance, the patient's sitting position may give some hints to his relationship with the physician: Does he take a frontal position. Does he look at me from aside in a sceptical way? Or does he remain standing in the door, looking to the floor when speaking?

Scratching plays a very important role in the behaviour pattern of atopic dermatitis patients. The physician can observe an instinctive gentle rubbing of the bridge of the nose which appears in cases of mistrust or uncertain topics. When speaking about emotional or stressful topics the perinasal skin usually turns pale due to paradoxical vascular reactions. Suppressed aggression and anger which cannot be acted out in an adequate way often provokes an autoaggressive scratching. In general, two patterns of scratching behaviour can be distinguished: a mere rubbing and chafing associated with an erythema of the predilected sites; and an excoriative scratching which can result in such a severe itch that patients would like to pull their skin off.

The physician should know that the patient feels helpless in a vicious circle of racking itch and apparently uncontrollable autodestructive scratching. You may ask the patient to assess the intensity on a 10-point scale and record the time and situation in a diary. Frequently, such a diary may provide further data for intervention.

Another approach involves an extended anamnesis of at least half an hour, which is reserved to talk with the patients about the way they cope with their disease. A favourable setting may be a group discussion about the various factors triggering their disease. A self-help group may develop out of this group, and the physician may take the role of a professional consultant only occasionally.

An important aim of individual interviews is to explore the patients' motivation for psychotherapy, which depends largely on their conception of the disease, their expectations about the outcome of different treatment approaches and the pressure of suffering from the disease. Also, the expression/awareness of emotions is important for the selection of patients for psychotherapy. In general, three subgroups of patients can be distinguished with regard to a differential indication for psychotherapy [38]:

1. Patients with a somatic conception of disease, low pressure of suffering from the disease and lack of expression/awareness of emotions (alexithymia);
2. Patients with a somatic conception of disease, high pressure of suffering from the disease and adequate expression/awareness of emotions;
3. Somatopsychic patients with a psychosomatic conception of disease, high pressure of suffering from the disease and good expression/awareness of emotions.

The last group of patients can easily be prepared for referral to a psychotherapist. It is helpful to seek contact with well-versed colleagues working nearby.

With the first two groups of patients a psychosomatic treatment is not promising unless the patient recognises the relationship between the symptoms and his or her own situation of life. A favourable insight may be enhanced by asking the patient about a possible temporal relationship of eruptions and changes in life situation. Further, the physician may also give a direct feedback about personal impressions if the patient has enough confidence. Soon the proposal can be made to participate in a relaxation training programme such as progressive muscle relaxation training or autogenic training to reduce itching [39].

According to personal experience [40] the patient may take several years before opting for psychotherapy. Since this step requires the willingness to try to change certain habits in daily life, it is important to let patients decide on their own and not to force them into this step.

15.2.6 Psychotherapy

As already mentioned, to find an adequate psychotherapeutic treatment also requires close contact with colleagues who are willing to cooperate and who have enough experience and knowledge about the problems of patients with chronic diseases, especially atopic dermatitis. In general, it will be helpful to join a Balint group which may provide the possibility of discussing problem cases with colleagues and trained psychotherapists.

The practitioner may be confronted with a host of psychological treatment methods. The following approaches are suggested to be effective in patients with atopic dermatitis: analytic psychotherapy and psychoanalysis, behavioural therapy, relaxation training, biofeedback training, hypnotherapy and multi-element approach.

Analytic Psychotherapy. Several reports have been published concerning the use of conventional psychotherapy as treatment for atopic dermatitis [41, 42]. Williams [43] posited that eczemic children conform to a specific personality pattern and that they almost inevitably were faced with rejection from their mothers. With this rationale Williams treated 53 children with chronic atopic dermatitis. Two groups were established: one of 33 children in whom the therapeutic emphasis was on management of the maternal rejection factor, and one of 20 in whom the treatment consisted solely of potential dietary and air-borne allergen elimination procedures plus the use of local topical medication.

The results indicated that at the end of a 24-month observation period, 15 children (45%) of the first group were symptom free. However, in the second control group only 2 (10%) had remitted. In addition, the successful 45% in the first group achieved remission 3–7 months after beginning treatment, while the 10% of the control group which improved did so only after 15 months.

Furthermore, several authors have presented impressive case studies which underline the efficacy of analytic psychotherapy [44, 45]

Behavioural Therapy. Behavioural approaches most often focus on modification of the scratching behaviour. Operant methods which aim at the reduction of the positively reinforcing consequences of scratching and at the enhancement of alternative behaviour (such as relaxation) may be useful to interupt the vicious circle of itch and scratching [46–49].

Relaxation Training and Biofeedback Training. Until now only a few studies existed about the effects of relaxation training or biofeedback training. Miller et al. [50] treated four patients with eczema in a pilot study involving the therapeutic use of galvanic skin response biofeedback applied to this type of skin disorder. The authors' premise was that eczema is characterised by increased epidermal hydration in the form of intercellular or intracellular oedema and, therefore, should be related to high skin conductivity.

Of the four patients studied, two had complete remissions within 4 weeks of biofeedback training. The other two individuals reportedly did not regularly practise the technique and showed only moderate improvement.

Haynes et al. [53] treated eight patients with frontal EMG feedback and relaxation training. Overall results indicated a 50% reduction in the affected skin areas' itching level within, but not across, treatment sessions.

Hypnotherapy. Although a paucity of research has used hypnotherapy as a treatment for atopic dermatitis, those studies that have been reported claim positive results [51–53]. Zhukov [54] conducted a study of patients with atopic dermatitis. The results indicated that a complete recovery was noted in 36% of the experimental group and in 16% of the control group. A marked improvement was seen in 28% of the experimental group and in 9% of the controls. A follow-up overwhelmingly testified to the permanent nature of the improvements.

Multi-Element Approach. Besides the treatment methods mentioned, psychotherapy approaches such as bioenergetics might also be promising since skin diseases are interpreted in psychoanalytic theories as early disturbances of personality development and can be characterised in this sense as preverbal. However, until now no investigations have been presented about either bioenergetics or other humanistic psychotherapies, such as gestalt therapy and client-centered therapy, which may be effective, too.

As demonstrated in the treatment of psoriasis [55], the combination of psychological and dermatological treatment including special patient training seems to be the most promising approach. Brown and Bettley [56] compared the efficacy of a dermatological therapy with that of a combination of dermatological and psychiatric treatment in 72 patients who were assigned to the groups at random. They found no significant differences between the groups. This result suggests that uncontrolled psychiatric treatment of atopic dermatitis patients regardless of indication or suitability of therapy is likely to fail.

To sum up briefly, atopic dermatitis is a skin disease with a genetic disposition, which is also triggered by psychological factors. Psychological treatment approaches may prevent the effect of these factors. Furthermore, psychotherapy is indicated in cases of inadequate, emotional, "somatopsychic" reactions to this chronic condition.

References

1. Braun-Falco O, Plewig G, Wolff HH (1984) Dermatologie and Venerologie. Springer, Berlin Heidelberg New York
2. Brocq L, Jacquet L (1891) Notes pour servir à l'histoire des neurodermatites. Ann Dermatol Syphiligr 97:193
3. Hanifin JM, Rajka G (1980) Diagnostic features of atopic dermatitis. Acta Derm Venereol [Suppl] (Stockh) 92:44–47
4. Rajka G (1986) Natural history and clinical manifestations of atopic dermatitis. Clin Rev Allergy 4:3–26
5. Vickers CFH (1980) The natural history of atopic aczema. Acta Derm Vernerol [Suppl] (Stockh) 92:113–115
6. Champion RH, Parish WE (1968) Atopic dermatitis. In: Rook A, Wilkinson DS (eds) Textbook of dermatology. Blackwell, Oxford
7. Wütherich G (1984) Immunpathologie der atopischen Dermatitis. Monatsschr Kinderheilkd 132:426–431
8. Rajka G (1986) Atopic dermatitis. Correlation of environmental factors with frequency. Int J Dermatol 25:301–304
9. Hanifin M, Lobitz WC (1977) Newer concepts of atopic dermatitis. Arch Dermatol 113:663–670
10. Stüttgen G (1981) Physiologie and Pathophysiologie des Juckreizes. Münch Med Wochenschr 123:987–991
11. Cormia FE (1952) Experimental histamine pruritus. I. Influence of physical and psychological factors on threshold reactivity. Invest Dermatol 19:21–29
12. Graham DT, Wolf S (1950) Pathogenesis of urticaria. JAMA 1396–1402
13. Ring J (1981) Atopic dermatitis: a disease of immuno-vegetative dysregulation. In: Ring J, Burg G (eds) New trends in allergy. Springer, Berlin Heidelberg New York
14. Slade JD, Hepburn B (1983) Prednisone-induces alterations of circulating human lymphocyte subsets. J Lab Clin Med 101:479–487
15. Faulstich ME, Williamson DA, Duchman EG, Conerly SL, Brantley PJ (1985) Psychophysiological analysis of atopic dermatitis. J Psychosom Res 29:415–417
16. Schwendner R (1986) Psychische Belastungen und Streßreaktionen bei Neurodermitikern und Psoriatikern. Dermatologie-Kongreß, Davos
17. Panconesi E (1984) Stress and skin disease; psychosomatic dermatology. In: Parish LC (ed) Clinics in dermatology. Lippincott, Philadelphia
18. Kaschel R (1987) Verhaltensmedizinische Aspekte der atopischen Dermatitis. Eine Pilotstudie. Dipl Psychologie, Universität Tübingen
19. Koblenzer CS (1983) Psychosomatic concepts in dermatology. Arch Dermatol 119:501–512
20. Wittkower E, Russel B (1953) Emotional factors in skin disease. Cassell, London
21. Brown DG (1972) Stress as a precipitant of eczema. J Psychosom Res 16:321–327

22. McLaughlin JT, Shoemaker RJ, Guy WB (1962) Personality factors in adult atopic eczema. Arch Dermatol Syphilol 68:506–516
23. Rajka G (1986) Natural history and clinical manisfestations of atopic dermatitis. Clin Rev Allergy 4:3–26
24. Schur M (1980) Zur Metapsychologie der Somatisierung. In: Brede K (ed) Einführung in die psychosomatische Medizin. Syndikat, Autoren- und Verlagsgesellschaft, Frankfurt/M
25. Marty P (1980) Die allergische Objektbeziehung. In: Brede K (ed) Einführung in die psychosomatische Medizin. Syndikat, Autoren- und Verlagsgesellschaft, Frankfurt/M
26. Medansky RS, Handler RM (1981) Dermatopsychosomatics: classification, physiology and therapeutic approaches. J Am Acad Dermatol 5:125–136
27. Rechardt E (1970) An investigation in the psychosomatic aspects of prurigo Besnier. Monographs of the Psychiatric Clinic Helsinki University, Central Hospital, Helsinki
28. Bosse K, Fassheber P, Hünecke P, Teichmann AT, Zauner J (1976) Zur sozialen Situation des Hautkranken als Phänomen interpersoneller Wahrnehmung. Psychosom Med Psychoanal 21:3–61
29. Fjellner B, Arnetz BB (1985) Psychological predictors of pruritus during mental stress. Acta Derm Vernerol (Stockh) 65–504–508
30. Klein JM (1982) Stress und Neurodermatitis: "Atopic neurodermatosis". A new concept. Stress 3:11–14
31. Böddeker KW, Böddeker M (1976) Verhaltenstherapeutische Ansätze bei der Behandlung des endogenen Ekzems unter besonderer Berücksichtigung des zwanghaften Kratzens. Z Psychosom Med Psychoanal 21:61–101
32. Bosse K, Hünecke P (1986) Der Juckreiz des endogenen Ekzematikers. Münch Med Wochenschr 123:1013–1016
33. Jordan JM, Withlock FA (1972) Emotions and the skin: the conditioning of scratch response in cases of atopic dermatitis. Br J Dermatol 86:579–585
34. Balint M (1964) The doctor, his patient and the illness. Pitman, London
35. Pines D (1980) Skin communications: early skin disorders and their effect on transferrence and countertransferrence. Int J Psychoanal 61:315–323
36. Spitz R (1967) Die Entstehung der ersten Objektbeziehung. Klett-Cotta, Stuttgart
37. Schröpl F (1984) Die Bedeutung psychischer Faktoren bei der Neurodermitis. Riedell, Frankfurt
38. Bosse K, Gieler U (1987) Seelische Faktoren bei Hautkrankheiten. Huber, Bern
39. Haynes SN, Wilson CC, Jaffe FG, Britton BV (1979) Biofeedback treatment of atopic dermatitis: controlled case studies of eight cases. Biofeedback Self Regul 4:195–209
40. Neraal A (1987) Therapeutischer Umgang mit Neurodermitispatienten. Dtsche Krankenpflege 2:78–80
41. Klein HS (1949) Psychogenic factors in dermatitis and their treatment by group therapy. Br J Med Psychol 22:32–45
42. Walsh MN, Kierland RR (1947) Psychotherapy in the treatment of neurodermatitis. Proceedings of staff meeting, Mayo Clinic 22:578–583
43. Williams D (1951) Management of atopic dermatitis in children: control of the maternal rejection factor. Arch Dermatol Syphilol 63:545–556
44. Thomä H (1980) Über die Unspezifität psychosomatischer Erkrankungen am Beispiel einer Neurodermitis mit 20-jähriger Katamnese. Psyche 24:589–624
45. Krichhauff G (1955) Bemerkungen zu genetischen und neurosenstrukturellen Faktoren bei endogenen Ekzemen. Z Psychosom Me 2:184–192
46. Allen KE, Harris FR (1966) Elimination of a child's excessive scratching by training the mother in reinforcement procedures. Behav Res Ther 4:79–84
47. Dobes RW (1977) Amelioration of psychosomatic dermatosis by reinforced inhibiton of scratching. J Behav Ther Exp Psychiatry 8:185–187

48. Melin L, Frederiksen T, Noren P, Swebilius BG (1986) Behavioral treatment of scratching in patients with atopic dermatitis. Br J Dermatol 115:467–474

49. Walton D (1960) The application of learning theory to the treatment of a case of neurodermatitis. In: Eysenck HJ (ed) Behaviour therapy and the neuroses Pergamon. New York

50. Miller R, Conger R, Dymond A (1974) Biofeedback skin conductance conditioning in dyshydrotic eczema. Arch Dermatol 109:737–738

51. Horan JS (1950) Management of neurodermatitis by hypnotic suggestion. Br J Med Hypnotism 2:43–49

52. Kline MV (1954) Psoriasis and hypnotherapy: the acceptance of resistance in the treatment of a long-standing neurodermatitis with a sensory imagery technique. J Clin Exp Hypnosis 2:313–322

53. Twerski AJ, Naar R (1974) Hypnotherapy in a case of refractory dermatitis. Am J Clin Hypnosis 16:202–205

54. Zhukow JA (1961) Hypnotherapy of dermatosis in resort treatment. In: Winn RB (ed) Psychotherapy in the Soviet Union. Philosophical Library, New York

55. Bremer-Schulte M, Cormane RH, van Dijk E, Write J (1985) Group therapy of psoriasis: duoformula group treatment as an example. J Am Acad Dermalol 12:61–66

56. Brown DG, Bettley FR (1971) Psychiatric treatment of eczema: a controlled trial. Br Med J 2:729–734

15.3 Chronic Urticaria

U. Stangier

A large number of known and unknown factors, including psychological stimuli, contribute to the aetiology of urticaria [1]. Advances in allergologic and immunologic research increased the knowledge about this disease but also produced complex data about its aetiology. However, these data have not yet been integrated into an adequate multifactorial and dynamic approach. Two simplifying concepts over-emphasizing single causes of urticaria are still widespread: that it is essentially an allergy, and that it is a psychosomatic response.

In practice, extensive diagnostic investigations often fail to find the cause for the recurrent attacks of chronic urticaria, leaving both the patient and the physician frustrated. Contrary to popular opinion about the disease, an allergic genesis for instance can be proved in only a small percentage of patients [2]. Even if skin testing produces positive results, symptoms very often persist despite the removal of the suspected triggering factor. The failure to detect any somatic, allergic or non-allergic factor in more than half of the patients in turn gives rise to the search for a possible psychogenesis. However, the fixation on a single cause is not a promising approach to a disease, in which multiple factors contribute to its manifestation. Especially in chronic urticaria, as Rees [3] pointed out, "various causal agents can exert summative or possibly synergic effects" (p. 185). It is evident that the existence of a somatic triggering mechanism does not necessarily exclude the simultaneous relevance of psychosomatic correlations.

The following literature review refers mainly to chronic urticaria, in which psychosomatic aspects are thought to be more important than in acute urticaria. Nevertheless, it should be noted that this differentiation is an artificial one. The definition of a chronic course varies from author to author, ranging from 2 weeks to several months.

Statistics regarding the relative importance of psychological factors diverge, depending on the different criteria and methods of investigation. In two earlier studies it was concluded from extensive interviews that in 83% [4] and 68% [3], respectively, of the patients psychological factors played an important part in the aetiology. In contrast, when simple questions about aggravating factors were presented to larger patient samples, emotional stress was less frequently found to be a contributing or main cause, the proportion ranging from 7% [5] to 35% [2] and 48% [6]. These conflicting results can be attributed above all to differences in assessment methods. Closer personal contact allows a more thorough investigation than anonymous questionnaires. On the other hand, the interviewer might influence the patients to respond to questions as they think is expected. In addition, retrospective reports of patients may be affected by an observer bias [7]. They may attribute the onset of their disease – due to a lack of clearly identifiable causes – to stressful events which they recall better.

Furthermore, it seems to be useful to discriminate different forms of urticaria. For instance, it could be demonstrated that stressful events were significantly more often associated with the onset of symptoms in patients with cholinergic urticaria and dermographism than in patients with cold urticaria [8]. It is reasonable to assume that different pathogenetic pathways could derive from different susceptibilities to stress.

15.3.1 Psychophysiological Aspects

For a more adequate understanding of the relationship between emotions and urticaria it is also necessary to consider the underlying psychophysiological mechanisms. As a reaction to psychosocial stimuli such as stress, activity of the CNS – as a somatic correlate of psychological processes – also involves the activation of autonomic, endocrine and even immunological responses. Apparently, these responses are organised into specific patterns, depending on the subjective perception of demand characteristics of a situation, and the personal ability to cope with them [9]. Prolonged or extremely intense activation of the physiological systems is suggested to act as a trigger on pathogenetic mechanisms in somatically predisposed individuals.

An important study many authors have referred to was conducted in 1950 by Graham and Wolf [10]. Thirty patients with chronic urticaria were interviewed about their life situations before the onset of the disease. Simultaneously, cutaneous vascular reactions were recorded in 13 of the patients. When talking about stressful aspects of the past, an increase in skin temperature and a decrease in the minute vessel tone could be observed in those 11 of the 13 who expressed resentful emotions. In addition, 5 developed urticarial wheals during the interviews. Furthermore, 29 of the total showed a common attitude in the situation preceeding the urticarial attack:

> [they] considered themselves wronged or injured (usually by someone in a fairly close relationship), and they regarded the traumatizing situation as one which precluded any action on their parts. They believed that they could neither retaliate nor run away. In this setting they became intensely resentful, and urticaria developed. (p. 1398)

The authors suggested that resentment may contribute to wheal formation by extreme vasodilatation and increased pressure in the vessels. However, it has been argued that vasodilatation is not necessarily associated with increased vascular permeability, exudation of fluid and formation of urticarial wheals [11]. Changes in permeability are mainly due to vasoactive mediators such as histamine and represent a mechanism different from vasodilatation [12]. Nevertheless, it could also be observed that the exudation of fluid in an artificially produced blister is influenced by emotional arousal [13].

Another approach to investigate the link between the CNS and urticaria is the use of suggestions to produce or suppress skin reactions under hypnosis. A remarkable series of controlled studies by Black and colleagues [14–17] demonstrated the suppression of different types of allergic skin reactions, including immediate-type hypersensitivity, by hypnotic suggestions. Despite the inhibition of wheal response and vasodilatation, the activation of the underlying immunological reaction – i.e. antibody formation and mononuclear cell infiltration – could be proved in two studies [14, 17]. Therefore, Black's results suggest the existence of a psychophysiological control mechanism by which the CNS may act on peripheral vascular reactions, especially the exudation of fluid, which may be relevant also to urticaria.

The central pathogenetic pathway responsible for all forms of urticaria is the release of vasoactive mediators, mainly histamine, serotonin, prostaglandins, platelet activating factor and leukotrienes, from mast cells and basophilic leucocytes. Data from experimental studies indicate that plasma levels of histamine [18], prostaglandins [19] and plasmin [20], which is involved in the activation of vasoactive kinins, are responsive to emotional stress. However, not all these observations apply to urticaria, and until now the release of mediators into the skin has not yet been studied in urticaria patients under stressful conditions.

The psychophysiological pathway resulting in mast cell degranulation can be explained by different mechanisms:

1. The stress-induced activation of adrenergic and cholinergic hormones may enhance the release of mast cell mediators [21]. For instance, the release of acetylcholine in the skin due to sympathetic stimulation of the sweat glands could be relevant for cholinergic urticaria. Recently, a new form of adrenergic urticaria triggered by noradrenaline was identified [22].
2. Neuropeptides may act as potent vasoactive mediators on mast cells, too. Substance P, which can be identified in the primary sensory nerve endings in the skin, is an important mediator not only of pain sensation, but also of inflammation and hypersensitivity, since it is capable of inducing mast cell degranulation [12, 23]. Furthermore, substance P is suggested to be responsive to emotional stress [24, 25].
3. Finally, evidence exists for another, as yet unidentified link between the CNS and the release of histamine which might be independent of stress-induced sympathetic stimulation. Similar to the remarkable series of animal experiments concerning behaviourally conditioned immunosuppression by Ader [26], it could be demonstrated that the release of plasma histamine can be triggered not only by antigen presentation, but also, through associative learning, by environmental stimuli [27]. This result suggests that symbolic stimuli may influence mast cell activity by a pathway which is not related to emotional stress.

However, more experimental data are needed to give more precise explanations of how psychological events contribute to the development of urticaria.

15.3.1.1 Personality and Stress

Until now Alexander's considerations about psychosomatic specificity have profoundly influenced psychodynamic concepts of the psychogenesis of various disorders, including urticaria. This theory links particular unconscious emotional conflicts to the activation of different autonomic reactions which in turn result in the development of specific psychosomatic diseases [27]. A modification of Alexander's theory was introduced by Graham, who attempted to find specific attitudes related to the onset of certain diseases. This refers to observable aspects of emotional behaviour instead of latent unconscious conflicts. As mentioned above, patients with urticaria were found to see themselves as being mistreated but could not express hostility [10]. However, most authors referred to Alexander's concept of a specific conflict configuration.

Saul and Bernstein presented a detailed case study of a woman with chronic urticaria [28]. Psychoanalytic treatment revealed that the urticaria attacks were associated with the frustration of intensified longings for love. The symptom seemed to take the place of repressed weeping which would have provided relief from anger. Other psychoanalytic authors found either a passive-dependent and immature personality [29] or anxiety and guilt connected with hostile aggressive impulses [30] as central psychodynamic factors in several cases of chronic urticaria.

A distinction between a passive-dependent, submissive and resentful subgroup of patients was made in several investigations with larger patient samples, based on psychiatric interviews [31–33] or projective test procedures [34]. Since no standardised diagnostic methods and control groups were used, these findings might be rather the consequence of the investigators' common starting point than the reflection of actually common patient characteristics. However, two studies at a later date using more reliable and objective personality inventories confirmed the hypothesis that increased *submission* and *resentment* are typical personality features of patients with urticaria [35, 36].

Other authors have underlined the importance of anxiety as a dominant affect in many patients with chronic urticaria [3, 33, 38]. Psychometric investigations found elevated levels of anxiety as well as depression [35, 37].

Indeed, a confusing number of personality traits have been suggested to be responsible for urticaria attacks, but they are scarcely specific. For instance, repressed hostility has been related to nearly all of the diseases which are often characterised as psychosomatic.

Furthermore, it is not quite clear by which mechanism personality characteristics are relevant for the induction of urticarial wheals. In contrast to Alexander [27] and Graham and Wolf [10] most psychoanalytic authors neglect psychophysiological aspects, considering urticaria as a conversion reaction in the sense of a symbolic solution of a particular unconscious conflict [33]. Thus, it is interpreted as a regressive attempt to discharge intense affects by physical symptoms. These speculations may be evoked by the fact that urticarial lesions are characterised by rapid and transient occurrence, reversibility and lack of secondary skin abnormalities.

Another, less speculative approach to explain the relationship between psychological characteristics and physical symptoms is the stress concept. Selye's theory of a non-specific stress response to any environmental stimuli requiring adaptation [39] resulted in the attempt to correlate accumulations of stressful life changes with the development of physical and psychological symptoms. Indeed, two studies indicate that patients with chronic urticaria experienced significantly more stressful life events before the onset of their disease than did control groups [35, 37].

However, life event research has been much criticised, since the amount of stress depends above all on the individual capacity to cope with life changes [7], and daily experiences of stress (daily hassles), which are suggested to be more important than extraordinary life changes (major life events) [40]. In accordance with these arguments, Reinhold [41] concluded from unstructured interviews with 27 patients with chronic urticaria that in most cases chronic stress and minor crises, but not major crises, preceded the onset of the disease. Her impression – which is in line with that of other authors [4, 42] – was that chronic urticaria represented "non-specific responses to non-specific stress in persons of widely differing personality".

To sum up the findings, the great variety of different personality traits (resentment and anxiety being the most prominent among them) which have been observed in patients with chronic urticaria does not suggest a specific urticaria personality. A promising research approach seems to be the formation of subgroups with different psychological characteristics related to specific psychophysiological response patterns. As already mentioned above, different emotional reactions to stressful demands such as anger, fear and depression appear to be closely related to the activation of particular autonomic, endocrine and immunological reactions [9]. This might increase the risk to develop urticaria in predisposed individuals. The attempt to identify *different* psychological characteristics which increase the susceptibility to a disease seems to be more appropriate than to look for common psychological features in individuals with a specific physical disease.

15.3.2 Psychological Treatment

The various forms of psychological therapy which have been reported in the research literature for urticaria can be classified into three principal approaches. In most studies, symptomatic treatment methods have been applied to modify underlying psychophysiological reactions. Less frequently the use of supportive psychotherapy focusing on problems of the actual life situation and of psychoanalytic treatment approaches has been described.

It is a well-known phenomenon that urticarial wheals can be produced and removed by hypnotic suggestions [43]. Two investigations could also demonstrate beneficial long-term effects of hypnotic treatment in larger samples of urticaria patients [34, 44]. The treatment included two elements that may both be effective: instructions for relaxation and suggestions that symptoms will disappear.

Closely related to the particular results of suggestion are placebo effects, which are not specific for any treatment approach, especially expectations concerning treatment outcome [45]. Indeed, it was shown that antihistamines could be successfully replaced by placebo in the vast majority of patients with daily eruptions of urticaria [46]. This remarkable result indicates that positive expectations may be an essential requirement of any treatment approach in urticaria.

Since the use of hypnosis is no longer common in psychotherapeutic practice, because of the vagueness of the underlying effect mechanisms and its limited applicability, relaxation methods represent an alternative widely used and extensively evaluated for a large number of psychosomatic conditions [47, 48]. Whereas autogenic training and progressive relaxation training aim at the reduction of general autonomic arousal, biofeedback training focuses on the modification of specific autonomic reactions, changes of which are recorded by apparatuses and reflected in optic or acoustic signals. For instance, the usefulness of galvanic skin response biofeedback training was demonstrated in a patient with chronic urticaria whose symptoms were maintained by increased general anxiety [49]. In another case study progressive muscle relaxation was successfully employed besides various other behavioural techniques, including systematic desensitisation and covert reinforcement [50]. This treatment aimed mainly at the reduction of tension associated with anxiety and anger.

Autogenic training may be effective, too, although it has not yet been evaluated in urticaria. However, positive results were reported in some cases of food intolerance, which is also often mentioned to be a factor in urticaria [42, 51].

A crucial point in the efficacy of relaxation training is the maintainance of regular home practice [44, 49, 50]. Further research should clarify whether relaxation is indicated only in case of psychological problems associated with increased autonomic arousal. Furthermore, additional measures such as behaviour therapy or supportive psychotherapy may be frequently necessary to enhance the patient's coping with actual life problems.

Supportive psychotherapy is characterised by the limited extent to which deeper personal conflicts are worked through, and by the limitation of time. Interventions focus on stressful aspects of the current life situation and may include behaviour therapeutic techniques [52], client-centered therapy [53] and short-term psychoanalytic techniques [54]. This approach should be taken into account when evidence exists for psychological problems, but subjective or objective circumstances (motivation of the patient, institutional context) preclude a more extended psychotherapy. Several reports suggest the effectiveness of short-term supportive psychotherapy, although they do not give detailed information about the methods [4, 29, 32, 41].

Finally, there have been very few reports on the psychoanalytic treatment of urticaria. As already mentioned, Saul and Bernstein [28] gave a detailed description of a patient with special reference to the analysis of dream material. Rechenberger [55] investigated 30 patients with chronic urticaria and also reported the clinical findings from psychodynamic treatment. In 26 patients it involved only 2–3 sessions, in the remaining four patients, 12–230 sessions. The basic conflict at the onset of urticaria was the threatening of a close, intimate relationship by a third person. In contrast to most psychoanalytic authors already mentioned, the patients in this study were characterised by a depressive personality structure. Rechenberger observed that they were clearly conscious of the situation preceding the attacks of urticaria. After this conflict had been worked through, the urticaria usually disappeared, but motivation for further psychotherapy also vanished.

Carefully controlled therapy studies are needed to evaluate the efficacy of various methods and to determine psychological criteria for differential indication (anxiety, depression). Furthermore, different treatment effects should be distinguished, especially itching and wheal formation [44].

Finally, an aspect not yet investigated is the secondary consequences of the disease. Due to the complete reversibility of the lesions, urticaria does not represent such an aesthetic problem to the sufferer as other chronic dermatoses, above all psoriasis. However, swelling, itchiness and pain may affect the patients' lives and result in certain kinds of illness behaviour. Psychological interventions should not only focus on the prevention of the disease but might also modify such unfavourable consequences.

To sum up briefly, two findings arise from the research literature about the efficacy of psychological treatment. First, suggestive as well as relaxation methods may be beneficial to provide symptomatic relief in a large number of patients in whom emotional problems associated with tension and increased autonomic arousal contribute to the manifestation of the disease. Secondly, clinical reports indicate that symptoms might be easily influenced by psychological treatment approaches focusing on actual problems. Therefore, short-term supportive psychotherapeutic interventions generally seem to be more promising than psychoanalytic treatment.

In practice, however, psychological treatment strategies are derived above all from the analysis of the psychological problem, not from the somatic diagnosis. The following case may illustrate which psychodiagnostical aspects determine clinical behaviour therapy.

A 50-year-old bank clerk with chronic recurrent urticaria of 2 years' duration had undergone extensive allergologic diagnostics with negative results. In addition, the patient complained of hypertension and arrhythmia. Since the physician observed a striking tension in the patient's behaviour during all consultations, he had asked him about present worries or stress. On the verge of tears the patient reported that for the past few years he had constantly been under pressure at work, where he had accepted an increasing deterioration of his position. He agreed to the suggestion that this might be a possible cause of the somatic symptoms and that psychological counselling might help him to cope with the difficulties.

The first contact with the psychologist to whom he was referred revealed submissive and defensive behaviour and a tendency to avoid any conflictive topic. In a personality inventory the scores in depression, nervousness and sociability were markedly elevated, and he reported multiple psychosomatic complaints.

Functional Analysis of Problem Behaviour. The target problem was defined as a deficit in social skills, i.e. learned helplessness in conflict situations and fear of confrontations. This behaviour pattern could be traced back to his parental home and characterised also the current relationship with his wife.

It occurred especially in challenging situations at work when he was unjustly charged with failures and removed to a lower position (antecedent conditions). The submissive behaviour was generated by a negative self-concept and the desire to please everybody (mediating cognitions).

His lack of assertive behaviour resulted in a constant social decline associated with increasing stress which contributed to the somatic symptoms (consequences).

Psychological Treatment. The therapeutic interventions aimed at the modification of cognitive, behavioural and psychophysiological aspects of the problem behaviour. An essential part of the therapy focused on the awareness and reevaluation of basic attitudes and their consequences. Furthermore, the rehearsal of assertive behaviour served to compensate for deficits in social skills. Finally, relaxation training was conducted to reduce the tension.

Although the patient adopted a passive attitude to the therapy and made only slow progress within the treatment of 15 months' duration, the urticaria disappeared soon after the beginning, recurring only twice within 3 years.

15.3.3 Patient Management

When taking into account psychosomatic aspects, the practising dermatologist is confronted with two main tasks: the integration of psychological aspects in the somatic treatment, and the indication and preparation of the referral to a psychotherapist.

Whereas general outlines of psychosomatic dermatology are referred to elsewhere [56], some special problems in the treatment of patients with chronic urticaria should be pointed out. As described in the introduction to this section, the common search of physician and patient for the triggering factor often remains ineffective.

Positive findings in allergic diagnostic procedures may reinforce the patient's rigid fixation on a single cause. Patient education, that is explanation of the multifactorial aetiology and of symptomatic and preventive treatment approaches (anti-allergic medication, avoidance of allergens, stress management, etc.), is an important didactic tool to modify the patient's inadequate conceptualisation of the disease and treatment [57]. Often unrealistic expectations are not due to a lack of information. Sometimes, patients look for a somatic diagnosis, especially that of allergy, to conceal emotional instability which is then attributable to a more acceptable somatic symptom [58, 59]. This might also concern a small proportion of patients with chronic urticaria who stick to a strictly somatic explanation of their symptoms, not aware of the close relationship to their personal life.

The physician should not adopt the pressure of responsibility the patient imposes on him or her in cases of unsuccessful but correct diagnostic and therapeutic measures. Empathetic understanding of the patient's frustration is important, but it does not mean that the physician has to become helpless, too. He or she should be aware that difficulties in the relationship may also reflect more general emotional disturbances of one person, in the sense of a transference and countertransference.

In general, a widely accepted criterion for the diagnosis of a psychosomatic aetiology is the evidence of a close temporal relationship to stressful life conditions (but not the absence of any identifiable somatic cause). Then, anamnestic inquiries provide more information about possible sources of chronic or acute stress (daily hassles, life changes), personality characteristics (anxiety, depression) or unspecific vegetative disorders, thereby clarifying the psychosomatic background. Poor expression of emotions, an extremely pessimistic way of thinking and lack of adequate abilities to cope with conflict situations are often found to be typical characteristics of psychosomatic patients.

If the anamnestic data give rise to a referral for psychological treatment, the patient should be prepared for this step. In this context, it is important to give a rational, simple and acceptable explanation of how tension and nervousness might contribute to the disease. Motivation for psychotherapy not only depends on the patient's suffering from the disease, but also on the level of information about psychotherapy, his or her personal concept of the disease and adequate treatment. Therefore, the principal goals and the procedure of psychological treatment should be illustrated. However, the final decision to refer to a psychotherapist should be taken by the patient on his own.

If there is no insight into psychosomatic aspects, the physician may instruct the patient to carry out self-monitoring, which means to record changes in symptoms over a certain period. Sometimes it is possible to detect particular events associated with emotional distress which might explain the worsening of symptoms.

The following case may demonstrate a typical example for the usefulness also of limited psychological measures in the management of urticaria.

A 38-year-old employee at the university consulted the dermatologic clinic with chronic recurrent urticaria which had first appeared 10 years ago. The tentative diagnosis of a cholinergic urticaria had been made on the basis of anamnestic data, and skin testing produced a positive result. However, specific medication had not resulted in symptom removal.

The patient's obliging and sociable behaviour was conspicous, and he gratefully complied with all diagnostic and therapeutic procedures which were proposed to him. Being asked about possible trigger factors, he spontaneously stated that his urticaria had nothing to do with emotional stress. However, he had noticed that wheals did not appear during exhausting bicycle tours on weekends but often on his short way to work. Furthermore, he felt that his skin condition improved when he was relaxed.

In order to enhance the patient's insight into possible stressful aspects of his life, the physician mentioned that according to his experience with many patients, urticaria often occurs under stressful, apparently desperate, unsolvable situations. The patients, however, suppress or fail to notice the emotional tension. This explanation given, the patient became aware that his employment was threatened and that this uncertainty about his future life exerted a subtle, but constantly paralysing strain on him. At the same time he recognised that the urticaria appeared for the first time in a similar situation when he left high school, 10 years ago, without having a job in prospect.

Willingly, he accepted the proposal to participate in relaxation training. No further therapeutic aids seemed to be necessary at that time, since the patient was obviously able to reflect the conflict situation on his own. After this contact the patient did not consult the clinic again. On a chance encounter after several months he mentioned that his urticaria had disappeared, and the relaxation training appeared no longer necessary to him.

Again, this case also illustrates that, in most patients with urticaria, the physician can refer to emotional problems *in a direct way*, and that some patients, thus becoming aware of the cause of their emotional distress, may develop their own capacities to deal with it more adequately.

Some authors [57, 60] recommend, in selected patients, the use of tranquilisers and antidepressants. Certainly, the psychopharmacological treatment may provide temporary relief, but in most patients, this might reduce motivation for psychological treatment. In addition, temporary administration is proposed as a test to determine whether the symptoms are related to emotional disturbances. However, except for patients with severe psychiatric disturbances, other diagnostic and therapeutic approaches exist which may be appropriate in most cases. As Keegan [57] pointed out, drugs (as well as relaxation training) reduce symptoms, but they do not solve emotional or other problems.

References

1. Warin RP, Champion RH (1974) Urticaria. Saunders, Philadelphia
2. Champion RH, Roberts SOB, Carpenter RG, Roger JH (1969) Urticaria and angioedema. A review of 554 patients. Br J Dermatol 81:588–597
3. Rees L (1957) An aetiological study of chronic urticaria and angioneurotic oedema. J Psychosom Res 2:172–189
4. Stokes JH, Kulchar GV, Pillsburg DM (1935) Effect on the skin of emotional and nervous states. Arch Dermatol Syph 31:470–499
5. Juhlin L (1981) Recurrent urticaria: clinical investigation of 330 patients. Br J Dermatol 104:369–381
6. Green GR, Koelsche GA, Kierland RR (1965) Etiology and pathogenesis of chronic urticaria. Ann Allergy 23:30–36

7. Cohen F (1979) Personality, stress, and the development of physical disease. In: Stone GC, Adler NE, Cohen F (eds) Health psychology. Jossey-Bass, San Francisco

8. Czubalski K, Rudzki E (1977) Neuropsychic factors in physical urticaria. Dermatologica 154:1–4

9. McCabe PM, Schneiderman N (1985) Psychophysiologic reactions to stress. In: Schneiderman N, Tapp JT (eds) Behavioral medicine: the biopsychosocial approach. Erlbaum, New York

10. Graham DT, Wolf S (1950) Pathogenesis of urticaria: experimental study of life situations, emotions and cutaneous vascular reactions. JAMA 143:1396–1402

11. Beall GN (1964) Urticaria: a review of laboratory and clinical observations. Medicine 43:131–151

12. Lembeck F (1983) Mediators of vasodilatation in the skin. Br J Dermatol 109[Suppl 25]:1–9

13. Kepecs JG, Robin M, Brunner M (1951) Relationship between certain emotional states and exudation into the skin. Psychosom Med 13:10–17

14. Mason AA, Black S (1958) Allergic skin responses abolished under treatment of asthma and hayfever by hypnosis. Lancet I:877–879

15. Black S (1963a) Inhibition of immediate-type hypersensitivity response by direct suggestion under hypnosis. Br Med J I:925–929

16. Black S (1963b) Shift in dose-response curve of Prausnitz-Küstner reaction by direct suggestion under hypnosis. Br Med J I:990–992

17. Black S, Humphrey JH, Niven J (1963) Inhibition of Mantoux reaction by direct suggestion under hypnosis. Br Med J I:1649–1652

18. Reimann JH, Meyer HJ, Wendt P (1981) Stress and histamine. In: Ring J, Burg G (eds) New trends in allergy. Springer, Berlin Heidelberg New York

19. Mest HJ, Zehl V, Sziegoleit W, Taube C, Förster W (1982) Influence of mental stress on plasma level of prostaglandins, throboxan B_2 and on circulating platelet aggregates in man. Prostaglandins Leucotrienes Med 8:553–563

20. Teshima H, Inoue S, Ago Y, Ikemi Y (1974) Plasminic activity and emotional stress. Psychother Psychosom 23:218–228

21. Bourne HR, Lichtenstein LM, Melmon RL, Henney CS, Weinstein Y, Shearer GM (1974) Modulation of inflammation and immunity by cyclic AMP. Science 184:19–28

22. Shelley WB, Shelley ED (1985) Adrenergic urticaria: a new form of stress-induced hives. Lancet 2:1031–1033

23. Payan DG, Levine JD, Goetzl EJ (1984) Modulation of immunity and hypersensitivity by sensory neuropeptides. J Immunol 132:1601–1604

24. Farber EM, Nicholoff BJ, Recht B, Fraki EJ (1986) Stress, symmetry and psoriasis: possible role of neuropeptides. J Am Acad Dermatol 14:305–311

25. Siegel RA, Düker E-M, Fuchs E, Pahnke U, Wuttke W (1984) Responsiveness of mesolimbic, mesocortical, septal and hippocampal cholecystokinin and substance P neuronal systems to stress, in the male rat. Neurochem Int 6:783–789

26. Ader R (1981) Psychoneuroimmunology. Academic, New York

27. Alexander F (1950) Psychosomatic medicine, its principles and applications. Norton, New York

28. Saul LJ, Bernstein C (1941) The emotional setting of some attacks of urticaria. Psychosom Med 3:349–369

29. Kaywin L (1947) Emotional factors in urticaria. Psychosom Med 8:131–136

30. Schneider E (1954) Psychodynamics of chronic allergic eczema and chronic urticaria. J Nerv Ment Dis 120:17–21

31. Wittkower ED (1953) Studies of the personality of patients suffering from urticaria. Psychosom med 15:116–126

32. Kraft B, Blumenthal DL (1959 Psychological components in chronic urticaria. Acta Allergol 13:469–475

33. Shoemaker RJ (1963) A search for the affective determinants of chronic urticaria. Psychosomatics 4:125–132
34. Kaneko DL, Takaishi N (1963) Psychosomatic studies on chronic urticaria. Folia Psychiatr Neurol Jpn 17:16–24
35. Lyketsos GC, Stratigos J, Tawil G, Psaras M, Lyketsos CG (1985) Hostile personality characteristics, dysthymic states and neurotic symptoms in urticaria, psoriasis and alopecia. Psychother Pschosom 44:122–131
36. Anasagasti JI, Peralta V, Harto A, Chinchilla A, Ledo A (1986) Estudio de la personalidad en pacientes con urticaria chronica. Rev Clin Esp 178:177–180
37. Fava GA, Perini GI, Santonastaso P, Fornasa CV (1980) Life events and dermatological disorders: psoriasis, chronic urticaria and fungal infections. Br Med J 53:277–282
38. Russell-Davis D, Kennard DW (1964) Urticaria. J Psychosom Res 8:203–206
39. Selye H (1956) The stress of life. McGraw Hill, New York
40. Kanner AD, Coyne JC, Schaefer C, Lazarus RS (1981) Comparison of two modes of stress measurement: daily hassles and uplifts versus major life events. J Behav Med 4:1–19
41. Reinhold M (1960) Relationship of stress to the development of symptoms in alopecia areata and chronic urticaria. Br Med J I:846–849
42. Teshima H, Kubo C, Kihara H, Imada Y, Nagata S, Abo Y (1982) Psychosomatic aspects of skin diseases from the standpoint of immunology. Psychother psychosom 37:165–175
43. Whitlock A (1976) Psychophysiologic aspects of skin disease. Saunders, Toronto
44. Shertzer CI, Lookingbill DP (1987) Effects of relaxation therapy and hypnotizability in chronic urticaria. Arch Dermatol 123:913–916
45. Bowers KS, Kelley P (1978) Stress, disease, psychotherapy and hypnosis. J Abnorm Psychol 85:490–505
46. Rudzki E, Borkowski W, Czubalski K (1970) The suggestive effect of placebo on the intensity of chronic urticaria. Acta Allergol 25:70–73
47. Luthe W (ed) (1970) Autogenic therapy, vol 4: Research and therapy. Grune and Stratton, New York
48. Tapp JT (1985) Multisystems interventions in disease. In: Schneiderman N, Tapp JT (eds) Behavioral medicine: the biopsychosocial approach. Erlbaum, New York
49. Moan ER (1979) GSR biofeedback assisted relaxation training and psychosomatic hives. J Behav Ther Exp Psychiatry 10:158–159
50. Daniels LK (1973) Treatment of urticaria and severe headache by behavior therapy. Psychosomatics 14:347–351
51. Ikemi Y, Nakagawa S, Kusano T, Sugita M (1970) The application of autogenic training to "psychological desensitization" of allergic discorders. In: Luthe W (ed) Autogenic therapy, vol 4: Research and therapy. Grune and Stratton, New York
52. Goldfried MR, Davison GC (1976) Clinical behavior therapy. Holt, Rinehart and Winston, New York
53. Rogers CR (1951) Client-centered therapy. Houghton Mifflin, Boston
54. Davanloo H (ed) (1978) Basic principles and techniques in short-term fdynamic psychotherapy. SP Medical and Scientific Books, New York
55. Rechenberger I (1976) Tiefenpsychologisch ausgerichtete Diagnostik and Behandlung von Hautkrankheiten. Vandenhoek and Ruprecht, Göttingen
56. Van Moffaert M (1982) Psychosomatics for the practising dermatologist. Dermatologica 165:73–87
57. Keegan DL (1976) Chronic urticaria: clinical, psychophysiological and therapeutic aspects. Psychosomatics 17:160–163
58. Brodsky CM (1983) "Allergic to everything": a medical subculture. Psychosomatics 24:731–742
59. Pearson DJ (1986) Pseudo food allergy. Br Med J 292:221–222
60. Sanger MD (1970) Psychosomatic allergy. Psychosomatics 11:473–476

16 Gynaecology, Obstetrics and Sexual Function

H. A. Ripman

The female genital tract, so important for the survival of the species, is suitably housed out of sight within the safe confines of the bony pelvis with access only through the vulval introitus, guarded by the powerful adductor muscles of the thighs. It is the object of religious law, ritual and myth, and in Western society is predominantly unseen, untouched and unmentioned. In many families, even today, modesty forbids the exposure of naked little girls to the view of little boys, and quite often the family has no name at all for the vulva, which being unmentionable seems to need none.

It is hardly surprising, therefore, that in the growing female, particularly after puberty when she cannot but be aware of the important functions of and feelings that derive from her pelvic organs, there develop inhibitions, phobias, feelings of guilt and disgust, and other emotions for which the genital tract is often the chosen avenue of expression. No one is more influential, for better or worse, in this respect than the mother by way of example of her attitude to her own physiology, her attitude towards her daughter's physiology and her response to any morbid symptoms that her daughter may develop. Topics relating to genital tract functions, even menstruation, are still distasteful to many people. Discussion of the problem in a relaxed interview, dragging the subject from shameful darkness into the light of unembarrassed conversation, may in itself be recognisably beneficial, while inappropriate levity or embarrassment can bury the matter even deeper. Examination, above all in younger patients, should not be undertaken until a measure of confidence has been established and must be carried out with extreme gentleness and continuing explanation. It is often wise to examine the hands first, possibly holding them a while and passing comment on the unbitten nails or conversely silently noting their bitten nature. If the patient has ascended the examination couch without removing her underwear, it is wise to leave the situation undisturbed until time for examining the genitalia arrives. It may well be that on the first occasion no more than a visual assessment of the state of affairs should be made, leaving digital and invasive examination to a subsequent visit. Anything but extreme gentleness and empathy on the part of the doctor may have serious and long-lasting consequences, particularly in young people. Very rarely, admission as a day case for examination under a general anaesthetic will be considered necessary, and this is preferable by far to a trial of strength between the gynaecologist and a little girl's gluteal and adductor muscles in outpatients.

16.1 Menstrual Disorders

It is difficult to identify those environmental circumstances which induce menorrhagia as opposed to amenorrhoea, and equally difficult to define what particular psychodynamic aberrations are conducive to one response as opposed to the other.

There are no specific personality profiles or underlying psychodynamics that appear to be determinant in this matter. It seems that overall, a gradually developing, repetitive, fluctuating, unresolved stress, often with underlying resentment or anger, is conducive to menorrhagia, whereas a radical change of environment, profound depression or absolute catastrophe leads to amenorrhoea.

16.1.1 Amenorrhoea

Primary amenorrhoea becomes pathological only when the menarche is significantly delayed. Every doctor has met patients in whom the menarche either at a normal age or at a late age followed some conspicuous life event. Such records form, by implication, an enormous volume of anecdotal evidence that a late menarche is frequently psychogenic, but the matter remains far from proven. When a young girl or her family are worried by what they consider to be the delayed onset of menstruation, a general physical examination, including the genital tract, should be carried out, and any abnormal findings should be acted upon. The age at which more profound investigations should be undertaken is variously considered to be anything from 15 to 18, earlier in the absence of normally developed secondary sexual characteristics, later in the presence thereof. If these investigations reveal no organic explanation, then psychogenic causes should certainly be considered. If unacceptable stress or undue vulnerability are uncovered, common humanity dictates that suitable measures should be adopted. When, in due course, menstruation commences (and the earlier the intervention, the more likely this is to follow), whatever management or treatment is currently being pursued will receive the credit, and a further piece of anecdotal evidence, more or less convincing, of psychogenic primary amenorrhoea will be recorded. Any subsequent amenorrhoea is termed secondary amenorrhoea.

A full general history and examination with particular consideration of the possibility of pregnancy is essential. (A pregnancy test is not reliable less than 4 weeks or more than 12 weeks after the last coitus, unless positive.) Symptoms and signs of abnormal thyroid or adrenal status should be sought, together with evidence of metabolic disorder (e.g. diabetes) and weight loss (particularly deliberate and excessive). A blood prolactin assay should be carried out, and if abnormal, pituitary tomography examination. If all the findings are normal, then the patient's oestrogen status may be defined by a 4-day course of norethisterone which, upon cessation, will induce endometrial shedding, if the endometrium is normally primed. This reassuring response will sometimes in itself produce psychotherapeutic benefit and will indicate the presence of ovarian and endometrial potential. Should no withdrawal bleed occur, ovarian failure (the menopausal state) must be excluded by a serum FSH assay. A diagnosis of psychogenic amenorrhoea may thus be suspected by a process of exclusion.

The association between amenorrhoea and major depressive illness is well documented by Fava [1], but in the case of major psychiatric disorder it is the preponderant illness that requires treatment rather than the failure to menstruate. Anti-depressants have the potential of reversing the amenorrhoea in many of these cases, and the resumption of menstruation can have a beneficial effect on the psychiatric illness.

While in general multiple hormone patterns of no special diagnostic or prognostic significance are found, in cases of psychogenic origin, the pathway of influence would appear to be through the hypothalamus, possibly by way of the adrenals [2, 3]. In particular there does seem to be a failure of cyclicity in gonadotrophin secretion. The response to antidepressant drugs by patients suffering from major depression has been mentioned. Fava et al. [4] have pointed out that a syndrome of depression, hostility and anxiety in women with amenorrhoea, frequently with loss of libido and sometimes with galactorrhoea, can be a manifestation of hyperprolactinaemia. The reduction of prolactin levels with bromocriptine in these cases has been found to relieve the depression as well as to induce menstruation.

The psychogenesis in many cases of secondary amenorrhoea is undoubted. Anorexia nervosa and pseudocyesis will not be dealt with here, but suffice it to say that in pseudocyesis the condition is frequently to some degree iatrogenic. The patient either passionately desires or passionately fears a pregnancy, and at some stage, almost always, the belief has been endorsed with professional support. The essential therapy is the establishment of negative conviction by any means, if need be including ultrasound examination, endocrine induction of endometrial shedding (withdrawal bleeding) or even uterine curettage.

Even the most stable, mature and well-balanced personality may, under certain circumstances, respond to stress with amenorrhoea. Such events as internment in concentration camps or prisoner of war camps were almost universally effective in this respect. Women recruited into the forces, entering religious life or a woman's college, or taking up nursing are similarly vulnerable. Incidents such as rape, bereavement, changes of life style or travel are all frequently associated with amenorrhoea. The greater the trauma, the more universal the breakdown, and extreme environmental conditions can induce this disability even in those who do not have social or personal deficits, individual variations being reflected only in the length of time between the trauma and onset, and the duration, of the symptom.

Other patients, however, develop amenorrhoea in the absence of conspicuous stress, intrapsychic vulnerability and unique sensitivity to events being the major determining factors. Rejection of the female role, conflict over pregnancy and motherhood, general repression of sexuality, infantile regression and fear of mutilation have all been considered as significantly psychodynamic, and none, one or several may be relevant in any particular case. It is often far from clear to what extent a woman's denial of her sexuality, as manifest by dislike of menstruation, sexual problems and a negative attitude towards her genital tract, contributes to the onset or the protraction of the symptom.

Therapy depends on the identification on the one hand of the precipitating stresses, and on the other hand of the patient's sensitivity, once the possibilities are realised.

The simple example is that of the wives and sweethearts of men killed in the Normandy battles in 1944. Many of these men posted as missing, believed killed had the opportunity of sleeping with their partners very shortly before proceeding overseas. When the disastrous news was received, amenorrhoea was an extremely common response. Under the circumstances it was not unnatural that the possibility of pregnancy should have been received with very strong emotion, either a great hope or a great fear. This tended to prolong the amenorrhoea at a time when exclusion of that possibility by pregnancy testing was far less easy. In due course, almost all these women returned to their previous menstrual habit.

A more complicated case was that of a 19-year old girl whose mother and father had separated when she was 3. She was brought up surrounded by hate, her mother attempting to induce in her a hatred of her father. In this, to some extent, she succeeded, and at the same time revolted her daughter by her exhibitions of alcoholic and sexual excesses. She complained of amenorrhoea which she thought was the cause of frigidity in her relationship with a 37-year-old man with whom she had fallen in love. On careful analysis it transpired that she had first menstruated at the age of 15 and very rarely each year thereafter, but never when living with her mother. She herself had not recognised this fact, and the possible significance of the disgust she had of her mother and the distrust she had of her father were discussed in some depth. She proceeded to menstruate regularly 4 weeks later despite being domiciled with her mother, but she continued to be liable to episodes of amenorrhoea related to stress, She required a caesarean section 12 years later for the delivery of her first child, her cervix being seemingly unable to dilate in spite of the presence of good pains. By then she was in her third marriage after two divorces, one miscarriage and the termination of an unwanted pregnancy.

Clearly in those cases in which the stresses can be relieved or even mitigated that should be done. Even their definition may be helpful. As regards the patients' psychodynamic conflicts, reassurance, counselling or more formal psychotherapy is indicated.

16.1.2 Menorrhagia

The patient complaining of menorrhagia or heavy periods inevitably presents to the doctor the problem of defining whether they are, in fact, heavy. It is important to exercise this doubt because much anxiety may be endorsed by erroneous assessment. A patient's attitude to her menses is very relevant. To a woman who regards menstruation with profound distrust or disgust, any period is excessive. For the most part a woman defines her periods as heavy largely on one of three grounds: by comparison with her previous menstrual habit, by comparison with her mother's habit, or because they cause social embarrassment or inconvenience. Clearly the first two are widely open to misinterpretation. Fraser et al. [5] showed that there were many major errors of individual perception in this matter, inability to distinguish day-to-day variations in volume, and a poor correlation between the number of pads and tampons used and the measured menstrual loss, with individuals showing extreme variations between blood loss and pad usage. He concluded that reliable assessment could only be obtained by objective measurement of the blood loss. As a research project this is worthwhile, but as a clinical procedure it is usually impracticable. For the most part, therefore, when a patient complains of menorrhagia, even when various features of the case suggest the loss is not unduly heavy, if the patient domestically, socially and athletically is unable to live with it, then she requires help. However, that being said, the foregoing should indicate that a number of patients complaining of menorrhagia need painstaking consideration and reassurance to relieve their anxiety rather than hormones and curettage in an attempt to reduce what is, in fact, a normal loss. In such cases the patient should be persuaded that she is misinterpreting the volume of flow rather than imagining or exaggerating it. Discussion and explanation, and on occasion practical advice concerning hygienic measures, if successful, should enable the patient to live with her habit. There will, however, inevitably be patients in whom a normal menstrual flow remains unacceptable and they will sometimes proceed through a succession of medical advisers, by way of hormone therapy, to dilatation and curettage and hysterectomy.

Nonetheless a diagnosis of menorrhagia may be perfectly valid and the loss truly excessive, while the cause is emotional. Blaikley [6] recorded eight instances of psychogenic menorrhagia.

Amongst them was a patient whose husband was a sexual pervert and whose menorrhagia was cured by a separation order; a patient who was married to a violent husband, who derived considerable improvement from separation and complete relief from divorce; a patient whose husband made excessive and occasionally abnormal sensual demands upon her, and to whom sexual relations had become repulsive. The family doctor took the matter up with the husband, and the patient's periods became normal. The husband subsequently reverted to his former habits including physical violence, and the patient's periods reverted to a lengthy loss and a short cycle.

While it had previously been recognised that emotional situations produced a single heavy period, it had not been appreciated that long continued menorrhagia could be entirely psychogenic. Many of the cases were normal women subjected to excessive emotional strain, and there was frequently a delay of 6–12 months from the onset of the strain before the menorrhagia developed. Blaikley attributed the heavy loss to vasodilatation and endometrial hyperaemia. If the cycle was shortened, he considered it likely that cerebral influences were affecting the hypothalamus which in turn controlled the pituitary. He quoted Fremont-Smith as describing a patient who bled almost continuously for 9 months, was subjected ineffectively to endocrine therapy and curettage, but whose bleeding ceased after a 3 h discussion with a psychiatrist and whose periods remained normal thereafter for 5 years.

In general the proof of an emotional origin for menorrhagia lies in the recovery that takes place when the emotional state returns to one of tranquillity. It was his experience (and mine) that menorrhagia is associated with an anxious, agitated state, whereas amenorrhoea is a response to depression and defeat. Stott [7], in a retrospective study, found that patients with menorrhagia were more likely to have had anti-depressant medication prescribed for them at some time previously than the patients in the control group. Elsewhere [8] he quotes Ballinger [9] as finding psychiatric morbidity higher than the norm in gynaecological outpatients, particularly high in patients complaining of menorrhagia and higher still in those selected for hysterectomy. Gath [10] stressed the particularly high levels of psychiatric morbidity in patients selected for hysterectomy because of menorrhagia.

It is not uncommon within the family circle for the mother's menstrual performance to constitute a monthly crisis, and at that stage in each month for the mother to be the centre of attention, sympathy and support. When finally the family persuade her to seek relief from her problem, and in due course a hysterectomy is performed, she may find herself postoperatively in a worse situation than she enjoyed before. There is no monthly crisis, no monthly sympathy and no monthly support.

Such a patient may lean on the aftereffects of "the operation" (as a substitute for menstruation) for months, years or on occasions a lifetime.

As has been indicated above, in a number of cases such an unhappy outcome can be avoided by painstaking exploration of the patient's history, environment and emotional state, suitable manipulation of the state of affairs and if need be psychotherapy.

Gath et al. [11] found that hysterectomy seldom led to psychiatric disorder, and indeed there was some evidence to suggest that the operation on occasion might alleviate pre-existing psychiatric disorder. Martin et al. [12, 13] found that almost all patients receiving psychiatric treatment after hysterectomy had received similar treatment before the operation. However, half the patients with prehysterectomy psychiatric disorder were found to be psychiatrically well after the operation. It was tentatively suggested (and my experience would support this) that those pre-operatively suffering from psychological illness and who have genuinely heavy periods, may receive from the operation some psychiatric benefit, while those whose periods are to the best of one's judgement not excessive would profit from psychotherapy rather than hysterectomy. These latter may be considered primary psychiatric menorrhagias, whereas the former are secondarily psychiatric menorrhagias. From this may be seen the importance of, at the least, attempting to define whether the menorrhagia is real or imagined.

16.1.3 Dysmenorrhoea

Painful menstruation is usually classified as primary (an inherent dysfunction of the uterus) or secondary (consequent upon some pelvic pathology).

16.1.3.1 Primary Dysmenorrhoea

The pain typically commences with or just before the flow is at its worst on the first day, then steadily eases. From the menarche the girl is usually pain-free, but within months or a few years, the dysmenorrhoea develops, becoming steadily worse over ensuing cycles. At least 50% of teenage girls have some uterine pain and 5% to 10% by their early twenties are incapacitated for several hours each month. The freedom from pain enjoyed in the initial cycles results from their anovular nature. The pain derives from muscular ischaemia due to excessive uterine contraction, and in severe cases is accompanied by contraction of smooth muscle elsewhere: in the vasculature, causing intense palor and sometimes fainting; in the stomach, causing nausea and vomiting; and in the large bowel, causing looseness of the stools. The condition is greatly, often completely, relieved by pregnancy, and even a first trimester miscarriage may confer benefit.

The aetiology of the severe cramping has in the past been attributed to a narrow cervical canal, to uterine malformation and immaturity, to retroversion, to hormone influences and to constipation. Currently it is regarded as a response to excessive prostaglandin production. Certainly the pain is not imagined. Most clinical gynaecologists have been under the impression, and very many have held the conviction, that the patient's personality and attitude to the pain could exacerbate to an unacceptable degree a discomfort which to the majority of women was a tolerable, biological phenomenon. The maternal influence appeared significant. A child brought up in a household in which menstrual days were black days had only a small chance of escaping that influence, and when her own periods commenced and some discomfort developed, apprehension led to tension, excessive contraction and pain. Severe dysmenorrhoea was apparently more common in migrainous, perfectionist, obsessional women, those liable to colon spasm, and in dark, hirsuit, slightly android women. When it occurred in the fairer, more feminine types, it seemed that the immature and parent dependent were over-represented.

Such has been the general opinion amongst practising gynaecologists, and while some research into the psychosomatic aspects of dysmenorrhoea, the extent to which it is personality determined and stress related, has supported these views, other research workers have found them unsupportable.

Amos and Khanna [14] found that recent life stress could increase the severity of spasmodic and congestive dysmenorrhoea, particularly the former. They did not investigate the effects of long-term stress.

Lundstrom and af Geijerstam [15] considered the disappointment of menstruation in the infertile patient to be an aggravating factor, and that the physical and social benefit of dysmenorrhoea (by way of justifying absence and attracting sympathy) should not be forgotten.

Lawlor and Davis [16], while discovering that one-third of adolescent girls did not know whether their mothers had dysmenorrhoea, found that of those who did know, 84% of dysmenorrhoeic girls had dysmenorrhoeic mothers, in contrast with 50% of girls with painless periods. Jay and Durant [17] quote Wood as finding dysmenorrhoea in 30% of the daughters of dysmenorrhoeic mothers, and in only 7% of the daughters of those with painless periods. Woods and Launius [18] found dysmenorrhoea to be significantly more common in more masculine types.

On the other hand Lawlor and Davis [6], concluding a comprehensive study of the relationship of primary dysmenorrhoea to personality and attitudes in adolescent females, commented:

> A certain percentage of teenage females probably do experience psychosomatic dysmenorrhoea just as a certain percentage of all teenagers experience various other types of psychosomatic pain. However, our results do not support the view so often found in the literature that psychogenesis is the probable cause of primary dysmenorrhoea because these girls have certain negative personality traits. ... the practitioner should provide reassurance for the normal teenager that her pain is neither contrived nor evidence of an inherent personality problem.

Iacono and Roberts [19], in a study of 31 women with severe dysmenorrhoea matched against 31 women with painless periods, found that "no dysmenorrhoeic personality as such can be demonstrated." Undoubtedly, recent research, making much use of statistics and attributing previous contradictory findings to faulty methodology, is coming to the overall conclusion that spasmodic dysmenorrhoea is an organic and not a psychosomatic complaint.

Management entails in the first place the exclusion of any underlying pathology, in order to establish the diagnosis. Thereafter, the use of analgesics, the induction of anovular cycles (usually with the contraceptive pill) or the prescription of prostaglandin inhibitors will render menstruation better than tolerable for the vast majority. It would be surprising if a bad pain, deeply seated, out of sight and impalpable, to be expected and experienced at regular monthly intervals, was not at least to some degree made worse by apprehension. All pain is aggravated by stress and tension, and certainly some people are more susceptible to suggestion than others. As Lundstrom [15] puts it, "psychological factors should always be kept in mind." As Lawlor [16] states, "management should include ... the acknowledgement of the normal emotional reactions accompanying any pain, and the correction of any misinformation that the patient may have received." Jay [17] comments "while psychologic factors may not be primary causes of primary dysmenorrhoea, various emotional traumas common to adolescence may sometimes aggravate menstrual discomfort."

Discussion, reassurance and efforts to procure a relaxed state of mind and body undoubtedly have a place. In favour of this, moderate physical exercise and a diet leading to regular bowel function are beneficial as, for some, are lessons in relaxation. The confidence induced by a few painless periods, the result of medication, can furthermore be beneficial in the long term particularly when supported by the assurance that repeat medication is available if needed.

16.1.3.2 Secondary Dysmenorrhoea

This is commonly felt a day or two before the onset of menstruation. It is not cramplike in nature but usually described as a severe protracted deep pelvic ache. It may be worsened by micturition and particularly by defaecation. Its cause may be diagnosed by clinical examination and if need be, laparoscopy. Its treatment is that of the primary pathology.

The presence of some abnormal pelvic finding does not necessarily indicate that the dysmenorrhoea is a consequence thereof. Modest islands of endometriosis are extremely commonly found and may well be irrelevant. Severe congestive premenstrual dysmenorrhoea, sometimes associated with menorrhagia, sometimes with dyspareunia, is not infrequently the result of sexual problems particularly anorgasmic coital experiences and sexual fantasies. Painstaking enquiry, explanation and sexual counselling are indicated and can prove extremely helpful.

16.2 Vaginal Discharge

Soon after birth a baby may exhibit responses to the stimulus of transplacentally acquired hormones such as a clear, mucoid, vaginal discharge, sometimes bloody, breast enlargement and sometimes secretion. Parental anxiety is commonly the most serious feature, and explanation and reassurance that resolution will occur spontaneously without treatment are all that is needed. Thereafter until puberty the vagina is unstimulated by oestrogen and vulnerable to infection, commonly with mixed organisms of low virulence. From puberty to the menopause the fluor of cervical mucus varies in nature and volume through the menstrual cycle and in response to erotic stimulation. At the menopause, oestrogen deprivation again renders the patient liable to bacterial vaginitis.

In the case of children it is necessary in the first instant to determine whether a significant vaginal discharge exists, and if so, its volume, nature and particularly whether it is blood-stained. Many mothers will present daughters with complaints of discharge where nothing more morbid exists than the mother's maladjustment to sexuality – her own, her daughter's or both. Inspection of the vulva and underwear may be unrewarding, it commonly being the case that the child is presented recently bathed and dressed in clean clothing. A second visit with instructions to attend with the child unbathed (since the night before) and wearing white underwear (unchanged since getting out of bed in the morning) will produce the necessary evidence.

A specimen of any discharge can usually be collected either with a platinum loop, a pipette or a swab, and such specific therapeutic measures as indicated by the findings can be undertaken. Sometimes the discharge is insignificant (it takes very little discharge to produce a great deal of worry in mothers of some children and indeed to become the focus of attention of a whole family). Often it is the vulval soreness (complained of as a "stinging" when the child enters the bath) that is the true problem. The standard of perianal hygiene may be relevant. Questioning may reveal that antiseptic solutions are being used in the bathwater, which commonly makes matters worse. Careful drying is important after bathing and the avoidance of hot, thick occlusive underwear or nylon tights.

When the discharge is blood-stained it will usually be necessary to perform an examination under anaesthetic; very rarely, a sarcoma botrioides may be found but much more commonly a foreign body. The removal of the foreign body with the introduction of a little oestrogen cream to encourage healing will relieve the symptoms. Unfortunately, there may be long-term consequences. It is of consummate importance that what the child has done should be allowed no greater significance than an indication of the healthy child's natural inquisitiveness. All too often it is interpreted by the family as having connotations of indecency, immorality, etc. and the family attitude of horror and disgust may induce a long-lasting sense of shame and guilt in the young child.

16.2.1 Teenage Discharge

In their late teens girls may present complaining of excessive vaginal discharge. When they are examined, no more than a free flow of healthy mucus is found. It can cause them great anxiety and offence and justifies very careful consideration. Frequently, the girl has started courting and may have indulged in love-play, or indeed, sexual intercourse. The erotic stimulation induces a physiological secretion of cervical mucus considerably in excess of anything that she has experienced before. This, in turn, induces firstly a morbid fear that the "sinful" activities in which she has indulged have led to a venereal infection, and secondly the embarrassing belief that the mucoid wetness in the region of her external genitals will prove offensive when explored and discovered by her consort. It is often necessary to arrange for the patient to have ready access to a gynaecologist in order to show him or her the condition in its most florid state. No reassurance will be effective if the patient leaves the consultation feeling that she has been examined on a good day, and thus the real merits of her case have not been considered. After examination, including a swab if necessary, if all is found to be normal, a comprehensive explanation of the nature and innocence of the condition is usually all that is needed. We have seen women in whom the mucoid secretion was so profuse that it stained through to the outer clothes, producing an observable damp patch. A nurse employed her best friend always to walk out of the classroom behind her when in midcycle, so that the others should not see a patch on her skirt. In such cases it is justifiable by diathermy cautery to the cervical canal to diminish the secretion. It should be stressed, however, that this is very rarely necessary, and if carried out when the discharge is excessive only in the patient's opinion, the cautery may, in due course, render the vagina unsatisfactorily dry for coital purposes.

16.2.2 Leucorrhoea

During the menstrual and childbearing years vaginal discharge may result from vaginal infections, cervical secretions or pathology in the uterus and above. Vaginitis may result from bacterial infection of neglected tampons or residual pieces of tampon, or from infection with *Trichomonas vaginalis, Candida albicans* and other sexually transmitted agents. The cervix may be the site of polypi or carcinoma. Discharge from within the uterus and above is often blood-stained and offensive, and results predominantly from retained products of conception, but less often from a variety of other pathologies that will not be dealt with here.

The secretions of the cervical mucus glands, when excessive, constitute the condition of leucorrhoea. Changes in its nature and volume through the menstrual cycle are normal, but even such normality may be the cause of complaint and disgust on the part of the patient. The use of tampons to control the flow is to be discouraged. The patient should learn to accept the state of affairs as being physiological; its biological implications should be explained and reassurance thereby afforded. Opportunity should be given for the expression of any fears or guilt feelings, which are not uncommonly present. When the mucoid discharge is excessive, it favours the growth of columnar epithelium over the portio vaginalis giving the area around the external cervical os a red appearance. This is a cervical erosion. It is a most unfortunate name which has caused much unnecessary worry to patients and doctors alike. It is frequently regarded as the cause of the discharge, which is not the case; it is the result of the discharge. It rarely produces symptoms although occasionally, when traumatised during coitus, some modest bleeding may occur.

It is not clearly understood why the mucus secretion from the cervix is sometimes excessive. Sometimes it appears to be in response to oestrogens, as in pregnancy or from the contraceptive pill. Sometimes there is an infectious element, usually very superficial and of low virulence. In these cases the discharge has a yellow purulent appearance. There is no doubt, however, that quite frequently excessive mucoid discharge, particularly when associated with cervical tenderness, premenstrual pelvic pain and sometimes menorrhagia, is the result of pelvic congestion consequent upon unresolved erotic stimulation. This stimulation may be produced by fantasy or by factual sexual contact.

A patient from a rigidly Presbyterian background was engaged to the only son of a widow who suffered a lengthy, predominantly neurotic, chronic illness. The widow was very possessive of her son, and his fiancée was not made welcome in the house. Their courtship was carried out mostly in cinema seats and parked cars. The woman complained of excessive mucoid discharge, giving her a sore vulva. She had acquired temporary relief when a gynaecologist had cauterised the cervical canal, but the trouble had returned. She suffered considerable premenstrual pelvic pain, and her periods were heavy, though not incapacitating. She had never had intercourse, so she did not know whether she had dyspareunia. She was advised that when she got married and led a full, uninhibited sexual life, her symptoms would resolve. In due course her fiancé broke loose from his dominating mother, and the couple were able to marry. There were some initial coital difficulties, including deep dyspareunia, but the woman accepted explanation and reassurance, and before long the dyspareunia and the leucorrhoea disappeared.

Weiss and English [20] described a patient who, as a result of intense repressed hostility, suffered severe colicky diarrhoea and leucorrhoea. Both these symptoms were relieved by intensive psychiatric treatment and readjustment of the personality. They interpreted the leucorrhoea, like the diarrhoea, as the "production from the body of something unpleasant, one purpose of which was to vent repressed ill feelings upon the environment" (p 576).

There is no doubt that in the absence of significant pathology, a careful psychosexual history is indicated in patients complaining of excessive mucoid vaginal discharge.

16.3 Irritable Colon, Colon Spasm, Spastic Colon

No consideration of psychosomatic gynaecological complaints would be complete without attention to the confusion caused by, and the misdiagnoses resulting from, colon spasm. The psychodynamics and aetiology of this condition are dealt with elsewhere in this book; suffice it here to define the many faces that it presents to the gynaecologist.

1. Pain in the right iliac fossa. Doctors have become wiser regarding the diagnosis of grumbling appendix, but there are still many innocent vermiform appendices removed. Too often at such an operation, in search of pathology, the inexperienced surgeon will remove a cyst from the right ovary. Such cysts are most commonly simple retention cysts of absolutely no morbid significance, and very rarely the cause of the pain from which relief is sought. The removal of such a small innocent lesion may, however, institute a protracted anxiety about the state of her ovaries. Pain in the caecum is less common in colon spasm than pain in the sigmoid colon. On palpation of the right iliac fossa an ill-definded mass that gurgles may be felt, and a similar gurgling or squelching sensation may be recognised in the right posterior quadrant of the pelvis on bimanual examination, the patient identifying this as the site of her pain. Right adnexal inflammatory disease may be misdiagnosed.

2. Pain in the hypogastrium and left iliac fossa. A spastic sigmoid colon may mimic salpingitis, ectopic pregnancy or ovarian cyst. On palpation a firm, tender, sausage-like mass will usually be felt in the left iliac fossa. The patient may, in the morning upon rising, when her bladder and rectum are full, be aware of and able to palpate it

herself. Not infrequently bimanual examination will enable the tender bowel to be followed in continuity from the upper rectum, past the pelvirectal junction, over the left adnexae, into the left iliac fossa. It can be exquisitely tender, far more so than the caecum in the pain previously described.

3. Dyspareunia. The pain resulting from colon spasm during intercourse is most commonly felt in the midline behind the uterus, but it may be felt to the left of the midline in the region of the adnexae. It may take protracted gentle and painstaking examination, and much co-operation from the patient, for the condition to be differentiated from an ovarian tumour in the pouch of Douglas, a hydrosalpinx, a sterile pyosalpinx or an ectopic pregnancy.

4. Pelvic pain. Colon spasm is a potent cause of pain deep in the pouch of Douglas. Sometimes it derives from the pelvirectal junction, sometimes from a loop of sigmoid prolapsed between the uterus and rectum. It is generally a protracted nagging pain with acute exacerbations, which are not unlike proctalgia fugax. If directly asked, the patient will often confirm that acute shooting pain is felt deep in the pelvis when she sits down smartly with both buttocks on a firm surface. (However, this sign may be found with any inflammatory lesion in the pouch of Douglas, e.g. ectopic pregnancy, endometriosis, infectious disease of the adnexac.)

5. Endometriosis. The inconsistent disparity between the symptoms induced by endometriosis and the extent of the pathology found on clinical examination or at laparotomy has long been recognised. Furthermore, small areas of endometriosis, apparently asymptomatic, are extremely commonly seen in patients undergoing laparotomy for fibroids, ovarian cysts, sterilisation, etc. Recently, inspection of the pelvis by laparoscopy has tended to become an almost routine part of any gynaecological examination in patients with pelvic pain. Small areas of endometriosis are consequently being very commonly found to which the pain is erroneously attributed, and to this protracted therapy is directed. In such cases colon spasm must be seriously considered as an alternative diagnosis.

6. Dysmenorrhoea. Many patients with colon spasm complain of cyclical exacerbation in thc prcmcnstrual phasc, and in consequence of its menstrual association, the pain may be considered as dysmenorrhoea. In some this appears to be related to increased irritability and tension, in others to a change in bowel function. Very many women experience some change in bowel habit in relation to the menses, most commonly a tendency towards premenstrual constipation and menstrual looseness. Jeffcoate [21] regarded unilateral dysmenorrhoea as deriving from colon spasm rather than the genitalia.

In the conditions described above there is both a need to exclude organic pathology and a need to take a positive attitude towards the diagnosis of colon spasm. Sometimes sigmoidoscopy will be necessary, less often a barium enema, and laparoscopy may be needed to provide the final conviction of the absence of organic disease. Jeffcoate's comment is worth quoting.

> To say that pelvic pain has no organic basis does not mean that the pain is imagined; the pain is real, but it is caused by a functional disorder of the genital or

extragenital organs, and more often the latter. Treatment of such a disorder calls not for surgery but for sympathetic analysis and understanding of the woman and her environmental problems.

16.4 Infertility

Conception is a random affair, successful only when a large number of influences are favourable at the same time. Advances in recent years have defined an increasing number of infertility factors. There remain, none-the-less, some childless marriages (variously assessed at anything from 5%–18%) in which no fault is found or explanation forthcoming. Such couples are frequently described as functionally infertile. If the investigations are carried out and unexplained infertility diagnosed early enough, 50% of these couples will have conceived within 3 years as Templeton and Penny [22] indicated. It is not uncommon for as many as 7% of patients attending an infertility clinic to be found pregnant at their first visit. With such a chance phenomenon it is inevitable that the occurrence of a pregnancy is occasionally attributed to the last measure taken in the pursuit of its achievement. Such anecdotal attributions when analysed often prove unjustified. Sandler [23] recorded a number of influences favourable to conception, i.e. making an appointment, having semen analysed, undergoing vaginal examination, accepting reassurance and applying for adoption. "The only common factor in all these antecedent events," he declared, "is the relief of tension." This, of course, is not so. There is another factor, namely, the passage of time. Almost everyone knows of some couple considered infertile who achieved pregnancy soon after adoption. Sandler [24] studied the matter and concluded that "adoption facilitates conception in those cases in which organic factors have been adequately treated and there is continuing emotional tension." The significance of the last half of this sentence must be stressed, for Mai [25], reviewing the literature on this topic, concluded that while it might not be a fact, it had not yet been proven a myth. Arronet et al. [26] analysing 534 infertile couples of which 133 adopted a child, concluded that the therapeutic value of adoption was speculative and without proof, and Lamb and Leurgans [27] studied 895 couples of whom 128 adopted a child and found that this did "not support the hypothesis that adoption affects subsequent fertility". If in fact it does, it would seem likely that it operates only in cases with a very particular psychotherapeutic requirement.

However, psychological influences are undoubtedly relevant, above all the coital aspect. (Psychosexual problems are discussed elsewhere in this chapter.) Intercourse may be too infrequent (or indeed too frequent), mistimed, incomplete or a total failure by reason of vaginismus or impotence, or may be followed by obsessional cleansings and douchings. It is not very uncommon to meet a couple complaining of infertility who apparently unknowingly have failed to perform the coital act and in whom the woman is still a virgin, sometimes very many years after marriage. The importance of taking a meticulous coital history from both the wife and the husband cannot be overestimated, and the disparity in the two stories provided may be both astonishing and revealing. An alert ear may pick up various nuances that indicate a degree of ambivalence in the desire for pregnancy. This is well illustrated by Sandler [23]. A suggestion of ambivalence may also be gathered from the woman's inability to record her menstrual dates or her morning temperatures or to keep her clinic appointments.

Many clinics decline to investigate infertile marriages of less than two years' duration, which is probably wise in view of the number of couples who conceive without intervention during the course of that time. A distinction should be drawn, however, between investigation and counselling. At no stage is it too early to take a careful history and make a thorough clinical examination, including the genitalia of both partners. Much anxiety and stress can thereby be allayed and much comfort afforded. The highly organised professional wife of today, having regulated her fertility by efficient contraception until an age when it is beginning to decline, can become very frustrated and angry with much loss of self esteem following her failure to achieve immediate conception when she wishes it. A full appraisal of her normality and expectations can be very beneficial to the happiness of her marriage, and all that follows therefrom.

When investigations are necessary they must be carried out with tact and sensitivity. Not only may they induce organic infertility by trauma and the introduction of infection, but through too obsessive and protracted temperature recording, mucus inspection, date watching and other analyses may translate the double bed into a laboratory bench, the act of making love into a process of "going in for a baby" and cause the occasions for coitus to become defined by the thermometer rather than the emotions. Furthermore, it is not uncommon for coitus to be confined to the wrong rather than to the appropriate day.

Ovarian function is regulated by the pituitary gland, controlled by the hypothalamus, which is influenced by the cerebral cortex. It was pointed out earlier in this chapter that anovulation and amenorrhoea may be of psychosomatic origin, the extreme examples being pseudocyesis and anorexia nervosa. Lachelin and Yen [2], in a very full investigation of 11 patients with amenorrhoea, found evidence of substantial follicular growth and activity, the functional defect being attributable to acyclic gonadotrophin release, resulting in failure of follicular maturation and ovulation. Psychogenic factors were identified, and reversal of the amenorrhoea followed after appropriate counselling.

Similarly influenced may be the unique changes of cervical mucus during the menstrual cycle, also under pituitary ovarian control. It is only in recent years that the importance of the mucus factor has been recognised, initially in respect of its physical properties but latterly also of its production of sperm antibodies [28]. The relation between psychological factors and immunity is described in Chap. 10, and fertility may also be affected. The inconsistency of tests for Fallopian tube patency have long been recognised. Generally the conclusion has been drawn that this is due to spasm. Considering the influence of stress on the function of plain muscle throughout the body, it would be surprising if the tubes were not similarly responsive. Stalworthy [29] pointed out 40 years ago that tubal spasm could be emotional in origin. Sandler [23] described a very evident case of tubal spasm, reasonably presumed to be due to stress and responsive to medication.

Nonetheless, as Humphrey [30] warns, to attribute childlessness to psychological causes needs more than a process of exclusion, and strong positive indications should be evident; techniques for investigating infertility are still being developed which may ultimately reveal pathology. Edelmann and Connolly [31], in an excellent survey of the entire subject particularly stressing the importance of defining psychosomatic causes from consequences, state:

> As biomedical knowledge increases, it is possible that an anatomical neuroendo-crinological or pathophysiological cause may eventually be found for all cases of infertility. However ... this would not rule out the possibility that a psychosomatic mechanism operates to mediate infertility in some cases.

16.4.1 Fertility Drugs and Fertilisation Techniques: Psychological Hazards

Because medical treatment can defeat a woman's (or a man's) unconscious psychosomatically mediated resistances to conception and parenthood, it is not surprising that reports [32, 33] are appearing of some harmful consequences. These include breakdown of marriages and syndrome shifts to other psychosomatic manifestations or to psychoneuroses or psychoses. However, it is often the children who are the main casualties, being either rejected, manipulated or indulged. The apt term *messiah* or *miracle children* has been applied to them [32].

These unfortunate occurrences start from a failure to recognise, investigate and diagnose psychosomatically based infertility *before* embarking on any of the type of interventions mentioned. Clearly, the first diagnostic requirement is a psychosomatically orientated history from both spouses but with special attention to the manner in which they present their plea, to the parent's attitudes to the children and to each other, whether their mothers had poor obstetric experiences or had suffered nervous illnesses, to their own attitudes to siblings, to their degree of emotional maturity [23] and independence, and so on.

Brahler has recommended a period of delay of 6 months before a final decision is reached. This seems sensible, and the time should be used by a psychodynamically orientated doctor or therapist to try to bring into consciousness any unconscious feelings the potential parents may have about pregnancy and parenthood. This was summed up by Sandler [23]: "We must beware of forcing these patients into a role for which they are unprepared."

16.5 Pregnancy and Labour

It would be surprising if the prospect of the experiences of pregnancy and labour, being of such magnitude, did not exercise considerable psychosomatic influences on the patient. She will never be the same again, nor will the relationship with her mother or her husband, her anatomy or her appearance. The very need to attend antenatal clinics will impress upon her that her course is fraught with hazards. Regarding labour she must wonder how so large a thing can come through so small a hole without inevitable pain and suffering, being cut open or torn, split apart and bleeding, possibly even dying. As men speak of their experiences at war, so she will have heard women speak of their labours. Those that have proceeded normally will have little to say; those to whom the bizarre has occurred, will speak endlessly. There may be fears of a deformed baby, the demands of motherhood, that their body will never recover, and that their sexual apparatus will be forever damaged. To see her through these stresses she needs stability in her life situation, the security of emotional support from her consort and a clear view of her nesting arrangements, not only as regards labour, but very particularly the home to which she will take her baby. These needs are paramount.

In recent years the agonies and hazards of pregnancy and childbirth have been significantly reduced with a consequent improvement in the reputation of both. The attitude of mind engendered by the concept of natural childbirth, the teaching of the National Childbirth Trust, etc. have enabled many women to proceed with enhanced equanimity, and as more find their childbearing an acceptable and rewarding experience, so they will preach with favourable influences to the next generation. It is true that in instances in which the labour has turned out to be not quite so natural, patients are at risk of a sense of failure. While the accoucheur should avoid giving the impression that a patient has had a hard and difficult labour, the mother should be encouraged to feel a sense of achievement, and triumph over such problems as did arise. It would be a pity if this progress towards the physiological were to be interrupted by universal expectation of an epidural anaesthetic as an essential prerequisite of acceptable childbearing and a caesarean section as an easy alternative. On the other hand, when used as necessary, such procedures are not only a blessing to the patient in question, but also to the generation next in line who will be spared lurid details of protracted and agonising labour.

16.5.1 Hyperemesis Gravidarum

Morning sickness is often regarded as a normal and inevitable concomicant of early pregnancy. It has become less common, and considerably less frequently serious, in the past 40 years, and one suspects that this is in part consequent upon the changed attitudes of women towards pregnancy, namely, that it is a physiological state and not an illness and now carries a much less significant degree of mortal hazard.

Many pregnant women have an exaggerated gagging reflex and find it difficult, for example, to clean their back teeth or even to wear their false teeth without retching. Nausea is also common in pregnancy, and worsened by fatigue, hunger and hypoglycaemia. Prophylaxis includes avoiding long intervals between meals and six o'clock exhaustion. There is no doubt a hormonal influence exemplified by the increased incidence and severity of pregnancy sickness in patients carrying twins or a hydatidiform mole. However, hyperemesis (which might be regarded as morning sickness developed to an exceptional degree) has undoubtedly a considerable psychosomatic content. Certain features in these patients are outstanding.

1. They appear to take a pride in their vomiting, meticulously recording the frequency and accounting the smallest emit as vomit.
2. They exhibit a determined reluctance to accept management or therapy. The patient under observation in hospital will claim to have vomited several times in the lavatory unwitnessed by the ward sister. When confined to her room the patient will claim to have vomited in the wash basin, again, unwitnessed. When confined to her bed, her vomit bowl may show nothing more than a few millilitres

of saliva and mucus. When instructed to eat, she will fail to do so and will fail to take glucose medication left by the bedside.

3. They will often concentrate their vomiting activities to the time that their husbands are available as witnesses.

The following is an example, in which the obstetrician is arranging by telephone a patient's admission to hospital:

Husband: I am afraid my wife is behaving exactly as she did in the last pregnancy, and being very sick.

D: I am sorry. How many times a day?

H: Oh, four or five, I should think.

P: (calling from upstairs in bed) No, 11 times, tell him 11 times.

And later, in hospital the husband, having been told by the Sister that it would be best for him not to visit until the vomiting had ceased, which would be soon, took offence at what he considered a punitive attitude. The obstetrician, on explaining that it was generally accepted that the presence of husbands had a detrimental effect on therapeutic success, after a lot of thought and a long silence, exclaimed,

H: By Jove, your're right, it had never struck me. She is only sick before I go out in the morning and when I get home in the evening.

The condition would seem to be one in which nausea leads to vomiting, and in some women, largely because of their failure to take food, ketosis develops. This aggravates the tendency to vomit, and if the process is not arrested, a vicious circle develops, which, if unrelieved, can lead to cardiac, hepatic or renal failure, and indeed, death.

Not all women claiming to be hyperemetic are, in fact, as ill as they would have the doctor believe. Some, and these cases are not confined to the first trimester and are sometimes referred to as hysterical vomiters, will claim to have eaten and drunk nothing for the past week or two; they do not look ill, their pulse and blood pressure are normal, and they do not have concentrated urine or constipated stools. Their story is manifestly untrue, but it is unshakable. Their urine should be tested for ketones. If there are no ketones they may be reassured and observed as outpatients. If ketones are present they should be admitted to hospital. Patients with hyperemesis may be treated as outpatients for as long as there is no ketosis, but frequent observation is necessary. They should be encouraged to take small items of a high calorie diet at frequent intervals. As always in early pregnancy, medication should, if possible, be avoided. If ketonuria develops, the patients should unquestionably be admitted to hospital. These patients are extremely difficult to treat at home. The pressure must be intense and the confidence in a favourable outcome to simple nutritional measures absolute. She is encouraged to take a high calorie, light diet in the first instance. If unable or unwilling to do that, she should take glucose in powder form and in liquid form half-hourly. If she fails to do this the nurses must, every time they pass the patient, give her a glass or spoonful of glucose. If this fails to clear the ketosis, then calories must be provided by intravenous glucose. This will always clear the ketosis, and thereafter the patient can advance step by step through glucose by mouth, to a light diet and to a full diet. These patients need to be treated with a very firm hand. Some do better in a single room, others in the company of other patients. They are best spoken to from the foot of the bed rather than the bedside. Failure to obey therapeutic instructions should be treated as undisciplined rather than understandable, with a straight face or a frown, rather than a smile and a squeezed hand. Confinement to bed is usually advisable. It reduces vomiting opportunities and unwitnessed records of vomiting. The granting of desirable privileges, such as visitors, radio, television, being allowed out of bed and leaving the room, as rewards for food retention can modify behaviour [34]. The patient should not be allowed out of hospital until a full diet is being taken. On discharge it should be pointed out that since they started eating normally they have not vomited, and if vomiting returns and they need to be re-admitted, it would be a clear indication that they have not been eating properly. Some of these patients will be admitted a second time, and even a third time. On each occasion the folly of their ways will be pointed out, they will be treated as before and discharged with the same advice.

Mrs. S. was admitted with hyperemesis, treated by the regime outlined above (including intravenous glucose), cured and sent home. She was re-admitted 72 h later, again treated in the same fashion, and on this occasion discharged to a convalescent home where her condition remained satisfactory. When home her hyperemesis returned. She was re-admitted. Once more she was treated routinely, and on this occasion was discharged to a convalescent home near where she lived. She was allowed to pay visits to her own home, which induced one or two minor vomits, but in due course she lived the rest of her pregnancy at home without sickness.

Opinion is none the less very divided regarding the importance of psychosomatic influences in hyperemesis gravidarum. Fairweather [35] found a high incidence of hysterical infantile and immature personalities and strong maternal dependence. Katon et al. [36], in a comprehensive review of the literature, similarly found a preponderance of immature personality and strong maternal dependence. The condition is now less commonly regarded as a manifestation of conscious rejection of the pregnancy. It is not common in women seeking abortion [37] or in unmarried mothers. Chertok et al. [38], studying 67 vomiters (none of them truly hyperemetic, however) amongst 100 primagravidae, found substantial ambivalence of attitude towards the child and referred to Deutsch's view that the woman who vomits has chosen to do so rather than to miscarry. By many it is considered as a consequence of anxiety, common factors being: (a) insecurity induced by the transition from being dependent (on the mother) to being dependable (to the child); (b) difficulty in coping with the concept of pregnancy and labour in general; (c) insufficient attention and reassurance from the husband; and (d) a conviction that vomiting through pregnancy is inevitable [39–41]. Weiss and English [42] state: "to regard vomiting in pregnancy as a physical ailment and to neglect it as a problem in behaviour is to fail to do justice to the patient" (p. 185). Priest [43] recommends that the ward staff be helped to understand the patient's distress and encourage sympathetic management. "The psychiatrist," he states "has little to offer in the management of this condition." (p 99). The immediacy of the illness makes that so. Urgent organic measures need to be taken. Some authors claim that sympathy and a warm relationship are an integral part of this therapy. We feel that a disciplinary attitude and a firm hand are essential. The stern, dominating midwife of yesterday was more successful with these patients than is her much gentler, sympathetic sister of today. It could be that the conviction with which the therapy is offered is the critical factor.

16.5.2 Premature Labour

There is a wealth of anecdote to support the concept that premature labour may be induced by acute mental stress, and many early onset labours have been attributed to psychological wear and tear or chronic stress. Newton et al. [44] set out to define to what extent psychological stress did in fact determine the onset of premature labour. Using a life events inventory modified for pregnant women, they found that those pregnancies resulting in premature labour were far more likely to have been stressful than those going to term, which was particularly striking because in the shortened pregnancy fewer major life events would have been expected. Such influences as age, gravidity, parity and social class were excluded. In 8 of the 30 women in the pre-term group, and in 8 of the 19 in the very pre-term group, a major life event actually seemed to precipitate labour, for the number of major life events in the 1 week immediately preceding the onset of labour was far higher in the pre-term groups. While it is unlikely on the whole that an antenatal preventive role could be adopted, an effort could be made to reduce some of the stresses created by giving either moral support or financial help. It surprised the investigators to find out how many women had been having continuous worry for many months during pregnancy without their attendants being aware of it.

16.5.3 Uterine Inertia

Protracted labour may result from organic or functional causes. The former include malpresentation, disproportion, hydramnios, twins, fibroids, etc. It may, however, occur inexplicably, in the absence of any underlying recognisable abnormality. A striking feature of many of these labours is the apparent ambivalence of the uterus, the upper segment forceful in its efforts to discharge the fetus, the lower segment and cervix rigid in their determination not to allow the fetus to proceed. The pains are protracted, unrelenting, unduly agonising, and in severe cases, almost constant. Colon stasis, gastric dilatation and retention of urine are accompanied by gross distention, vomiting, ketosis and dehydration, with consequent increase in morbidity and even mortality to both mother and fetus.

No experienced obstetrician has any doubt that anxiety and fear are detrimental to the progress of labour, while confidence born of understanding and adequate support exercise a favourable influence. There is almost inevitable emotional stress before labour in picturing what is to come, based on hearsay or previous experience in multigravidae, or simply the prospect of the unknown. As labour develops the painful contractions themselves induce a secondary, anxious and fearful state as they confirm the patient's apprehensions. Lederman et al. [45] measured plasma adrenaline, noradrenaline and cortisol levels during labour and studied their relationship to self-reported anxiety and length of labour. They found a significant correlation between the level of anxiety and the adrenaline level; when the adrenaline level was high, there was a significant protraction of labour. It was postulated that adrenaline was associated with increased contraction of the lower segment, reluctance of the cervix to dilate and hence delayed progress. Higher plasma cortisol levels were also found in association with higher levels of psychological stress. Burns

[46] examined ACTH and subsequently cortisol levels in plasma during late pregnancy and related these to the duration of the first stage of the subsequent labour. A direct correlation was found, high levels of both being associated with longer labour. He considered that this added "further support to the proposal that a relation exists between psychological stress and human difficulty in labour." Buchan [47] assessed the consequences of stress by plasma 11-hydroxycorticosteroid levels and found that although the threat of epidural analgesia and internal fetal monitoring increased the emotional stress before labour, the relief from pain afforded by the epidural eliminated the progressive rise of corticosteroids during labour. This explains the finding that adequate analgesia is a significant therapeutic agent in the treatment of hypertonic uterine inertia.

It is extremely difficult if not impossible to forecast accurately the way in which any one patient will respond to the prospect of, and the experience of, labour. The prevention of nervous inertia must therefore depend to a large extent on the management during pregnancy and labour afforded to all patients. The following points are important:

1. Confidence in staff and unit resulting from reputation
2. Example set by staff at the antenatal clinic, some of whom will be encountered during labour
3. Level of success of antenatal classes in providing understanding and relaxation
4. Standard of care of the patient in labour and the provision of companionship, either nursing staff or relatives
5. Adequate analgesia in labour
6. Adequate explanation of all findings, normal and abnormal, and all interventions during labour
7. Comprehensive review of labour post-partum, uncovering and correcting misunderstandings and erroneous conclusions

The merit of company in labour has been clearly shown by Sosa et al. [48]. One is led to pass comment that an attendant constantly checking the fetal heart rate with a stethoscope has significant merits lacking in an electronic monitor.

16.6 Breast Feeding

Every herdsman knows that a locum milker, however skilled, will usually record less than the full expected yield, and that such distractions as children playing around in the hayloft overhead will reduce the let-down and consequently the volume recovered. The effect of stress is well recognised.

The physical factors that determine successful breast-feeding relate to the adequacy of the glandular tissue, protraction of the nipple, durability of the nipple and areola, laxity of the breast skin, adequacy of secretion by the gland tissue after delivery and the thrust forward of milk from the glands to the collecting area beneath the areolar during breast-feeding.

An outstanding influence, however, is a desire to succeed. To some extent this is a desire to establish a relationship. A mother's capacity to enjoy cuddle and contact with her child, which is the very essence of a passionate will to breast-feed, is determined to a large degree by her experience of this relationship with her own mother.

An appreciation of the merits of breast-feeding is also relevant. In a scientific era the evidence of the formula on the tin and the volume entering the baby can exert an overwhelming influence in favour of the bottle.

Finally, however well-motivated the mother is, she may lose this motivation in the face of painful breast engorgement, cracked nipples and a screaming baby.

Prolactin is the primary stimulus for the initiation of milk secretion post-partum. For the milk to be made available to the baby the ejection reflex, which is dependent upon the secretion of oxytocin, is essential. That oxytocin secretion is a response to suckling is very evident, but it has long been recognised that spontaneous ejection occurs independently of suckling, and McNeilly [49] has shown that oxytocin secretion rises 3–10 min before suckling in response to such stimuli as a baby crying or becoming restless, or to the mother making up the feed. I personally have vivid recollections of milk pouring from a mother's breast when the air-raid sirens sounded while she was in the corner shop and her baby was in her home. Voogt [50], studying the influence of anxiety, embarrassment, stress, etc. on the milk ejection reflex, found that adrenaline and noradrenaline reduced the secretion of oxytocin and hence the ejection reflex and enhanced the production of prolactin and hence the secretion rate; thereby the problem of congestion was compounded. Sjolin [51] thought those factors of most immediate importance to early termination of breast feeding, were connected directly with the mother's "immediate environment, with her personality and her emotions, her relations to her husband and family, and with her response to all kinds of minor everyday problems," and that her failure to continue breast feeding despite a strong wish was often "due to a lack of access to prompt and adequate support".

The necessary prerequisites of successful breast feeding are evident from the above. Besides the will to succeed, confidence, skilled sympathetic supervision, tranquillity before and during breast feeding, privacy and protection from embarrassment, and physical comfort, must be added ready availability and freedom of access between mother and baby. This is particularly important in the very early stages of lactation when the infant registers its nutritional needs to the maternal breasts which normally respond adequately. It is much more difficult to accommodate an increased demand for milk at a later stage if earlier the production has been at a low level.

An extremely narcissistic only child, who had used contraception for the first 6 years of marriage, thereafter complained of subfertility; the finding of infrequent intercourse was deemed to indicate considerable ambivalence about childbearing. When, on advice, coital frequency was increased, conception soon occurred. She was adamant from the beginning of the pregnancy that she would not breast-feed and proceeded through pregnancy hiding the cyesis as much as she could. In labour she vomited, otherwise it progressed straightforwardly. She failed to lactate, absolutely; indeed, she produced more tears than milk and was full of unhappy complaints. Uterine involution was very markedly retarded. She was subsequently seen dressed in ivory white leather, pushing an ivory white pram, with her daughter kitted up in ivory white clothes and coverings. She was never again pregnant.

16.7 Disorders of Sexual Function

K. C. Draper

In the foregoing section the management of patients presenting with gynaecological and obstetrical disorders in which a substantial psychosomatic component is present in their pathogenesis is given. This part describes a way of working with patients who present with sexual difficulties, many of them determined psychosomatically.

The boy, because his sexual organs are outside the body, becomes aware of any perceived deficiency earlier than the female, and such feelings may be the cause of agonising self-consciousness. Once again family attitudes towards sexuality and a boy's relationship with both his father and mother and the example that they set with each other, will influence his ability to achieve adult sexual relationships. The reproductive system and sexual functioning are not only susceptible to psychoneurotic anxieties, fantasies and phobias but also to psychosomatic presentations, which are our primary concern here.

16.7.1 Female Disorders

Increased openness in the discussion of sexual matters now enables more men and women than in the past to speak freely to a doctor about difficulties related to intercourse. However, doctors still have to be aware that many such problems are still not expressed verbally. This inability to talk of sexual matters, usually a symptom of a failure to accept their own sexuality, leads many women to present their problem psychosomatically as dyspareunia, pelvic pain or a discharge, or, psychoneurotically as difficulty with birth control.

Men who do not reveal their sexual difficulties openly sometimes present with genitourinary complaints, such as penile or varicocele pain, or even haematospermia or other psychosomatic symptoms. Having excluded an organic condition by appropriate examinations, the doctor often feels at a loss as to how best to help the patient whose problem appears to have a "nervous" basis. The first essential is not to say anything which leaves a patient feeling that it is his or her fault, that they are considered mentally unstable or that they are imagining their symptoms.

16.7.1.1 Management

As discussed in Chap. 5 traditional teaching on history taking is ill-designed to uncover emotional factors which are not fully conscious. The standard method involving much direct questioning is unhelpful. Enquiries such as, "What are you worried about?" are usually met with the answer, "Nothing." A very different approach is needed to reach any underlying anxiety.

For many women it was at a family planning clinic [52] that they first felt free to complain of sexual difficulties. Feelings of inadequacy when faced with such patients led a group of doctors to persuade the late Dr. Michael Balint [53] to lead a seminar to explore their predicament. By listening and thinking rather than questioning, they acquired a modified way of working, becoming aware of the subtleties of the relationship between doctor and patient. By offering insights thus gained, their patients were able to make progress where they had had difficulties previously. From experience of working in Well Woman Clinics and clinics for psychosexual difficulties they found that satisfactory results can be obtained in a comparatively short time by focussing on the here and now of the consultation [54]. A retrospective analysis [55] of the treatment of 1768 consecutive cases by 26 doctors who had been trained to use this method showed that there was a substantial improvement in 50% of all cases seen (or 65% of 1373 completed cases). The average time spent on each case was 2 h. Unfortunately, a control series is not available.

16.7.1.2 Listening and Observing

It is not easy for a doctor used to asking questions and giving opinions to decide to abandon control of the interview and observe the events that take place, e.g. the way in which the patient has presented to the doctor at that particular time, the manner in which the problem is described, and the emotional atmosphere generated; all these may be relevant.

It was during a busy family planning clinic that a 21-year-old student stumped in, picked up the chair and moved it back a yard, sat down and demanded that she be sterilised. Asked to talk about herself, it was soon apparent that she was in the throes of a divorce and wanted to concentrate on her musical career. Consciously, she wanted to be rid of her sexuality and all its implications, but showed this by the way she distanced herself angrily from the doctor whom she suspected was concerned with her sexuality and the likely long-term consequences of acquiescing to her request without first finding out about her unconscious motives.

Diffidence and hesitation while talking about sex, requests for birth control advice or presentation of a physical symptom may be the only indications of an underlying psychosexual problem.

Mrs. O., a well-dressed woman of 48, attended a menopause clinic complaining of pain in her joints which she felt was exacerbated by her period being overdue. Her GP had prescribed for her arthritis and hot flushes. However, in the clinic, encouraged by the type of facilitating approach already described, she admitted that she really wanted advice on birth control. She had never been able to discuss anything with her husband, who had started using a sheath, which had led to occasional impotence, and she was worried for her marriage. After clinical assessment a progesterone-only pill was prescribed. Two months later her periods had become regular, her joint pains less distressing, and she felt well. She said her husband had taken a while to realise that he could now have normal intercourse without risk of pregnancy, but everything was now fine.

Doctors short of time and faced with embarrassed or inarticulate people often feel driven to ask questions but will usually learn more by waiting and tolerating silences. Facilitations such as "you seem to have difficulty talking about this" can free someone to share their thoughts, whereas a question is more likely to drive them further into themselves. Allowing an interview to develop in this way initially worries some doctors, leaving them feeling confused. It takes a little time for a young doctor to tolerate feelings of confusion and impotence.

Allowing Expression of Emotions. When given space to talk in this way a patient may reveal strong feelings such as despair, anger, pain or sorrow; again the doctor needs to encourage patients to express their feelings by facilitations, etc., as described in Chap. 5.

Mrs. X was having a routine cervical smear in a Well Woman Clinic when she also mentioned that severe abdominal pain, undiagnosed after two laparoscopies, was making her life a misery. Her notes showed that she had no children, but had had two late miscarriages. It was suggested she must also have had a lot of pain (emotional) from the loss of her two pregnancies. Her brittle smile collapsed, and she began to weep softly, saying that the baby would have been 10 the following Saturday. She was allowed to weep further, and while holding her hand the doctor suggested that she come back for a longer appointment. At the next consultation she suddenly asked, "How long do you grieve?" Weeping, she told about the second miscarriage when the baby had lived for 4 h. After it died it was taken away by her husband and mother, and they never told her where it was buried. She felt unable to ask them and had never been able to weep for the baby. On the birthday anniversary she had nowhere to lay her wreath. A month later she came back looking brighter and although still suffering abdominal pain she said she had not felt so well for years. She talked with pleasure of events in the future, and it seemed at last that she had begun to accept the tragedy of her loss. Four months later she was symptom free. (See also Chap. 6 on phobic IBS cases for similar histories.)

16.7.1.3 Doctor-Patient Relationship

During interviews doctors may notice that some patients evoke from them very different emotional responses. For example, it was easy to accept feelings of sympathy towards Mrs. P., who is small and slight and burdened with two small children, household chores and a busy husband. On the other hand Mrs. Q. aroused irritation when she *demanded* removal of the IUCD inserted only recently at her request, saying that she now thought she would like to try something else, especially as she and her husband did not have sex very often! [I wondered if the husband felt as irritated as I did. If so it was possibly not surprising that they did not make love very often!]

While feelings of empathy for a patient's suffering are easy to accept, other feelings which doctors may have about patients, such as annoyance or dislike, are more difficult to recognise. Expression of these sentiments at an early interview is, of course, not only unprofessional but potentially damaging to a patient. Doctors have to learn to recognise feelings in themselves and refrain from acting upon them, and use that experience to learn more about the patient. These insights are invaluable in psychological management. See Chap. 4 on working through transference and counter-transference.

Mrs. Y. My heart sank as I read the referral letter. Mr. and Mrs. Y. had seen the marriage guidance counsellor and had been to another sex therapy clinic: they had not been helped but were determined to stay together. At the first appointment, with their two children aged 2 and 4, the

younger sat on his father's knee while the elder child explored the room and climbed onto my lap. While listening to Mrs. Y's recital of her husband's shortcomings I offered the child a sweet and was then taken aback to hear Mrs. Y. say sharply, "I'd rather she didn't accept sweets from strangers, she is trained not to." How, I thought in my annoyance, can she expect me to help improve the intimate aspects of the marriage when she cannot trust me enough to give her child a sweet? However, I accepted the admonition with discretion, took a deep breath and retrieved the situation, turning it to advantage with the enabling suggestion that Mrs. Y. must find the world a very hostile place, and it seemed as though no one could really help her, not her husband, neighbours or professionals. Seen alone at the next session Mrs. Y. said, while discussing birth control methods, that her periods had started when she was only 10.
D: That must have made life very difficult at primary school.
P: That was the least of my worries.

She went on to describe her clever, pretty twin sister, always surrounded by a crowd of friends, while she was lonely and excluded. She was only 6 months old when her father left home, saying that she and her sister were not his children. His subsequent visits to the family always ended in quarrels. As she grew up her three elder brothers took over father's role and were bullying and oppressive. From then on she was much less hostile, and it was possible to explore what she felt about her unhappy childhood. Her prickly and untrusting manner melted in parallel with my initial feelings of irritation.

Learning to use the doctor-patient relationship in this way can provide a short cut to understanding a patient's difficulties. It would have been easy for any doctor to wallow in the satisfaction of caring for Mrs. P., thereby perhaps losing sight of the best way of helping her, whereas Mrs. Y might well have evoked the opposite response from doctors trained only in standard history taking and not able to recognise their anger in time.

16.7.1.4 Genital Examination

It is during the physical examination of the genitals that patients commonly reveal through non-verbal behaviour much about their feelings for their own sexuality [56]. Sometimes the examination is avoided as long as possible with excuses such as menstruation even when the appointment has been booked ahead with that in view. While observing such avoidance it is not helpful to challenge the woman, rather it is necessary to find the *reason* for the avoidance.

Mrs. J. had attended the clinic for 2 years, but her notes revealed that she had never a vaginal examination because she had said at her first attendance that she was a virgin. When next seen she said she was menstruating, the following time she was in a hurry to keep a dental appointment, and again on another occasion she was menstruating. When it was suggested that she must be worried about being examined, she responded by bursting into tears, saying that she had never been able to have sexual intercourse.

The technique [56] of vaginal examination requires doctors to be confident in themselves while at the same time sensitive to a patient's normal reluctance to submit to this invasion of her privacy and the important recognition that the presence of observers or interruptions should be avoided if possible. If a chaperon is present she must be unobstrusive. Clutching a woman's hand and comforting her implies that she is going to be submitted to a traumatic procedure. Much may be learned by the way a woman approaches the examination. Sometimes she may stand chatting half-way to the couch, delaying undressing or even lying down fully dressed in boots and trousers. Telling her to hurry up is pointless, but a remark such as, "This seems to make you nervous", often enables her to express her feelings. Women with severe sexual problems may arch their backs to try to escape over the end of the couch, while others appear to develop severe adductor spasm of their legs. When vaginismus is severe, there may appear to be no vaginal orifice, or it may be so small as only to admit the insertion of one finger. In some circumstances a contraction may be felt while the patient is relating a traumatic experience.

Offering check-lists for all possible reasons of nervousness to young doctors only closes minds and gets in the way of listening.

Mrs. I. is an Italian aged 27 who made an appointment to see that she was fitting her contraceptive cap properly. Despite everything being all right, she was quivering with nervousness.
D: It seems as if something is really worrying you?
She began to weep while rolling over and pointed to a small scar at the base of her spine. As her tears subsided, she said she had had an operation when she was 2 years old but had never dared to ask her parents about it; she had always assumed that it must have been for spina bifida, which she thought was hereditary. She was longing for a baby and although she knew tests were available to exclude spina bifida, she realised that abortions would be out of the question because her husband was a Catholic. She had never dared to share these anxieties with her husband.

On other occasions it is not nervousness but a stony detachment about the whole procedure which will alert the doctor that the patient may think sex is all rather dirty, especially if accompanied by a remark such as "I don't know how you can do this all day, doctor."

Thus the vaginal examination may reveal much about a woman's fantasies, or feelings of inadequacy, and her doctor should attempt to understand possible symbolic meanings of what is said or what is going on, and not take them only at face value.

16.7.1.5 Decisions on Further Treatment

There will be occasions when a doctor has to decide whether to offer a patient a further consultation or to let matters rest. The following case study is illustrative.

Mrs. A. brought an urgent referral letter from her GP. She was over 50, mousy, drably dressed and scuttled into the room like a frightened rabbit. The letter said that her GP had tried to take a smear but had found it too difficult. She had been married 20 years, but intercourse had been erratic for 2 years and was always painful so she and her husband had stopped bothering. She said they would have liked to have had children but thought her husband never really wanted any, and now it was too late. None the less she had heard about sexual problem clinics but she had been too shy to talk to her husband about it. Then she mentioned how she and her husband both had jobs they really enjoyed and shared hobbies, and that they were very lucky. Although nervous, the patient did not have vaginismus, and a decision was made not to disturb the accommodation the couple had made with each other. However, it is wise in such cases, when there is doubt, to give the patient the opportunity of making a further appointment if necessary.

16.7.2 Male Disorders

Although women were the first to present at clinics dealing with sexual problems, nowadays half the patients attending are men. It seems that they feel less threatened by a woman doctor and more willing to admit impotence to her rather than to another male. Male sexual complaints are usually made in terms of performance; difficulty in achieving an erection, impotence and problems with control of ejaculation, both premature and retarded. While there are neurological and toxic causes for such complaints, such as MS and diabetes on the one hand, or excess alcohol intake or certain drugs on the other, by far the most common are emotionally based and psychosomatically mediated. When men complain of lack of interest in sex it is usually a cover up and a rationalization for feelings of inadequacy. Male sexual difficulties can be managed in the same way as described for women, with special emphasis on the doctor-patient relationship [57]. It is possible that a woman doctor may have some advantage in this respect and that a man's unconscious feelings for women in general may become manifest at the first consultation. As emphasised for the management of every other disorder described in this book, the physical examination is essential, and male psychosexual disorders are no exception. Many of these patients have hidden fears that their penis or testes are too small or have been damaged in some way, for example, subsequent to mumps. For a full description of working with male difficulties the reader is referred to Berry and Yorsten [58] reporting on a series of 50 impotent male patients. They found that 20 had had an enthusiastic recovery, 14 had had some improvement, 8 no improvement, and 8 had defaulted.

Not infrequently, male sexual difficulties are presented by a spouse or partner as, for example, Mrs. F., who came asking for a cervical smear but saying she did not need contraception any longer as her husband had developed diabetes and was impotent. Early in his illness he had asked a young doctor if he should know any more about it. "Not really," was the reply, "but you may become impotent," and so he did. After several years he told another doctor what had happened and he and his wife were referred with high hopes to a sex therapy clinic [59]. Sadly, however, he was unable to make use of the behavioural therapy and became even more downcast than before. The wife was asked by K. D. to come back and talk about it, and she spoke of the great worry she had about the instability of her husband's diabetes with any mild exertion precipitating a coma. He said when he first came out of hospital they had made love a few times, and she had then laid awake all night watching him, fearing that he would go into coma and die in the night. Her fear spread to him and soon all sexual activities stopped. She returned a fortnight later and to K. D.'s surprise she said that during a rare weekend alone together her husband had had an erection, and they had been able to make love.

Summary. This is a cautionary tale of how a doctor's innocent advice undermined the balance of emotional security and confidence upon which adequate sexual performance depends and emphasises how delicately it is poised and how narrow the gap between success or failure.

16.7.2.1 Impotence

Impotence is defined by Main [60] as "the failure of men to please their partners and themselves". It emphasises the point that the achievement of mutual sexual satisfaction depends on being concerned with the feelings of the other person and is not just a behaviour of organs. It is rare for an impotent man to fail to have an erection when he masturbates or wakes from an erotic dream. Impotence involves his inability to achieve an erection with a partner or being able to maintain it so that he can penetrate. This inability will be influenced by the conceptions he has about women formed during his childhood relationships and his subsequent experience.

Mr. M. was referred by a GP because, "He is having problems with intercourse. There is no physical abnormality." He sat down nervously and stared straight in front of him, avoiding eye contact. His girlfriend had sent him because although he could get an erection when she masturbated him it did not last. When he was 25 he had had a previous experience with a timid divorcee which had ended in failure, with him becoming angry and shouting; he was much ashamed of the memory. Asked about his family he said that his mother had died when he was 3 years old, and his father had spent the whole of each weekend in pubs. He had had to hang about outside and found it degrading. Now he lived with his sister and her family. For the past 3 years there had been quarrelling because his brother-in-law drank, and he dreaded going home from work. "I have come full circle, it reminds me of the way my drunken father used to beat me." Apparently the only woman in his life who had offered him any warmth was the girlfriend who had persuaded him to attend. He was seen 14 times over the following 18 months, and his manner became gradually easier as he worked through his feelings about demanding, damaging women who made him shake with anger at his own inadequacy. After taking out other girls without much success he gradually began to talk about one who was interesting him and whom he had taken out several times. At his penultimate visit he described rather sadly how on a bank holiday he had watched crowds enjoying themselves in the sun. He stayed away for a while, but at the next visit was seen sitting in the waiting room clutching a large bouquet for me. He had met a girl as lonely as himself but at last had felt relaxed and easy, and it had "just happened". He talked with confidence, and the change in his whole demeanour was striking.

Summary. The image Mr. M. had of women which dominated his fantasies was that they were terrible creatures who "take all". For some men, however, it is the fear of their own damaging aggression which prevents them from being effectively assertive.

16.7.2.2 Premature Ejaculation

Some men ejaculate before or as they enter, suggesting fears of being trapped, engulfed or overwhelmed by women as already discussed. Some degree of premature ejaculation is almost inevitable in early attempts at intercourse, enhanced now a days by higher expectations fed by the media or uncomplementary comparisons by a partner who has had previous experience. Failure to weather these early insecurities will depend not only on the context of the first relationship but also on the deeper unconscious attitude to women in general. Premature ejaculation can be a powerful way of disappointing a woman and a sign of passive aggression towards her and women in general.

Mr. O. Significantly, this man's appointment was made by his wife's social worker. The wife claimed that after 3 months of marriage Mr. O. had begun only to think of his own pleasure and that she was unable to reach orgasm. The patient himself did not realise he had a problem, but recalled when he was 15 how his mother had caught him and his girlfriend together. The mother had said he would tell his father but she never did because "he would have killed me". The patient had felt protective of his mother because of his father's rages, and although he too had a temper, he diverted it in aggressive and competitive sports. At school he had been teased and called "one ball" because he had lost one testicle in an accident when he was 11 years old. At sessions over the next few months he would sit sulkily, say he was improving and had made intercourse last 10 min, but his wife still complained that other men could last half an hour. I said, "You make me feel very angry with your wife and yet I have never met her." Laughing, he said he must make her sound like a bitch, but he was getting fed up with his marriage. He had wanted someone to love but had ended up having to do the housework. This important admission was not made until he had been seen for 4 months. He said he seldom played football and had given up training and that his wife had decided that he should diet. "You don't get many hot dinners at our house." She was always telling him that he was inferior, picking him up on grammar mistakes and his use of words. Two months after owning up to these feelings of anger, they decided on a trial separation. At the next interview, looking much fitter after being back in training, he said he had met a girl who was much in love with him but that he didn't want to be tied down. After a brief affair on a holiday abroad in which he said that sex had been fine because he did not care, he remained still nervous of what might happen if he was in a serious relationship. Six weeks later all was well with the new girlfriend who was fun and came to watch him play football; however, he was rather worried when he realised that he loved her, but found he could still last for ages".

Summary. The patient had been referred to be made a better sexual partner for his wife, but his childhood insecurity had been compounded by his suppressed resentment at her repeated denigrations. When a couple are united by reciprocal difficulties then improvement of one may sometimes be only attainable at the expense of the relationship.

16.7.2.3 Retarded Ejaculation

This must not be confused with somatic retrograde ejaculation due to a deformity in the valve of the urethra. The psychosomatic form of this disorder chiefly leads to problems when they want a child. In a study [61] of 22 men who presented with this complaint, 5 had been referred from subfertility clinics, and 7 were twins (13 times the national average), and the complaint had developed always in the less successful twin. It seemed that they felt that they had always lost out in competition for their mother's care, attention and appreciation. Now although their love-making pleased their partners, it seemed that they were unconsciously denying them the chance of conceiving a baby who would be a rival. The study found that men who were brought to the clinic by their wives had a poor prognosis, but those who attended themselves and were asking for assistance with sexual pleasure and not just conception could be helped when they were put in touch with their suppressed anger and resentment against women.

Mrs. P., aged 33 years, said while attending an infertility clinic that her husband could sometimes ejaculate but it never seemed to happen at the fertile time of the menstrual cycle. When she wanted intercouse at the time of ovulation, he was always "too tired". Mr. P was offered a separate appointment at which he told of his agonising childhood. Father had gone off before he could remember, leaving him with his paranoid schizophrenic mother. She would talk and shout at night, and he was the only one who could deal with her and keep the peace with the neighbours and landlord. Ashamed of his mad mother he never felt able to ask friends home but tried to find escape in cycling and dancing. He had been a reluctant husband, breaking off the engagement and meeting again before drifting into marriage. Shortly before the wedding he had a detached retina and was afraid that intercourse would precipitate a recurrence. Consciously, he said he wanted children, but angry remarks about the way neighbours indulged their children suggested ambivalence. First he resisted any suggestion of feeling two ways about parenthood but gradually was able to admit to his own fear of responsibility resulting from always having to be the responsible person since infancy. He always booked the last appointment (no competition!), and the consultation would go on and on. Gradually, he became able to give off his real thoughts and anger and in time was also able to give to his wife, i.e. ejaculate. Three years after the first appointment, the clinic received a card announcing the birth of a son.

16.7.2.4 Conclusion

Most patients go to their doctor to be "made better". Those described in this section are no exception and are at first reluctant to accept that they need to work with the doctor to gain understanding that, although their complaint may feel somatic to them, it is the fears and fantasies that lie behind it that have to be understood and worked through if they are to obtain relief. The approach needed to reach any underlying anxieties is very different from the standard medical interview.

References

1. Fava GA, Trombini G, Grandi S, Bernardi M, Evangelisti LP, Santarsiero G, Orlandi C (1984) Depression and anxiety associated with secondary amenorrhoea. Psychosomatics 25:905–908
2. Lachelin GC, Yen SS (1978) Hypothalamic chronic anovulation. Am J Obstet Gynecol 130:825–831
3. Aksel G (1979) Psychogenic amenorrhoea: diagnosis by exclusion. Psychosomatics 20:357–359
4. Fava M, Fava GA, Kellner R, Buckman MT, Lisansky J, Serafini E, de Besi L, Mastrogiacomo I (1983) Psychomatic aspects of hyperprolactinaemia. Psychother Psychosom 40:257–262
5. Fraser IS, McCarron G, Markham R (1984) A preliminary study of factors influencing perception of menstrual blood loss volume. Am J Obstet Gynecol 149:788–793
6. Blaikley JB (1949) Menorrhagia of emotional origin. Lancet 2:691–694
7. Stott PC (1983) The outcome of menorrhagia: a retrospective case control study. J R Coll Gen Pract 33:715–720
8. Stott PC, Teague L, Walker D (1983) Menorrhagia and the doctor-patient relationship. Practitioner 227:855–859
9. Ballinger CB (1977) Psychiatric morbidity and the menopause: survey of a gynaecological outpatient clinic. Br J Psychiatry 131:83–90
10. Gath D, Cooper P, Bond A, Edmonds G (1982) Hysterectomy and psychiatric disorder: demographic and physical factors in relation to psychiatric outcome. Br J Psychiatry 140:343–350

11. Gath D, Cooper P, Day A (1982) Hysterectomy and psychiatric disorder. Levels of psychiatric morbidity before and after hysterectomy. Br J Psychiatry 140:335–342

12. Martin RL, Roberts WV, Clayton PJ (1980) Psychiatric status after hysterectomy. JAMA 244:350

13. Martin RL, Roberts WV, Clayton PJ, Wetzel R (1977) Psychiatric illness and non-cancer hysterectomy. Dis Nerv Syst 38:974–980

14. Amos WE, Khanna P (1985) Life stress in spasmodic and congestive dysmenorrhoea. Psychol Rep 57:216–218

15. Lundstrom V, af Geijerstam G (1983) Treatment of primary dysmenorrhoea. Acta Obstet Gynecol Scand [Suppl] 113:83–85

16. Lawlor GL, Davis AM (1981) Primary dysmenorrhoea. Relationship to personality and attitudes in adolescent females. Journal of Adolesc Health Care 1:208–212

17. Jay MS, Durant RH (1983) The patient with dysmenorrhea. Postgrad Med 73:103–111

18. Woods DJ, Launius AL (1979) Type of menstrual discomfort and psychological masculinity in college women. Psychol Rep 44:257–258

19. Iacono CU, Roberts SJ (1983) The dysmenorrheic personality: actuality or statistical artifact? Soc Sci Med 17:1653–1655

20. Weiss E, English OS (1949) Psychosomatic medicine, 2nd Edn. Saunders, Philadelphia

21. Jeffcoate TNS (1969) Pelvic Pain. Br Med J 3:431–435

22. Templeton AA, Penney GL (1982) The incidence, characteristics and prognosis of patients whose infertility is unexplained. Fertil Steril 37:175–182

23. Sandler B (1968) Emotional stress and infertility. J Psychosom Res 12:51–59

24. Sandler B (1965) Conception after adoption. Practitioner 194:505–510

25. Mai FM (1972) Conception after adoption – myth or fact? Med Aspects Hum Sexuality 7:162–168

26. Arronet GH, Bergquist CA, Parekh MC (1974) The influence of adoption on subsequent pregnancy in infertile marriage. Int J Fertil 19:159–162

27. Lamb EJ, Leurgans S (1979) Does adoption affect subsequent fertility? Am J Obstet Gynecol 46:37–43

28. Elstein M (1982) Cervical mucus: its physiological role and clinical significance. Adv Exp Med Biol 144:301–317

29. Stallworthy J (1948) Facts and fantasy in the study of female infertility. J Obstet Gynaecol Br Commonw 53:171–180

30. Humphrey M (1984) Infertility and alternative parenting. In: Broom A, Wallace L (eds) Psychology and gynaecological problems. Tavistock, London, pp 77–94

31. Edelmann RJ, Connolly KJ (1986) Psychological aspects of infertility. Br J Med Psychol 59:209–219

32. Brahler C, Meyhofer W (1985) Psychologische Aspekte der Fertilitätsstörungen. Med Welt 36:230–241

33. Brahler C, Meyhofer W (1986) Zur Bedeutung von Partnerschaft und Körpererleben bei heterologer Insemination. Fertilität 2:161–168

34. Henker FO (1976) Psychotherapy as adjunct in treatment of vomiting during pregnancy. South Med J 69:1585–1587

35. Fairweather DBI (1968) Nausea and vomiting in pregnancy. Am J Obstet Gynecol 102:135–175

36. Katon WJ, Ries RK, Bokan JA, Kleinman A (1980) Hyperemesis gravidarum: a biopsychosocial perspective. Int J Psychiatry 10:151–162

37. Nordmeyer K (1946) Zur Aetiologie der Hyperemesis Gravidarum. Dtsch Med Wochenschr 71:213–214

38. Chertok L, Mondzain ML, Bonnaud M (1963) Vomiting and the wish to have a child. Psychosom Med 25:13–17

39. Ringler M, Krizmanitz A (1983) Zur Psychosomatik der Emesis Gravidarum: Wahrneh-mungs- und Einstellungsmuster von Frauen in der Frühschwangerschaft. Z. Geburtshilfe Perinatol 187:246–249
40. Ringler M, Krizmanits A (1984) Zur Psychosomatik der Emesis Gravidarum: die somatische und psychosoziale Situation von Frauen in der Frühschwangerschaft. Z. Geburtshilfe Perinatol 188:234–238
41. Zechnich R, Hammer T (1982) Brief psychotherapy for hyperemesis gravidarum. Am Fam Physician 26:179–181
42. Weiss E, English OS (1949) Psychosomatic medicine, 2nd Edn. Saunders, Philadelphia
43. Priest RG (1985) Psychological disorders in obstetrics and gynaecology. Butterworth, London
44. Newton RW, Webster PAC, Binu PS, Maskrey N, Phillips AB (1979) Psychological stress in pregnancy and its relation to the onset of premature labour. Br Med J 2:411–413
45. Lederman RP, Lederman E, Work BA, McCann DS (1978) The relationship of maternal anxiety, plasma catecholamines and plasma cortisol to progress in labour. Am J Obstet Gynecol 132:495–500
46. Burns JK (1976) Relation between blood levels of cortisol and duration of human labour. J Physiol 254:12P
47. Buchan PC (1980) Emotional stress and childbirth and its modification by variations in obstetric management. Epidural analgesia and stress in labour. Acta Obstet Gynecol Scand 59:319–321
48. Sosa R, Kennell J, Klaus M, Robertson S, Urrutia J (1980) The effect of a supportive companion on perinatal problems, length of labour and mother-infant interaction. N Engl J Med 303:597–600
49. McNeilly AS, Robinson ICAF, Houston MT, Howie PW (1983) Release of oxytocin and prolactin in response to suckling. Br Med J 286:257–259
50. Voogt JL (1978) Control of hormone release during lactation. Clin Obstet Gynaecol 5:435–455
51. Sjolin S, Hofvander Y, Hillervik C (1977) Factors related to early termination of breast feeding. Acta Paediatr Scand 66:505–511
52. Tunnadine LDP (1970) Contraception and sexual life: a therapeutic approach. Tavistock, London
53. Balint M (1964) The doctor, his patient and the illness, 2nd edn. Pitman, London
54. Draper KC (ed) (1983) Practice of psychosexual medicine. Libbey, London
55. Mears E (1978) Sexual problem clinics: an assessment of the work of 26 doctors trained by the Institute of Psychosexual Medicine. Public Health 92:218–223
56. Tunnadine P (1980) The role of the genital examination in psychosexual medicine. In: Elstein M (ed) Clinics in obstetrics and gynaecology. Saunders, London, pp 283–291
57. Tunnadine P (1983) The doctor-patient relationship with men. In: Draper KC (ed) Practice of psychosexual medicine. Libbey, London, pp 132–135
58. Berry J, Yorsten J (1983) Study of doctor seeing 50 patients with male impotence. In: Draper KC (ed) Practice of psychosexual medicine. Libbey, London, pp 136–144
59. Masters WH, Johnson VE (1970) Human sexual inadequacy. Little Brown, Boston
60. Main TF (1976) Impotence. In: Milne H, Hardy S (eds) Psychosexual problems. Bradford University Press and Crosby Lockwood Staples, London, pp 101–112
61. Lincoln R, Thexton R (1983) Retarded ejaculation. In: Draper KC (ed) Practice of psychosexual medicine. Libbey, London, pp 151–155

17 Anorexia Nervosa, Bulimia, Induced Vomiting and Purging

The publicity in the press and on TV given to the other manifestations of AN may have been the cause of recent increased frequency of these among older women. Many of them have learned that they may eat normally without exceeding their magic weight through vomiting or purging.

According to Halliday's and our own definition (Chap. 2) AN is not psychosomatic. That is because the mechanism through which the psyche affects the soma is wholly conscious and external. However, we have included it here because it is usually regarded as psychosomatic and because it is common, difficult to treat, may break marriages and threaten other members of the family. Although the management required is not easy to arrange in general practice, GPs by making an *early diagnosis* and by knowing the most suitable form of treatment for a particular patient can make an important contribution to the outcome.

The name AN itself is misleading because sufferers are *hungry*. Most eat large amounts of vegetables, lettuce, lean meat and cheese. What they do not eat is carbohydrates or only minutely, the exception being the vomiters and the purgers. A better name for the condition would be carbohydrate deprivation, but as millions of words are written on the subject every year, and an endless round of conferences are devoted to it, at which the doctors seem to eat well, it is too late to change. Early diagnosis may depend on recognising presentations other than weight loss or amenorrhoea, e.g. depression, constipation, lanugo, carotenaemic colouring as in myxoedema or a chance finding of hypokalaemia in the purger. Groups particularly at risk are athletes and ballet dancers.

17.1 Psychopathogenesis

Little has been added to our kowledge of the psychopathology of AN since the detailed reports of Bruch [1], Thomae [2] and Selvini [3]. Even earlier, Naudeau in 1789 [4] observed: "Both the patient and her family form a tightly knit whole, and we obtain a false picture of the disease if we limit our observations to the patients alone." Selvini [5], Minuchin [6] and Russell et al. [7] have emphasised the need to involve the whole family and to treat a patient's illness as a response of the patient's and the other members' relationships to each other.

For accounts of the *typically* provocative childhood and *typical* pattern of family relationships readers are referred to the above authors. Robot children is an apt description for the premorbid compliant behaviour of these patients, and it is their inability for a variety of reasons to establish separate identities and independence which is at the core of the psychopathology. We recall many mothers saying, "If this had happened to any of my other children I could have understood it, but not this one who has always been so good and never caused any trouble!" Families of AN patients are usually very caring yet insensitive to a vulnerable child's need for a separate identity, partly because it is not voiced, or if voiced, passes unheeded. There are exceptions to the caring background in AN, and as in MS (Chap. 9) some parents may be overtly coercive or suppress emotional expression as stupid or irrational. Parents of AN patients are often from the caring professions such as medicine, nursing, teaching and social work. Reasons for only one child in a sibship adopting such a destructive coping mechanism naturally vary, but present with such consistency as to constitute *typicality*. However, whatever the nature of the influences,the result is always that the relationship between the affected sib and the mother is such that a separate identity has not been established, and the mother is rejected as a model for the girl's developing femininity. Not for nothing has it been called the Peter Pan syndrome. Like Peter, the patients do not want to grow up physically, yet despite their childlike behaviour and appearence they yearn subconsciously to be accorded the separate identity which has eluded them throughout childhood and adolescence, but which they see their siblings and friends attain.

While genetic factors such as inherited timidity may play a part, a major factor is a sense of insecurity acquired through experiences in childhood which prevent them gaining a separate identity. For example, the child may be deterred by seeing a sibling behaving outrageously and causing great parental distress, or if circumstances during the mother's pregnancy or after the birth result in a tightly bonded relationship with that child. The role of fathers in psychopathogenesis has been much neglected. Fathers of anorexic children are often belittled by the mother and are, or appear to be, inert emotionally. This encourages the enmeshing [6] relationship between mother and other members of the family to develop. Enmeshment is close to the engulfment or entrapment described in MS in Chap. 9; indeed, we have four patients with MS who had previously suffered from AN [8]. The following is an example of circumstances in infancy predisposing to an enmeshing relationship.

Mother was a caring and organised person who decided she needed 4 years between each child so that she could look after them properly. The patient, the second of three sisters, was born in 1942 at her mother's sister's house while her father was abroad. Mother, anxious for her husband's safety during the pregnancy and puerperium, developed facial neuralgia when the patient was 10 months old. That she was still breast feeding suggests she was insecure, but her doctors told her to stop feeding at once. The baby then developed eczema, which was claimed to be an allergy to cow's milk but may well have been psychosomatic. She itched for the next 3 years, lost her hair, felt she was unattractive, and her skin was always too messy with ointments for her to be cuddled. From the age of about 18 months the patient recalled the need for ritualistic behaviour, without which she felt insecure. She had to look into the corners of the room from her cot and perform a sequence of acts before she could go to sleep. Some of the rituals persisted into adult life, which she recognised as her way of assuaging continuing feelings of insecurity. Envy of her elder sister who was cleverer, and of her younger sister who was pretty, filled early memories; this envy persisted into adolescence and beyond, and was a constant source of guilt. Her mother was religious and a disciplinarian; she never thought of doing anything at variance to what she felt her mother wanted, although she did not realise it until her sisters later pointed it out.

17.2 Psychological Management

Management of AN began to improve about 35 years ago when it was recognised that measures seen as punitive by patients were counter-productive. Before then, AN patients accustomed to parental anger at not eating, lying and deceit met comparable hostility again from nurses, dietitians and doctors, but they knew how to defeat it. If tube fed, they only had to vomit, and they did.

Recognition that AN patients were ill and as phobic about putting on weight as someone else might be for heights or enclosed spaces resulted in the empathetic yet firm approach by doctors and nurses which remains the basis of the standard behavioural approach.

17.3 Behavioural Management

Many, but not all, anorexics initially require admission to hospital which temporarily removes them from the cockpit of the family meal and enables their activity to be restricted until they attain a mutually agreed weight. Essentially this is a behavioural approach of reward and punishment. Privileges such as bathing, sitting out of bed, and going for walks which are initially removed, are gradually restored as rewards for gains in weight.

Simultaneously, individual or family therapeutic sessions are instituted, and these continue after the patient has reached the contract weight and gone home.

17.4 Outpatient or Inpatient Management or Both

An added advantage of using family therapy is that fewer children need be admitted to hospital, and many can be treated successfully in this way [6].

An example of a successful outpatient management alone was a girl who was at boarding school. At the first interview with both her parents they were asked if they would agree that, as she was nearly adult, she might be treated accordingly and come to subsequent interviews on her own. She had three brothers and no sisters. Most of the family pursuits were masculine, and the mother appeared to use her daughter as an ally in a long-running but tacit irritation with the males. Psychotherapeutic sessions enabled the patient to talk about her feelings about family and friends in a way she had not been able to do before. She said her AN started when a girlfriend at school had suddenly become interested in boys and discarded her (almost as common a trigger as competitive dieting with a friend or being teased for early signs of femininity).

After about six interviews she was still short of her contract weight, and it was re-affirmed that if she had not reached this by Christmas, she would have to come into hospital until she had reached it. At the same time she was asked if there was any carbohydrate she liked, and surprisingly she answered: "chocolate!" She was told she could eat as much as she liked. Two days later an irate mother telephoned.

M: My daughter has asked me to take 20 lbs (8 kilos) of chocolate to her at school – I have never heard such nonsense.

D: Well, you must decide, but I would have thought that it was good news that she was prepared to eat anything.

The receiver was slammed down, but the girl got her chocolate and recovered. She later married and had children, and to date has not relapsed. The chocolate episode was the first time she had won against her mother.

Sadly, most cases of AN are more difficult.

17.5 Family Therapy – The Systems Model

Recent work on psychological management using the systems model has improved the outlook for the younger patients with less than 3 years' history. A recent study by Russell et al. [7] confirmed the superiority of family therapy for younger patients but those over 18 did better with individual psychotherapy, as was to be expected.

Minuchin wrote, "In the systems model the locus of pathology is the individual in *context* ... of family members or with other significant people." By contrast he claimed that for the dynamically orientated psychotherapist, "the locus of pathology is the patient". We feel this is an exaggeration. The clinical chapters of this book emphasise that interaction between patients and key figures and surrogates is integral both to pathogenesis and to effective management of all psychosomatic disorders. What the application of family therapy has done has been to make it possible to treat more children with AN effectively and without bringing so many as previously into hospital. This success owes much to the technique which Minuchin has developed and described, and we regard his book [6] with its instructive transcripts as essential reading for anyone who has to treat anorexics.

At the first session, at which as many members of the family as possible are present, the therapist develops

> the therapeutic system: assumes therapeutic leadership, develops family trust, supports areas of competence of family members, and in general ... prepares for the stress ... of the following session which is the lunch session. [At this,] food which members have ordered arrives and lunch starts. [In this way] issues are enacted instead of talking about them.

(Minuchin recommends the use of one-way screens for observing interactions but lack of one does not matter). In the case of a particularly resistant 19-year-old, father, mother, sister and fiancé had been invited and sat down to their meal with the patient and took no notice of one of us, or the social worker, and dietitian, eating in the corner of the same room. Minuchin wrote: "A frequent and surprising result of the first lunch session is that directly afterwards, the anorexic begins to eat." That is just what occurred in the above case.

Not everyone will wish, or be able, to follow Minuchin's *over-focusing* on the issue of the risk of death from starvation by which he intentionally raises tension at the early lunch sessions, and by confronting members with what they are unconsciously doing to each other by manipulation and collusion. Tension is increased when the therapist gives an interpretation or instruction and then disappears behind his one-way screen, leaving the family to get on with it, only to return when he observes something that merits another intervention. The strategy of over-focussing on immediate life-threatening symptoms usually starts the patient eating, but as Minuchin points out, it should be short or the old (pathological) parental control reasserts itself. Therefore, over-focussing has soon to be followed by moving therapy "beyond the symptom bearer ... to the family interactions that supported the systems ... The goal is to shake the family system and facilitate ... alternative modalities of transacting." This is termed *under-focusing*, i.e. on food and eating. Other pithy comments worth mentioning are "disengaging from the parental triangle [triangulation] ... exposure of ... conflict avoidance patterns ... reinstatement of the absentee father."

Dare has stressed how important it is for the therapist not to *feel* that any one is to blame for the patient's AN because if he or she does, the family will sense it and oppose intervention.

The following case illustrates the value of this and may be considered an example of under-focusing. She was 20 and had just married. Three years previously she had become anorexic and had responded to the behavioural approach at another hospital. Even so, she still regarded herself as fat, and a never relenting fear of putting on even a few grams of weight and of losing *control* persisted. Two weeks after her wedding she took an overdose of anti-depressants, and the ensuing admission enabled the diagnosis of unresolved AN to be made. She said she was very close to her mother and expected the close bond to continue despite her marriage. In therapy it was pointed out that even those who love us most can also hurt and frustrate us. She said her mother was worried about her, and she feared that she would be visiting and telephoning even more than ever when she left hospital. Asked what happened when she and her mother went out shopping or visiting, she replied: "Mother says we'll go out this afternoon, visit Auntie Joan and buy the Christmas things. *She just says it* – sometimes I think I would like her to ask me, but I have never said anything because I like being with her so much." Her husband confirmed this. It was suggested that her mother was probably unaware of this behaviour, and that both parents and husband be invited to the next session. She gave her permission for her mother to be asked tactfully whether she realised what she did.
D: (to mother) You have both liked doing things together for so long, I wonder if you may not
   tend to take her for granted?
M: I don't think I do, do I dear?
P: Well, sometimes I feel I would like you to ask me whether I want to go out, instead of assuming
   I do.
M: (taken aback) Do I do that?
Husband and father: Yes, I think you do.
   From then on mother asked if she could visit, instead of just arriving, and she asked her daughter's opinion about things in general. Having at last gained a separate identity and *control* of the relationship with her mother, her obsessional need to control her weight was no longer necessary, and she remitted.

17.6 Prognosis

Whatever the therapy pursued, the results are disappointing, and a substantial number (30%–50%) of patients enter a chronic form of anorexia, no longer endangering life, but leaving them psychological and social cripples. A few who remit during the childbearing years relapse after menopause.

Key Words: Power and Control. Doctors and nurses, when first treating patients with AN, are usually struck by their power and the unrelenting refusal to give it up.

Patients themselves do not see themselves as powerful but they will acknowledge that control is of paramount importance. It is their overwhelming terror at losing control that leads to their implacable refusal to give in to their hunger and put on weight, which conveys the impression of power.

Two Pieces of Advice. Anorexics should be told by their doctors early on that they know they are always hungry although they do not eat, and second that control is vital to them. Patients soon acknowledge that both are true and realise that the doctor understands their dilemma, which helps to reduce their initial hostility and distrust, for few anorexics consult doctors voluntarily, and most do not think they are ill.

Whichever therapy is pursued, the first move is to persuade the patient to eat by any means. Usual strategies include agreed contracts to reach a particular weight by a certain date, reinforced by a hospital admission for failure to do so. The behavioural approach in hospital starts treatment by removing privileges, which are subsequently restored one by one as rewards for gains in weight.

The patient quoted above was an exception, and it was possible to move straight away to under-focusing [6] away from the symptoms of weight and food. In most cases, whether being treated by family therapy or individual therapy, under-focussing should be pursued simultaneously with any behavioural treatment. The aim of this is to enable patients to establish a separate identity, and to control both interactions with significant key figures and themselves emotionally and physiologically, e.g. weight and menstruation, which they had not been able to do until they discovered they could do it, albeit unsatisfactorily, by not eating. Only when they have attained a measure of separate identify and some control of inter-relationships by normal means of expression are they able to forego the inappropriate and damaging means they felt previously was the only way open to them.

Summary. "*My weight is the only thing that I can call my own – that I control –* it gets on top of me that I think about it so much." This first statement was volunteered by a patient when it was suggested at her second interview that her presenting symptom of constipation might be due to underlying AN.

References

1. Bruch H (1962) Perceptual and conceptual disturbances in anorexia nervosa. Psychosom Med 24:187–194
2. Thomae H (1963) Some psychoanalytic observations on anorexia nervosa. J Med Psychol 36:239–248
3. Selvini Palazzoli M (1962) Anorexia nervosa. Chaucer, London
4. Naudeau J (1789) Observations sur une maladie nerveuse accompagnée d'un dégoût extraordinaire pour les aluments. J Med Chir Pharmacol 80:197
5. Selvini Palazzoli M (1974) Self starvation. From intrapsychic to the transpersonal approach to anorexia nervosa. Chaucer, London
6. Minuchin S, Rosman BL, Baker L (1978) Psychosomatic families: anorexia nervosa in context. Harvard University Press, Cambridge
7. Russell GFM, Szmukler GI, Dare C (1987) An evaluation of family therapy in anorexia nervosa and bulimia nervosa. Arch Gen psychiatry:44:1047–1050
8. Paulley JW (1985) Psychosomatic aspects of multiple sclerosis. In: Wise TN, Trimble MR (eds) Advances in Psychosomatic Medicine, vol 13. Karger, Basel, pp 85–110

18 Ear, Nose and Throat and Eye Disorders

We do not have sufficient experience in these fields to do more than offer the reader some key references:

Vasomotor rhinitis	See Chap. 7 Holmes TH, Goodell G, Wolf S, Wolf HG (1950) The nose. Thomas, Spingfield Wolf S (1952) Causes and mechanisms in rhinitis. Laryngoscope 62:601–614
Menières disease	Hinchcliffe R (1967) J Laryngol Otol 81:471–485 Groen JJ, Schmidt PH (1986) Psychosomatic aspects of Menière's disease. In: Lacey JH, Sturgeon DA (eds) Proceedings of the 15th european conferences on psychosomatic research. Libbey, London, pp 309–314
Tinnitus	Hallam RS (1987) Psychological approaches to the evaluation of and management of tinnitus disorders. In: Hazell TWP (ed) Tinnitus. Churchill-Livingstone, Edinburgh, pp 156–175
Tonsillitis	Binning G (1950) The influence of perturbations of childhood life events on the occurrence of appendectomy. Canad Med Assoc J 63:461–467
Glaucoma	Swelheim I (1955) Emotion and intraocular pressure. Acad. Proefschrift (in English), University of Amsterdam Cohen SI, Hajioff J (1972) Life events in relation to glaucoma. J Psychosom Res 16:335–341 Shaheen O, El-Rifai M, El-Hoshy M (1975) The family of the primary glaucoma patient. Bull Ophthalmol Soc Egypt 68:185–197

Retinal detachment (central subserous chorio retinopathy)
Gelber GS, Schatz H (1987) Am J Psychiatry 20:331–338

Styes	Inman WS (1946) Br J Med Psychol 20:331–338
Disease of the eyelids	Inman WS (1938) Med Press 196:96–99
Retrobulbar neuritis	See Sect. 9.2
Sjögren's Syndrome	See Chaps. 6, 10

19 Psychosomatic Medicine: Past, Present and Future

19.1 Distant Past

The world literature suggests that a causal relationship between emotional stress and physical illness has long been acknowledged. The Bible is a particularly rich source. For example, Nabal (1 Samuel:5, 4–38) has been regarded as the first recorded psychosomatic death from MI [1]. This churlish but vulnerable man was humiliated verbally by his wife flaunting her independent behaviour and infidelity whereupon, "His heart died within him, and he became as a stone." That is an entirely *typical* life event for MI (Chap. 8). Another example is Job [2] whose symptoms suggest that he had an immunological disorder while in a state of pathological mourning. It also provides an example of incompetent psychological management by his comforters, compared with competent management by Elihu.

Job's sins were pride and self-righteousness and then disillusion with God for allowing his flocks to be stolen and the deaths of his servants and children, including his eldest son. Initial shock and grief were soon replaced by bottled-up anger and bitterness so clearly described, "Yet still did not Job sin with his lips." Three friends (Job's comforters) came to mourn with him and to comfort him, but he did not acknowledge them and they sat in silence. Job then developed boils from head to foot and was racked with rheumatism and boiling of the bowels. At last Job began to express his sense of injustice and feelings of martyrdom. However, when his friends suggested that instead of trying to justify himself he should acknowledge that he was not without guilt, he turned on them for being cruel. He complained how often it was that wicked men prospered while good men (like himself) were punished, a complaint often voiced by patients suffering from pathological mourning, especially eldest daughters ("little mothers" see Chap. 10).

His friends (comforters) then lost patience and withdrew emotionally by not answering him saying: "He was righteous in his own eyes."

A younger man, Elihu, neither a friend nor relative, told Job's friends that they had not been helpful because when he had not accepted their suggestions they had become angry and withdrawn from him. In psychotherapeutic terms they had behaved like unskilled psychotherapists who did not recognise their own counter-transference or, if they did, failed to work through it with Job. Elihu on the other hand behaved like a competent psychotherapist, speaking honestly but quietly (meekly) to Job and not withdrawing when he made little headway. In the end Job was able to accept his guilt and was rewarded (by God) by a return to normal health and prosperity and the birth of many more children.

Another lesson to be drawn from this account is that friends and relatives of patients are often too emotionally involved and may make things worse. In the same way, some care givers, for reasons of their own psychology, infantilise their patients/

clients and reject them when they decline the passive role, just as Job was rejected by his comforters, and with equally damaging results.

Some 2500 years after Job, the merchant of Prato's physician, Maestro Lorenzo Sassoli [3], believed in treating *l'animo e lo corpo,* and wrote to his patient in Avignon:

> To get angry and shout at times pleases me, for this will keep up your natural heat [i.e. to avoid bottling up emotions]; but what displeases me is your being grieved and taking all matters so much to heart. For it is this, as the whole of Physic [Medicine] teaches – which destroys your body more than any other cause.

Had the "whole of Physic" continued to teach doctors to pay as much regard to their patient's emotional feelings as they have increasingly paid to their bodies, this book might have been unnecessary.

19.2 Past

Fifty years ago Halliday [4], the father of British psychosomatic medicine, wrote: "The reluctance of the profession to adopt a psychological outlook cannot be dissociated from the growth of unorthodox cults which continue to flourish and impress where orthodox medicine fails." Halliday expected a change in outlook but died disappointed in 1982. Then as now there was dissatisfaction with the remoteness of some orthodox practitioners, their overdependence on drugs and technology, and their dismissive attitude to common afflictions which they were unable to relieve and called *functional. Illness behaviour or somatoform,* are the labels currently in favour. It may make some doctors happier, but it is as useless to patients as previous portmanteau terms. What worried Halliday, and still worries us, is that most alternative medicine practices are obscurantist and do not attempt to help psychosomatic patients change damaging coping mechanisms; instead, these tend to be compounded.

19.2.1 Years of Promise

Following Cannon's seminal work on the fight or flight response [5] the years 1930–1960 saw the flowering of psychosomatic medicine. It was a time of great promise. Competent research showed that emotional factors were playing a decisive causative role in patients suffering from a range of common painful afflictions to crippling or lethal diseases, and these were usually those resistant, or only partly responsive, to drugs or other physical treatment.

The pioneers were Flanders Dunbar, Halliday, Alexander, Wolff and Wolf, Sullivan, Wittkower, Grinker, Daniels, Engel, Graham, Groen and others. Meetings were attended by people from disciplines as widespread as psychoanalysis, epidemiology, biology, philosophy, physiology, medicine, surgery and animal ethology as well as psychiatrists and were immensely stimulating and resulted in contributions of outstanding merit.

Flanders Dunbar's book entitled *Psychosomatic Dagnosis* [6] was published in 1943 and detailed 8 years of work in the Departments of Medicine, Surgery and Psychiatry at the Presbyterian Medical Center, New York. Her explanation of the taking of a psychosomatic history and of special techniques of investigation, like other good things, have been buried in the sand of time instead of being used as the basis on which medical students and doctors of today could be helped to learn about the psychological management of psychosomatic disorders (see also Chap. 5).

She and Alexander [7] also pointed out that many psychosomatic disorders could be treated effectively by brief psychotherapy. "We were impressed by the quick response of most general medical patients to relatively superficial psychotherapy" ([6], p. 29). This important fact has been largely ignored or disbelieved. Case histories in this book strongly support Dunbar and Alexander on this point.

Other important contributions made at that time were books by Weiss and English [8] and Halliday [9], and in a brief but effective article Daniels [10] summarised questions which remain unresolved to this day, for example " Should the general medical man do psychotherapy?" He suggested it would be more suitable to ask: "To what degree can the doctor make his general medical treatment more psychotherapeutically effective, and to what degree if any should doctors utilise psychiatric technique?" To sceptics who maintained that all that is necessary in personality problems is common sense he pointed out, as we have done, that common sense is always valuable, but that it was an error to think that without knowledge of psychodynamics one was in a position to manage psychosomatic patients. He went on to illustrate the point by quoting the management of cardiac neurosis, cancer phobia and UC.

Measurement of Somatic Responses to Emotion. The 1940s and 1950s was also the era of important psychophysiological research. Physiological responses were measured in parallel with experimentally induced emotions. The leaders in this field were Wolf, Wolff, Grace, Holmes and Goodell [11–13]. Studies were carried out in the United Kingdom at the same time on colonic motility during interviews and/or pictorial presentations, structured to contain both psychologically traumatic and non-traumatic material based on prior knowledge of the subjects' sensitivities and provocative life situations [14, 15], while in Amsterdam [16] of skin resistance, respiration, pulse rate, blood pressure and blood flow were simultaneously recorded in patients and controls while exposed to the same form of stress of sitting for 10 min in silence and without explanation.

Follow-up Studies After Psychotherapy. The 1950s and early 1960s also saw the first follow-up studies after psychotherapy and psychological management in UC [17–19] and Crohn's disease [20]. More recently there have been studies on migraine [21] asthma [22, 23] and IBS [24, 25].

19.2.2 Years of Confusion

During the years of promise, however, there had always been some antipathy to psychodynamic concepts and psychodynamically orientated skills in therapy. Unfortunately, some of these opponents seized on work by Mirsky [26] on multicausality in the pathogenesis of DU (see Chap. 6) as a pretext for a prolonged (and we consider quite unjustified) attack on the earlier formulations of Dunbar, Alexander and others. The most immediate response to this was made by Wittkower [27], himself a pioneer, in his presidential address to the American Psychosomatic Society in 1960 when he said: "The concept of psychogenesis as far as psychosomatic disorders are concerned has been debunked ... and time honoured concepts attacked." He added wistfully: "Is it really true that we have struggled for so many years and that the contributions made by psychoanalysts amount to nil?" But as many case histories in this book show, success of psychological managements or psychotherapy for many psychosomatic disorders depends on the appreciation of a few of the most important of the psychodynamic concepts and mechanisms gleaned from interpretative psychotherapy, which are described in Chap. 4, e.g. resistances and transference, and indeed on the application of the hard-won experience of the pioneers.

The "Debunkers". Debunkers, first mentioned by Wittkower [27], have rarely repeated the work they criticised, or if they did, in such a superficial way that the results have been meaningless. Yet it is those results which when published are acclaimed and used selectively to discredit former studies. For example, gastroenterologists opposed to psychosomatic concepts always quote the negative but methodologically flawed [28–31] studies on the psychopathogenesis of UC and Crohn's disease by Feldman et al. [32, 33] but do not mention earlier numerous and more extensive studies to the contrary (Chap. 6). It is by such means that generations of students and young doctors have been, and continue to be, misled. However, this does not apply to psychosomatic medicine alone; for example, from 1932 until 1952 it was taught that the jejunal mucosa was normal in sprue and coeliac disease because one book [34] had stated categorically that previous reports of abnormality had been due to autolysis. Various considerations led J.W.P. 20 years later to question this accepted wisdom and some of the data in the original monograph, and then by means of jejunal biopsy at laparotomy [35, 36] to show that the pioneers had been right all along.

Rosch [37] has given other examples of important advances suffering at the hands of influential but uncritical debunkers. Goldberger's observation that pellagra was due to nicotinic acid deficiency was ridiculed by the Thompson McFadden report (1916) in order to advance the aetiological claims of the stable fly. Palomir's discoveries on immune defence were derided as they were not in accord with existing concepts, and like Semmelweiss, who discovered the cause of puerpural fever, he was persecuted and rejected by his colleagues and later committed suicide.

The examples quoted suggest that it is time that teachers in all medical and scientific disciplines, including psychosomatic medicine, imposed on themselves and their students a greater critical faculty, and discouraged parrot-like recitation as reprehensible and a threat to scientific advance. However, whereas the debunked pioneers on the jejunal mucosa were restored to respectability in 1952, the pioneers in psychosomatic medicine are still awaiting rehabilitation.

19.3 Recent Past and Present

19.3.1 The Retreat from Patients

Many debunkers also distanced themselves as far as possible from clinical involvement. Kubie described this phenomenon in 1971 [38] as the retreat from patients, summarising the reasons for it as follows:

> work with patients is painful; a tendency to undervalue clinical skills; a general failure to realise how long it takes to acquire clinical maturity; the emphasis on research for tomorrow's medicine at the expense of service for today's needs; propaganda for service to the "community" as though this did not require the highest degree of knowledge of individual human need ...

This retreat was also reflected in the decline in numbers of non-psychiatrists attending meetings on psychosomatic medicine and publishing articles in psychosomatic journals [27]. Increasingly, these non-psychiatrists, including psychoanalysts, found that the topics chosen for discussion, which had first drawn them into psychosomatic medicine, especially clinical research and treatment of patients with real psychosomatic disorders, seemed of less interest to the psychiatrists and liaison psychiatrists, who from 1960 onwards began to dominate the psychosomatic scene. Meetings and journals became increasingly repetitive, and overburdened eith personality inventories.

More recently, the monotonous publication of inventories has been replaced by equally monotonous measurements of type A behaviour, but little about its psychopathogenesis. Other deterrents to those who were primarily interested in clinical aspects and the management of patients have been incursions into proceedings by advocates of diverse group techniques, and alternative practitioners of various –opathies and –isms sheltering under the holistic umbrella.

19.3.2 Personality Inventories: An Unhelpful Diversion

As already mentioned, reports on the results of inventories filled both the pages of psychosomatic journals and the sessions at meetings for at least 15 years. Psychosomatists keen to rebut criticsm from academic colleagues in the "hard" sciences felt that they could now be seen to be collectors of "hard" data instead of the allegedly "soft" material presented earlier. Unfortunately, the tools used were mostly designed to investigate the psychoneuroses. Many such investigators seemed unaware that what they were measuring was wholly or partly irrelevant to the psychosomatic disorder(s) under examination. Graham [39] pointed this out in a trenchant analogy. It was, he said, as illogical to conclude that a disorder was not psychosomatic if such inventories and tests were negative as to conclude that there was no biochemical abnormality in diabetes or asthma on the basis of a multitude of tests if these did not include the two that mattered, i.e. blood glucose and pCO_2.

Another common error was for the investigator to think that the tool being used was measuring something when it was not. This was either because the inventory was too crude, or because the subject's typical defence of denial was not recognised. Had these workers seen more psychosomatic patients beforehand, or had had a better understanding of psychodynamics, many of these errors could have been avoided. However, it is inevitable that questionnaire/inventory techniques will always fail to uncover deeply repressed and subconscious feelings in patients whose very disability centres on their poverty of emotional expression. Examples of this are quoted in Chap. 6 on Crohn's disease and Chapter 9 on MS.

19.3.3 Behavioural Science: Another False Lead

From 1970 onwards Western medical schools saw a spectacular increase in the number of behavioural science teachers and the hours allotted to the subject. At various points in this book we have criticised aspects of behavioural science concepts and teaching, for example *non-compliance, sick role* and *illness behaviour*. On the other hand we have commended the increasing sophistication of life event research while pointing out its limitations, e.g. the need for much more sensitive interviewing techniques in some disorders such as MS and the AI disease, and the extension of the concept of an event to cover an emotional situation, as for example struggling against deadlines in migraine, and "fence-sitting" over some problem of decision in IBS. Medical educators, who had been under attack for some time for turning out too many doctors who know too little about their patients as people, at first supported the entry of behavioural science. Even today when asked why they are not doing more about teaching psychosomatic medicine some quote, in aggrieved tones, the number of behavioural scientists they employ, and the hours of curriculum time allotted to them. They appear to think that behavioural science and psychosomatic medicine are the same thing! However, as Tait [40] pointed out, disillusion was not long in coming, both among students who felt that much of the course was irrelevant to the management of patients, and among other faculty members who felt that the result did not justify the money and time allocated to it. Winefield [41] has written a clear account of behavioural science in the medical curriculum, some of which we could support. Unfortunately in an otherwise excellent chapter she fails, as behavioural scientists usually do, to mention or even acknowledge psychodymanics, or the consequences of disruption of an individual's psychological development on subsequent coping responses to environmental as well as internal emotional stresses.

Wolf, a notable pioneer, in his Samual Novy lecture in 1982 [42] discussing problems and pitfalls in behavioural approaches, said: "The epidemiological method, with its reliance on standard criteria and relatively large numbers, tends to blur the characteristics of individuals that may be significant." His conclusion was that biobehavioural studies had been "restricted to a Procrustean mould" unsuitable to people functioning in their social milieu. Graham, another pioneer, was equally outspoken: his criticisms in a presidential address [39] were directed at the fatuity of many personality inventories, but also at fellow members of the American society who had failed to acquaint themselves with earlier work and at many liaison psychiatrists who seemed to believe the patients referred to them for treatment were psychosomatic, but actually were not. He also deplored the abandonment of the concept of *specificity (typicality)* without sufficient reason, and felt that psychosomatic medicine had not progressed as it should have done.

Euphoria: But Not for patients. Despite the debunking and subsequent confusion the end of the 1970s found the mood of the American Psychosomatic Society enthusiastic and optimistic. Lipowski [43] observed that the "rapidly expanding field of psychosomatic medicine is far more diversified, scientifically rigorous, methodologically resourceful and therapeutically relevant than ever before." Had these claims been true, why have not more people with psychosomatic disorders benefited by now? The mortality rate for asthma has not changed over the last 30 years, so why is it that despite Lipowski's claim, very few of them receive any psychological help? The same is true of UC, hypertension, RA and migraine, all of which continue to kill, maim or distress their sufferers. Yet few psychiatrists are prepared to take on these people, or to acquire the necessary management skills when they do.

Psychosomatic medicine's most grievous self-inflicted wound has been its departure from its original raison d'être – the patient. Indeed, it has allowed itself to become so diversified that both research and training for clinical care have become too diffuse for much progress to be made. It has even become customary to use the term *psychosomatics* to cover social medicine, medical psychology, psychophysiology, etc., thus ensuring more confusion. By so doing the definitions of psyche and soma are stretched beyond all reason and are as damaging to these other disciplines as to psychosomatic medicine proper.

As opposed to unhelpful diversions, there have been good developments. The important researches of Weiner, Ader, Hofer and co-workers have brought neuro-psycho-immunology and neuro-psycho-endocrinology to a point of central relevance to the future of psychosomatic medicine [44–46]. Another field in which there has been substantial progress is epidemiology, notably of ischaemic heart disease by Bruhn and Wolf [47] in the secluded community of Roseto and by Marmot [48] in Japanese immigrants in California, both described in Chap. 8.

19.3.4 Resistances to Psychosomatic Medicine

Before discussing the future we shall mention briefly obvious and conscious reasons which have to date prevented psychosomatic medicine taking its place in the mainstream of medicine, but also suggest unconscious reasons likely to be even more potent because they are unrecognised. Some of these were summarised in 1986 [15].

First, some clinicians have an aversion to undertaking psychological management because they fear emotional involvement, and second, they are averse to requesting a psychotherapist to intervene because they fear reduction of their own status with their patient. Third, uncertainty is felt by some liaison psychiatrists and psychotherapists about their competence in the somatic area, which these patients often question, as well as doubts about the effectiveness of their therapies for psychosomatic patients, which is a possible reason for the paucity of outcome studies to date, which in turn has discouraged many doctors from embarking on psychotherapy or psychological management.

Another resistance; young doctors especially may be frightened by the idea that repressed emotional feelings can lead to disease because it implies that they would have to apply it to themselves as well. In order to protect themselves from such conscious or subconscious fears, they commonly use flat denial of the whole concept, while others make use of selective references to support prejudice. Another commonly voiced objection (resistance) to the psychosomatic concept is that emotional feelings as such cannot be measured. While this is scientifically correct, it is not scientifically defensible for opponents to conclude, as they usually do, that emotional feelings may therefore be *ignored* in experimental physiological or psychophysiological research. How some trained scientists are able to blind themselves to their own everyday experience that people and animals react differently according to how they perceive threats and respond to them is truly remarkable. When for example, four individuals are kicked or insulted, one may grovel, one may run away, another will attack physically or verbally and another may feel he has deserved it and ignore what has happened. It is not surprising therefore that such scientists find it even more difficult to accept that what an individual feels inwardly, whether it be guilt or loss or rage, if unresolved over a period of time may lead to a psychosomatic disorder or disease.

Equally, the refusal of doctrinaire psychotherapists to try to measure anything or perform outcome studies has done little to reduce the scepticism of scientifically trained doctors or psychiatrists about the usefulness of psychotherapy.

Ultraspecialisation and Closed Minds. As little as 50, even 30 years ago a surgeon such as Wilfred Trotter could be as eminent in other fields as in his own. He was the originator of the herd instinct. Arthur Hurst [49], one of the greatest physicians of this century, was able to write about the emotional aspects of asthma as follows:

> Like Floyer, I also suffer from asthma, so I have the advantage, which few writers on the subject possess, of 30 years of observations on a single case ... asthma may be caused by an idea, or an emotion ... Many patients who learn to rely on certain remedies are sure to become asthmatic if they discover they have forgotten to take their powder, inhalation, or injection with them. Some asthmatics have an attack with any little excitement, business worry or annoyance, but a severe fright is more likely to stop an attack than cause one.

None of three journals to whom this gem from the past was recently sent thought it worth publishing. The minds of those representing the asthma establishment have been closed to the emotional factor for many years.

Compared with 30 years ago today's specialists' outlook is narrower. Many of these men and women, even the most eminent, are noticeably uncomfortable if they find themselves involved in discussion about matters peripheral, or even tangential, to their own speciality. First, there may be an uncharacteristic silence, then a glassy look, followed by shuffling feet when an escape route is espied, and then: "Please forgive me, but I really must have word with Eric". Specialists now outnumber generalists in the medical and scientific establishment, and they control the direction and funding of research, of teaching, and of examination requirements. They read fewer journals outside their own specialities than was the case 30 years ago. At meetings nowadays sessions are arranged by the organisers in order to gratify the restricted interests of those attending, and to spare them the discomfort of having to listen to someone who might broaden their knowledge. Many ultraspecialists seem to be as frightened of new ideas as were religious bigots of old, and we should consider possible reasons for this.

Specialisation; Certainty and New Uncertainty. People trained in precision and certainty tend to find feelings of which they are not in control disturbing. Medical scientists may be visibly shaken when uncertainty is introduced into a world in which scientific advances have reduced fears of the unknown. Unfortunately, new uncertainties have a habit of arising just as man has allowed himself to think that he has mastered – *controlled* – his old enemies and abandoned previous stand-bys in time of trouble, e.g. the family, the community and religion. Frightened, vulnerable and defenceless, he finds that his new god, Science, has let him down. This may explain why the strongest antagonists to the relevance of unconscious feelings and psychodynamic concepts are to be found among doctors and scientists whose areas of study have become increasingly narrow, and including some psychiatrists and behaviourists who are among the most virulent opponents.

It is first necessary to pinpoint resistances which are logical and conscious, and then those which are emotional and subconscious. Such resistances are felt by doctors and non-medical scientists on the one hand, and by psychotherapists on the other. Not until sufficient people on each side of the gulf are prepared to try and understand their own feelings, as well as those on the other side, can progress be made. We can no longer allow resistances to be brushed under the carpet, instead, they will have to be confronted and worked through.

19.4 The Future

For psychosomatic medicine to take its place in the mainstream of medicine as was expected of it 50 years ago, one premise and some inspired action will be necessary. The premise is that specialisation in medicine will continue but that uncontrolled ultraspecialisation will have to be curbed, and measures taken to ensure a more broadly based training, continuing education and practice. This is because medicine is at a point of crisis. Ultraspecialisation is strangling it, and disillusion grows with the failure to meet expectations in the treatment of a large group of common disorders, many of which have been listed in this book. Doctors are increasingly regarded by the public and governments as technicians rather than as the professional men and women of the past. A likely result is that they will soon find themselves being paid as such. Over-specialisation has also led to some loss of job satisfaction for all but the most eminent. Restricted horizons and a daily diet of sameness are contributing to some of the boredom and cynicism now evident in a profession previously renowned for its devotion to patients and the absorbing interest it found in its work. Doctors who blame public ingratitude and the growth of litigation for much of this rarely recognise the extent to which their own behaviour has been responsible for much loss of esteem.

The Art of Medicine. At its best much of the art of medicine was the clinical application of psychosomatic medicine, but the skills took many years to acquire and were rarely as honed or precisely directed as we have found necessary if substantial numbers of patients with differing psychosomatic disorders are to receive the help to which they are entitled. For 40 years *the art of medicine* has been used as a term of derision by medical scientists and most professors of medicine so that the few clinicians who continued to practise it had to do so surreptitiously for fear of being accused of not being scientific.

The art of medicine not only requires skills, but first of all respect for the patient as a human being, and not solely as a medical, surgical or psychiatric "problem". Good manners in medical practice are of the utmost importance but have become rather rare.

There is an urgent need for action by universities and medical schools throughout the Western world to recognise the dangers outlined above and not only to take measures to help restore the lost art of medicine, but to refine the ways in which it can be learned and deployed. An essential part of such a programme must be to ensure that students and young doctors are trained in some of the skills of psychological management for psychosomatic disorders as described in this book.

Whatever is done, we must recognise the reasons why previous endeavours to achieve this objective have failed, and not repeat mistakes. For example many imaginative, combined medical-psychiatric teaching programmes in the United States of America and Europe over the past 30–40 years have not attained their goal. An important reason for this has been a *failure to provide a convincing model of the comprehensive physician.* Engel et al. [50] expressed this clearly:

> the student who has been urged to deal with his patient "as a whole" actually is treated to the spectacle that it takes two experts, an internist and a psychiatrist (and sometimes a social worker and psychologist as well), to do the job that he as a student is being asked to accomplish himself ... a factor of identification with the model physician which is so important in the learning process is blocked by the reality that there is no figure who is able to comprehend the patient in his totality. In the end students identify with either the psychiatrist or the internist, and only rarely with the still abstract symbol of the comprehensive physician.

If Engel's students had that problem 30 years ago, it is even greater today with more cooks in the kitchen, notably behavioural scientists of various persuasions, behaviourists and practitioners of holistic and alternative medicine.

It has also been assumed that the teaching of psychosomatic medicine could be done in centres also carrying out psychosomatic research. This policy has so far failed, and alternatives should now be tried; research workers in psychosomatic medicine, as in other disciplines, rarely have the time or inclination to care for a sufficient number of patients and thus provide the right models for students seeking to acquire clinical skills.

Some students and medical educators have become dissatisfied with the results of behavioural science teaching [40]. Behavioural scientists, not being clinicians treating patients, have the same problem as many psychosomatic medicine research workers, of not being able to provide the model which the student needs. The other hazard is that the students are prone to become infected with the idea that nothing is worthwile doing medically as long as society is not subjected to revolutionary reform.

Departments of Consultant Liaison Psychiatry (CLP) have been established for some time in North America and more recently in Europe. Such departments undoubtedly have an important role to play in any future programme for psychosomatic medicine. Not all liaison psychiatrists, however, even those dually trained in internal medicine and psychotherapy, have been able to remain sufficiently up to date in medicine itself to be able to provide the model physicians we and Engel consider to be so necessary, and in whom clinical colleagues are likely to have sufficient confidence to entrust their patients.

19.4.1 Holistic Medicine Is Not Psychosomatic Medicine

Recent enthusiasm among students and young doctors for a hotch potch of alternative medical techniques hiding under the banner of holistic medicine must be recognised for the mumbo jumbo which most are, and resisted. The main reason for this damaging diversion has been the failure of psychosomatic medicine to take its place in the mainstream of medicine, just as Halliday [4] warned 50 years ago, and it has led frustrated patients and doctors increasingly to look for alternatives, however unsatisfactory. The holistic approach advocated today [43] is no different from the "whole person medicine" which was the clarion cry 25 years ago. It sounded good but achieved little. Both overplay the importance of environmental stress like the rat race, as opposed to intrapsychic stress, and this led doctors to think that all they must do is to listen, empathise and occasionally confront: admirable, but dangerously simplistic. Like reassurance, the above is rarely enough and relieves few psychosomatic disorders for long. The holistic approach lacks the therapeutic precision that only competent psychological management provides in helping patients to change hitherto damaging coping mechanisms.

19.4.2 A Plan for the Future: New Departments of Clinical or Applied Medicine

Apart from trying to avoid errors we have listed as contributory to the lack of success of previous attempts to give young doctors the essential skills of psychological management, we will now consider additional measures which we think are necessary if psychosomatic medicine is to be brought into the mainstream of medical practice.

First, because the label *psycho*-deters many patients with psychosomatic disorders from seeking the help they need, we suggest that departments to which they are referred should be given names other than Department of Psychosomatic Medicine or Liaison Psychiatry, for example Department of Clinical or Applied Medicine. These *superstable* patients (see Chap. 2) are particularly sensitive to any suggestion that they need psychiatric referral. They *know* that they have physical symptoms and resent what they see as an implication that they are imagining them or are mental. Those who rightly are trying to persuade the public that there is no stigma in psychological illness may feel that our suggestion is a retrograde one, but we would urge them to try to understand the psychosomatic patient's dilemma, and not regard them as the same as psychoneurotics, who usually feel psychologically ill and are willing to accept psychiatric help.

Doctors of patients with psychosomatic disorders have the same problem. They are often aware that the aetiology of a patient's disorder or disease has a large emotional component, but they avoid making a psychiatric referral in case their patient resents it and leaves. However, a physician or GP who, unknown to the patient, is psychosomatically and psychodynamically orientated does not suffer the disadvantage of being regarded as a "trick cyclist", "mind bender" or "soul pincher" (translated from a well-known Dutch comic strip). Even so, as we have stressed in Chap. 3 and 5 it is only after taking a full medical history and making a full examination that the patient will be able to accept something like the following: "I wonder whether you would be surprised if I were to suggest that emotional factors might be playing a part in your trouble?" To subsequent enquiries about family and interpersonal relationships the patients may need reassurance that all doctors wishing to help their patients have to know about what sort of people they are and what makes them "tick". The reply is usually, "Well, that's alright then, but some of your questions sounded rather like a psychiatrists', and when my doctor suggested I see one, it annoyed me because I felt he thought I was imagining my symptoms which I know are real." For some time the term psychosomatic has been criticised for semantic and philosophical reasons. It is generally agreed that it is too late to change it because of the difficulties it would involve in retrieval of source material in the literature and also because there is no general agreement on a better name, but Lipowski thinks that the term psychosomatic disorder (illness) should be discarded altogether because it is incompatible with multicausality. On that basis it would also mean giving up speaking of an infectious or AI disease without adding, "by which we mean the major factor in this person's illness is virus X (or antibody Y), but he might not have been affected had he not been genetically disposed, malnourished, unhappy at her work, or unable to get over his mother's or spouse's death," and that would obviously be absurd. Psychosomatic disorder is a useful term like the others providing it is clearly defined and understood.

We envisage that the proposed Departments of Clinical or Applied Medicine would be places in which any clinical skill shown to have a value beyond placebo effect could be learned and practised. At the present time that would apply to various relaxation techniques, including autogenic training and the Alexander Principle [51]. It might well be that various manipulative techniques could be added later. Widening the range of therapies available in such departments and making psychological management of psychosomatic disorders only one of them would be one way of avoiding the inhibitory effect which the name Department of Psychosomatic Medicine has had hitherto on patients and doctors alike at the point of referral. Most of the therapies mentioned are practised on outpatients. That also applies to many psychosomatic disorders, but a few inpatient beds would be required for severely ill or incapacitated people with asthma, accelerated hypertension, UC, AI disease, etc.

There may be better names than Department of Clinical or Applied Medicine, and it does not matter much what they are as long as psycho-, holistic, whole person, behavioural and alternative are not among them. Whatever the title, its orientation towards patients should be manifest, hence the suggestion of "clinical", while "medicine" would reassure patients with psychosomatic disorders that the somatic aspect of their complaint remained in the forefront *even* if possible emotional factors were being looked into at the same time.

Staffing. Clearly, some of the techniques we have mentioned would require people with a variety of skills, particularly from physical medicine, physiotherapy and probably behavioural medicine, but the most important of all for inpatients is *nursing*. However, with regard to the medical staffing of that area of the department engaged in teaching and practice of psychological management of psychosomatic disorder, we suggest recruitment initially on a voluntary basis from departments of general practice, medicine and its subspecialties, surgery, psychiatry and liaison psychiatry. Applicants or seconded members would require sufficient dual medical and psychological training, or evidence of sufficient experience in the field, to satisfy an appointments committee. After a few years staff applicants would require accreditation to show that they had spent 2 years training in such a department. Examinations in this field would seem inappropriate, but in-course assessment would be useful.

Length of Courses. We suggest a course of 8 h per week for graduates, either as one whole study day or as two half-days over 2 years. It would seem that the most appropriate form of teaching would be in small groups and seminars, with the use of videotape and combined with supervised case management.

Initially the departments would almost certainly have to be in teaching hospitals or in affiliated hospitals, but in the longer run district hospitals might be even more suitable.

Students. At present many doctors who qualify and reach resident posts having never seen a patient with a psychosomatic disorder treated by psychological management alone, or in combination with standard methods of treatment, which, of course, are often necessary. This handicap could be obviated by arranging for students to attend for as little as 1 h per week in such a department as we suggest throughout their clinical years where they would be able to participate in seminars, case conferences, etc. Clinical skills of this sort cannot be learned in short slots of intensive instruction; what is needed is prolonged if dilute exposure.

Funding. The money saved by reducing the size of Departments of Behavioural Science might be diverted to such new departments. Secondly, Departments of Medicine and Psychiatry might be expected to contribute as they would both be beneficiaries. It is also a project which would appeal to liberally-minded Foundations unhappy with the present medical climate and neglect of emotional determinants in such disorders as RA, AI diseases, MS, hypertension, migraine, IBS and asthma.

Ultimately, realistic fees would be charged for graduates accepted for courses leading to accreditation.

19.5 Summary

Although psychosomatic illness has been recognised for thousands of years, it had to wait for Dunbar and the formation of the American Psychosomatic Society in 1939 to become a subject worthy of scientific interest.

We have touched upon this early promise and the pathfinders' belief that it should by now have taken its place in the mainstream of medicine. Why it has not done so is a matter of opinion, and we have discussed the grounds for our own view that if the clinical application of psychosomatic medicine is to advance to the benefit of the large number of patients who need it, then past mistakes in the teaching and training of doctors will have to be avoided, and false trails identified before they do too much damage. As observers peripheral to much of the academic skirmishing which has taken place over the past 25 years, our views may possibly be more detached than if we had been directly involved in the fray.

The doldrums into which psychosomatic medicine has drifted have been due first to its failure to build on the relevant and least controversial insights gained by orthodox psychotherapists, and second, to its failure to build on much of the early research. The reluctance of the psychoanalysts to modify their strict standards of working to take on sufficient numbers of verbally and emotionally restricted people with psychosomatic disorders was largely responsible for the disillusionment of clinicians who had initially been enthusiastic [52], and we are sure that this cannot be corrected until the reality of *specificity/typicality* is accepted, taught, learned and practised. Another hindrance to progress has been the conscious or unconscious resistance of many people, not least of psychiatrists untrained in, and uncomfortable with, even elementary psychodynamic concepts, but without which relevant research cannot be done, and effective, as opposed to ineffective, management/therapy is made widely available. Instead, there has been a retreat from patients. Drugs, behavioural techniques and methods of research which fail to take into account subjects' perception of what is being asked of them or their interrogators, have all served to keep patients at a safe emotional distance.

We have questioned the wisdom of leaving so much of the training of students and young doctors in psychosomatic medicine to behavioural scientists not equipped to be able to provide the essential model of the comprehensive clinician. We also feel that some social psychologists and liaison psychiatrists are unrealistic in thinking that changes in the patient's psychosocial environment are ever likely to make much impact on the totality of psychosomatic disorder, once established. As we have pointed out in the clinical chapters, a "managed" environment or approach which is one man's meat is often another man's poison, and if subjected to it some patients' condition will worsen. Another reason why recent enthusiasm for the psychosocial approach is ill-conceived is that anything beyond short-term engineered support as in a ward, group or family serves only to compound the patients' damaging coping mechanisms and discourages attainment of self-awareness. "Know thyself," said the Delphic admonition in the Temple of Apollo. A greater part of the effort of those currently engaged in sociological research and intervention should be directed to the causes of *emotional* deprivation in infancy and childhood when coping mechanisms are initially laid down [53] and which, when defectively inflexible, are the seed bed for all psychological disturbances, including psychosomatic disorders.

We have looked at the future of training of doctors so that the delivery of effective psychological management may be provided for the many and not just the few.

Finally, we have drawn attention to the deterrent effect that anything prefixed by "psycho" has on this *superstable* group of people, especially at the point of referral. Serious consideration should be given to the suggestion of changing the name of departments in which psychosomatic medicine is learned and practised, and eventually we hope they would be accommodated within Departments of Medicine, where they really belong.

References

1. Groen JJ, van der Valk JM, Treurniet N, Kits van Heyninggen H, Pelser HE, Wilde GJS (1965) Het acute Myocardinfarct, een psychosomatische studie. Bohn, Haarlem
2. Job:1, 10–42
3. Origo I (1957) The merchant of Prato. Cape, London
4. Halliday JL (1938) The rising incidence of psychosomatic illness. Br Med J 2:11–14
5. Cannon W (1929) Bodily changes in pain, hunger, fear and rage. Appleton Century Crofts, New York
6. Dunbar F (1943) Psychosomatic diagnosis. Hoeber, New York
7. Alexander F (1950) Psychosomatic medicine. Norton, New York
8. Weiss E, English OS (1949) Psychosomatic medicine. Saunders, Philadelphia
9. Halliday JL (1948) Psycho-social medicine. Hyman, London
10. Daniels GE (1941) Practical aspects of psychiatric management in psychosomatic problems. NY State J Med 41:1727–1732
11. Wolf S, Wolff HG (1943) Human gastric function. Oxford University Press, London
12. Grace WJ, Wolf S, Wolff HG (1951) The human colon. Heinemann, London
13. Holmes TH, Goodell G, Wolf S, Wolff HG (1950) The nose. Thomas, Springfield
14. Paulley JW (1950) Ulcerative colitis: a study of 173 cases. Gastroenterology 16:566–576
15. Paulley JW (1986) Psychosomatic medicine: a forward look. In: Lacey JH, Sturgeon DA (eds) Proceedings of the 15 th European conference on psychosomatic research. Lilley, London
16. Van der Valk, JM (1965) The role of psychosomatic disorder in adult life. In: Wisdom JO, Wolff H (eds) Proceedings of a conference held by the society for psychosomatic research in London. Pergamon, London, pp 120–132 (Discussion to Session 3)
17. Groen J, Bastiaans J (1955) Studies on Ulcerative colitis personality structure, emotional complications and effects of psychotherapy. In: O'Neill D (eds) Modern trends in psychosomatic medicine. Butterworths, London
18. Grace WJ, Pinskey RN, Wolff H (1954) Treatment of ulcerative colitis. Gastroenterology 26:462–468
19. Paulley JW (1956) Psychotherapy in ulcerative colitis. Lancet 2:215–218
20. Paulley JW (1971) Crohn's disease. Treatment by antibiotics, corticosteroids and psychotherapy. Psychother Psychosom 18:111–117
21. Paulley JW, Haskell DA (1975) Treatment of migraine without drugs. J Psychosom Res 19:367–374
22. Groen JJ, Pelser HE (1959) Experiences and results of group psycho therapy in patients with bronchial asthma. Ned Tijdschr Geneesk 103:65–75
23. Groen JJ, Pelser HE (1960) Experiences with, and results of, group psychotherapy in patients with bronchial asthma. J Psychosom Res 4:191–205
24. Hislop IG (1980) The effect of very brief psychotherapy on the irritable bowel syndrome. Med J Aust 2:620–622
25. Svedlund J, Sjodin I, Ottoson G, Dottervall G (1983) Controlled study of psychotherapy in the irritable bowel syndrome. Lancet 2:589–592
26. Mirsky IA (1958) Physiologic, psychologic and social determinants in the aetiology of duodenal ulcer. Am J Dig Dis 3:285–314
27. Wittkower ED (1960) Twenty years of North American medicine. Psychosom Med 22:308–316
28. West R (1967) Psychological factors and ulcerative colitis. Br Med J 2:56
29. Engel GL (1967) Psychological factors and ulcerative colitis. Br Med J 2:56
30. Paulley JW (1968) Emotion and ileitis. Br Med J 1:180
31. Brown D (1968) Emotion and ileitis. Br Med J 1:179–180

32. Feldman F, Cantor D, Soll S, Bachrach W (1967) Psychiatric study of a consecutive series of 19 patients with regional ileitis. Br Med J 4:711–714

33. Feldman F, Cantor D, Soll S, Bachrach W (1967) Psychiatric study of a consecutive series of 34 patients with ulcerative colitis. Br Med J 3:14–17

34. Thaysen TEH (1932) Non-troprical sprue: a study in idiopathic steatorrhoea. Oxford University Press, London

35. Paulley JW (1952) Discussion. Trans R Soc Trop Med Hyg 46 [6]:594–595

36. Paulley JW (1954) Observations on the aetiology of idiopathic steatorrhoea. Br Med J 1318–1321

37. Rosch PJ (1983) Miracle cures: misplaced faiths? Mod Med 51(9):253

38. Kubie LS (1971) The Retreat from Patients. Arch Gen Psychiatry 4:98–106

39. Graham DT (1977) What place in medicine for psychosomatic medicine? Psychosom Med 41:357–367

40. Tait IH (1973) Behavioural science in medical education and clinical practice. Soc Sci Med 7:1003–1011

41. Winefield HR (1981) Behavioural science in the medical curriculum. In: Christie MJ, Mellett PG (eds) Why and how in foundations of psychosomatics. Wiley, New York

42. Wolf S (1982) Psychosocial forces and neurol mechanisms in disease: defining the question and collecting the evidence. Johns Hopkins Med J 150:95–100

43. Lipowski ZJ (1977) Psychosomatic medicine in the seventies: an overview. Am J Psychiatry 134:233–244

44. Ader R (1980) Psychosomatic and psychoimmunology research. Psychosom Med 42:307–321

45. Hofer MA (1983) Relationships as regulators. A psychological perspective on bereavement. Psychosom Med 46:183–197

46. Weiner H (1983) What the future holds for psychosomatic medicine. Proceedings of th 7th world congress of psychosomatic medicine, Hamburg

47. Bruhn JG, Wolf S (1979) The Rosetan story. University of Oklahoma Press, Norman

48. Marmot MG, Syme SL (1976) Acculturation and coronary heart disease in Japanese Americans. Am J Epidemiol 194:225–247

49. Hurst AH (1924) Medical essays and addresses. Heinemann, London

50. Engel GL, Osler WL, Reichsmann R, Schmale A, Ashenberg N (1957) A graduate and undergraduate teaching programs on the psychological aspects of medicine. J Med Educ 32:859–871

51. Barlow W (1981) The Alexander Principle. Arrow, London

52. Karstens R (1972) Psychosomatic medicine: difficulties of integration. Psychother Psychosom 22:196–199

53. Rutter M (1985) Resilence in the face of adversity: protective factors in resistance to psychiatric disorder. Br J Psychiatry 147:598–611